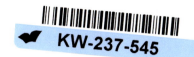

Understanding Dental Caries

1 Etiology and Mechanisms

Basic and Clinical Aspects

Gordon Nikiforuk

Understanding Dental Caries

1 Etiology and Mechanisms

Basic and Clinical Aspects

133 figures and 32 tables, 1985

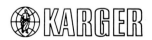

S. Karger · Basel · München · Paris · London · New York · Tokyo · Sydney

Gordon Nikiforuk

Professor of Preventive Dentistry and Immediate Past Dean, Faculty of Dentistry,
University of Toronto;
Senior Staff of The Hospital for Sick Children, Toronto, Canada

National Library of Medicine, Cataloging in Publication
Nikiforuk, G. (Gordon)
Understanding dental caries/
G. Nikiforuk.–Basel; New York: Karger 1985
Contents: v. 1. Etiology and mechanisms, basic and clinical aspects
1. Dental Caries   I. Title
WU 270 N692u
ISBN 3-8055-3906-1   (set)
ISBN 3-8055-3864-2   (v. 1)

Drug Dosage
  The authors and publisher have exerted every effort to ensure that drug selection and dosage set forth in this text are in accord with current recommendations and practice at the time of publication. However, in view of ongoing research, changes in government regulations, and the constant flow of information relating to drug therapy and drug reactions, the reader is urged to check the package insert for each drug for any change in indications and dosage and for added warnings and precautions. This is particularly important when the recommended agent is a new and/or infrequently employed drug.

Contents

Contents

Contents Volume 2

Contributors and Reviewers of Chapters

Early in the genesis of this book, it became apparent that one person cannot assimilate all the literature on dental caries. However, the visible fragmentation and isolation of chapters, one from the other, in many multi-authored books led me to a decision to write most of the text myself – an exercise in masochism. Subsequently the chapters were submitted to chapter reviewers*, listed below, for a critical evaluation. Some chapters or parts thereof were written de novo and these authors are designated as contributors**. The works of the contributors and reviewers has been vital and I gratefully acknowledge their assistance. Collating their contributions has been an arduous but rewarding task.

*Anders Bennick**
Professor, Department of Biochemistry, Faculty of Medicine and Faculty of Dentistry, University of Toronto, Toronto, Ont., Canada
Chapter 9: Saliva and Dental Caries

*Colin Dawes**
Professor of Oral Biology, Faculty of Dentistry, University of Manitoba, Winnipeg, Man., Canada
Chapter 9: Saliva and Dental Caries

*Richard P. Ellen***
Professor, Faculty of Dentistry and Department of Microbiology, Faculty of Medicine, University of Toronto, Toronto, Ont., Canada
Chapter 5: Formation, Structure and Metabolism of Dental Plaque; Chapter 6: Caries as a Specific Microbial Infection

*Thorild Ericson**
Professor, Department of Cariology, Faculty of Odontology, University of Umeå, Umeå, Sweden
Chapter 1: Clinical Features and Classification of Dental Caries

*John D.B. Featherstone***
Chairman, Department of Oral Biology, Eastman Dental Center, Rochester, N.Y.
Chapter 10: The Caries Process – Morphological and Chemical Events

*Ronald J. Gibbons***
Senior Staff Member, Forsyth Dental Center; Clinical Professor of Oral Biology and Pathophysiology, Harvard School of Dental Medicine, Boston, Mass.
Chapter 5: Formation, Structure and Metabolism of Dental Plaque; Chapter 6: Caries as a Specific Microbial Infection

G. Neil Jenkins(*)(**)
Emeritus Professor of Oral Physiology, Dental School, University of Newcastle upon Tyne, England
Chapter 7: Nutrition, Diet (Local Substrate) and Dental Caries; Chapter 8: The Role of Sucrose in Dental Caries

*George H. Nancollas**
Professor of Chemistry, Faculty of Natural Sciences and Mathematics, State University of New York at Buffalo, Buffalo, N.Y.
Chapter 4: The Nature of Tooth Substance

*Leon M. Silverstone***
Associate Dean for Research, School of Dentistry, University of Colorado, Health Sciences Center, Denver, Colo.
Chapter 10: The Caries Process – Morphological and Chemical Events

*John W. Stamm**
Professor and Chairman, Department of Community Dentistry, Faculty of Dentistry, McGill University, Montreal, Que., Canada
Chapter 2: Epidemiology of Dental Caries

*John A. Weatherell**
Head of Department of Oral Biology, School of Dentistry, University of Leeds, Leeds, England, U.K.
Chapter 4: The Nature of Tooth Substance

*R.A. Young**
Professor, School of Physics, College of Sciences and Liberal Studies, Georgia Institute of Technology, Atlanta, Ga.
Chapter 4: The Nature of Tooth Substance

Acknowledgements

Many individuals have contributed and assisted in the writing of this textbook. I cannot list them all but I express thanks to my colleagues at the Faculty of Dentistry, University of Toronto for their assistance and support.

Professor *G.N. Jenkins*, Rosenstadt Visiting Professor at the University of Toronto, contributed generously of his time and energy in editing the entire book in addition to writing several sections. His congenial temperament, editing skills and scholarly criticisms did much to lighten the load in writing this text.

Thanks are due to Professors *A.M. Hunt, D. Smith, H.J. Sandham, E. Fillery, N. Camerman,* from the University of Toronto; *B. Bibby* (Rochester University), *G.M. Whitford* (Georgia Medical College) and *B. Krasse* (University of Göteborg) for many useful suggestions and for reading portions of the draft manuscripts. The administrative support of Dr. *D. Kenney*, Chief of Dentistry of the Hospital for Sick Children, Toronto, over several years of writing is gratefully acknowledged.

Mrs. *M. Hearn*, Mr. *S. Burany*, Mrs. *R. Bauer* helped greatly in the artwork and photography and Mrs. *M. Shaw* started the word-processing ordeal.

Members of ORCA (European Organization for Caries Research) have played an important role in providing a forum for numerous discussions on the subject. I am grateful to each and all for numerous ideas and suggestions.

Ms. *Slavka Murray* typed and retyped the manuscript, mastered the word-processor, and in an untiring manner persevered until the textbook was totally assembled.

The staff of the publisher and Dr. *T. Karger* have been most helpful in offering and accepting suggestions. I am grateful for the manner in which they have expedited this publication.

Gordon Nikiforuk

Preface

This is an age of specialization, the age of the expert, the pursuit of a narrow field without universalizing. Compartmentalization of knowledge into specialties is a natural outgrowth of the knowledge explosion. Specialization has the advantage of permitting one individual to master the intricacies of a specific problem. It has the disadvantage of producing an expert who knows 'more and more about less and less'. As specialization increases the need to transcend it becomes even greater.

During the past 25 years there has been an increasing tempo of papers and symposia on dental caries resulting in a large amount of fragmented information. Facts and concepts from such diverse fields as crystallography (hard tissues), immunology, microbiology, physiology, nutrition and diet, epidemiology, spectroscopy, and others are available in unmanageable numbers. These disciplines have contributed important information but the total picture cannot be more than gleamed at unless the different pieces are properly fitted together. That is what this book will attempt to do.

Rather than produce a single voluminous book this work is divided into two shorter volumes. In Volume 1, the basic aspects of the etiology and mechanism of dental caries are presented; Volume 2 deals with clinical aspects of prevention. While each volume stands alone, Volume 1 is a desirable companion to Volume 2. In Volume 1 the nature of tooth substance, the role played by oral and plaque microflora and the contribution of diet and nutrition, as well as secondary factors such as saliva, fluorides and nutrition are presented. In Volume 2, the synthesis achieved in Volume 1 is applied to the practical, clinical aspects of prevention of caries.

The contents and the sequence of chapters in this textbook have formed the basis for the teaching of the subject of Caries at the University of Toronto. This has led to a more unified teaching of the subject and has eliminated the fragmentary approach characteristic of past efforts. It is hoped it may assist others in developing a course in Cariology. Although this book is primarily designed for undergraduate students of dentistry, the comprehensive nature of its contents should appeal to graduate students as well as to students of dental hygiene and dental assisting who wish to augment their knowledge of the caries process.

Undergraduate students too often ignore historical aspects of a subject, and feel massive bibliographies are asphyxiating. While references have been winnowed, and historical aspects compressed, some history and bibliography is essential for growth of learning. The subject of caries should be an exciting learning experience.

Caries, because of its uniqueness as a disease, its ubiquitous nature, and its stubborn resistance to resolution remains as one of man's most common, oldest, and singly costliest ailment. The total health handicap due to dental caries is staggering. In western countries there has been a dramatic decline in caries over the past decade but in the economically developing countries caries prevalence is increasing as dietary habits of industrialized nations are adopted. For this reason, it is important that the subject of dental caries is given as broad a readership as possible. Recognition of the enormity of the problem should spur efforts to reduce the ravages, the pain and the cost of this disease.

This book is obviously not the last word on the subject, nor is it the first. I hope it may compete with the best. The French philosopher *Montaigne* said it best: 'I have gathered a posie of other men's flowers and nothing but the thread which binds them is mine.'

Gordon Nikiforuk

To Marge Jordis, Andrew and Christian
for making intellectual pursuits a way of life

To my Saskatchewan farm heritage
where the love of learning was always nourished

1 Clinical Features and Classification of Dental Caries

Unique Aspects of Dental Caries

Teeth are tools that have evolved to ensure survival of species. Survival of all higher forms of life is dependent upon ingestion of food to fuel life's processes. Food comes in many forms and different consistency. Teeth serve the function of gathering, cutting, grinding and admixing food with saliva in order to prepare it for swallowing and its journey through the alimentary digestive system and conversion into energy for bodily needs. To serve this function nature fashioned the hard enamel covering of teeth and a suspensory mechanism (periodontal ligament) that withstands trituration forces of up to 300 lb. per square inch. Enamel tissue is ectodermal in origin, and is the hardest biological substance, having a density of about 3. The enamel cap is supported by dentin – a hard tissue of mesodermal origin. The tooth is the only hard organ in the biological kingdom that is comprised of two tissues of different embryological origin. It has evolved uniquely to fulfill its function. But even nature has to pay a price for creating so specialized a grinding and cutting tool. Enamel tissue by virtue of its unique biological properties is highly susceptible to environmental agents.

Enamel, in its adult state, is acellular, avascular and has no nerves or vital elements. The ameloblast cells which form enamel atrophy after completing their enamel-forming function, leaving behind only a thin organic coating over enamel. Enamel tissue is incapable of any natural defense mechanism based on cellular activity. Unlike soft tissue, enamel cannot usher an inflammatory reaction against microbial invasion, nor can it heal itself by cellular repair. Adult enamel tissue being acellular is incapable of any vital function such as glycolysis or respiration. It is metabolically inert but is capable of undergoing important physico-chemical exchange reactions such as remineralization. It is a paradox that enamel, a tissue so benign in its ability to mobilize biological defense mechanisms against noxious agents, should be positioned in the relatively hostile environment of the oral cavity.

The tooth erupts into the oral cavity with its complex ecology. The environment of an erupted tooth includes saliva, epithelial cells, the oral flora, foods and drinks, crevicular fluid, blood cellular elements that exude into the oral cavity, chemicals that may be ingested, chemicals that may be regurgitated from the stomach and other substances. Some environmental factors, as saliva, serve as a natural defense mechanism against dissolution of teeth by acidic foods or metabolites. Other factors, as microbial metabolites, can be potentially hostile to the teeth. The only other tissues exposed to such a diverse environment are the skin and gut. The skin and gut possess cellular mechanisms to regenerate themselves – enamel does not.

In view of the unique characteristics of the tooth it may be anticipated that dental caries does not fall into any of the well-recognized pathological classifications of diseases. A hard, noncellular, unyielding tissue will not succumb to the usual processes that destroy soft tissues. The carious process cannot illicit an inflammatory reaction in enamel; caries is obviously not a neoplasm or a degenerative condition. Dental caries is a peculiarly local disease which involves destruction of the hard tissues of the teeth by metabolites produced by oral microorganisms.

Dental caries is unique not only in terms of the pathological mechanism; other aspects, social and economic, are also worthy of note. Caries is a biosocial disease rooted in the technology and economy of our society. As living standards improve the severity of the disease usually increases. In the industrialized countries dental caries is one of the most ubiquitous and costly illnesses. Dental caries together with periodontal disease and malocclusion constitutes a very real personal problem to virtually every man, woman and child. While it is true that diseases of the teeth and their supporting tissues do not normally kill humans they certainly affect the person's efficiency and they can, if neglected, provoke serious conditions elsewhere in the body. Their contribution to the general fund of human misery is legendary.

In addition to the personal pain and discomfort the almost universal presence of caries in industrialized society presents a financial burden of major proportions. The impact of oral diseases varies according to the customs, attitudes and economics of a particular country or population. In developing countries where the basic, everyday needs of the population are not provided for, the problem of dental disease receives low priority. In the more developed countries where many of the basic human needs are being met, oral dental disease proportionally receives a greater emphasis. Except for mental health services it is the most costly single disease entity. Billions of dollars are spent annually in repairing damage to teeth from decay. This figure represents only the cost of treating dental caries. It is known that only approximately 40% of the population in North America regularly avail themselves of dental services. Hence, if all dental needs were looked after the cost would escalate. It is reasonable to conclude that the total cost of treating oral diseases would exceed the cost of treating any other single disease entity. Further, treatment alone does not confer immunity from subsequent attack. It is becoming increasingly clear that the only hope for reducing the burdens of dental ills is through prevention. Until recently dental caries has stubbornly resisted efforts at reducing the prevalence of the disease. More recent studies indicate a dramatic reduction in caries prevalence in populations benefiting from water fluoridation and from use of fluoride-containing dentifrices and rinses (discussed in chapter 2).

The uniqueness of dental caries makes it a fascinating study from a scientific standpoint. In the succeeding chapters (volume 1) the prerequisites for the development of dental caries will be delineated and the process by which teeth are destroyed at morphological and molecular levels discussed. In volume 2, the prevention of caries is presented in detail. The clinical features, classification and epidemiology of dental caries are presented first.

Classification of Dental Caries

Students in the beginning courses in dentistry will discern that dental caries is not a disease that randomly attacks all surfaces of teeth. A superficial examination of carious teeth reveals that the lesions have a predilection to specific anatomical sites. Even though dental caries has been studied exhaustively from clinical and basic science aspects there is currently no universally accepted classification of the disease. On the basis of clinical features and patterns, dental caries may be classified according to three basic factors:

- Morphology, i.e. according to anatomical site of lesions.
- Dynamics, i.e. according to severity and rate of progression of lesions.
- Chronology, i.e. according to age patterns at which lesions predominate.

In all probability, the different clinical types of caries have the same underlying etiology, but the susceptibility of the anatomical sites and the rate of progression of the lesions vary widely from one tooth to another, and from one individual to another. The anatomical configuration of a tooth and its position in the arch determines, to a significant degree, its susceptibility to a carious attack. Caries prevalence varies greatly as a function of age. What emerges is a definite pattern of caries in individuals. It is important to emphasize that a classification of caries according to its clinical features does not imply different etiologies. The mechanism of formation of the different clinical forms of caries is similar but may be affected differently by various factors (fluoride, saliva, oral hygiene) at different sites. As an example, fluoride exerts more of a cariostatic action on smooth than on occlusal surfaces of teeth.

Classification Based on Morphology (Anatomical Site of Lesion)
Occlusal (Pit and Fissure) and Smooth Surface Caries. The most common and simplest classification of dental caries is based on relative susceptibility of surfaces of teeth. The different surfaces of a tooth may be divided into two morphological types. Type I refers to pit, fissure and occlusal surfaces and type II refers to smooth surfaces of which there are two variations, interproximal and cervical or gingival (fig. 1/1a, b). Pit and fissure caries are limited to the occlusal surfaces of molars and bicuspids, the buccal pits of molars, and lingual surfaces of maxilliary anterior teeth (fig. 1/1a). These irregular surfaces are inherently more prone to dental caries due to their mechanical characteristics which result in poor self-cleansing features. Occlusal caries usually occur early in life before smooth surface lesions appear. Carious lesions located on surfaces other than pits and fissures are classified as type II, smooth surface lesions. Smooth surface lesions may be further subdivided as interproximal, occurring at mesial or distal contact points, or cervical, occurring on buccal or lingual surfaces near the dentin-enamel junction (fig. 1/1b).

Black's well-known classification of cavity preparation for operative dentistry is based on morphological considerations. Class I preparations involve the occlusal surface; classes II and III involve interproximal surfaces of posterior and anterior teeth, respectively; class IV involves the incisal corners of anterior teeth, and class V cavity preparations involve the labial or buccal enamel near the dentinoenamel junction. This classification was proposed specifically for cavity preparation; however, the system has relevance to the morphological classification of dental caries since *Black's* class I preparations are associated with pit and fissure caries, while class II–IV types are associated with smooth surface lesions.

Root (Cementum) Caries. Most but not all caries initiates at the enamel surface. Carious lesions that initiate at the dentinal-root portion of a tooth are called root caries. This type of caries is predominantly found in dentitions of older age groups with significant gingival recession and exposed root surfaces. In the 50- to 59-year age group almost 60% of patients examined had root surface lesions [*Banting and Ellen*, 1976]. Root caries initiates on mineralized cementum and dentin surfaces which have a greater organic component than enamel tissue. For this reason the bacterial flora causing root caries may be different from the flora that initiates enamel caries. Root surface caries in contemporary populations occurs

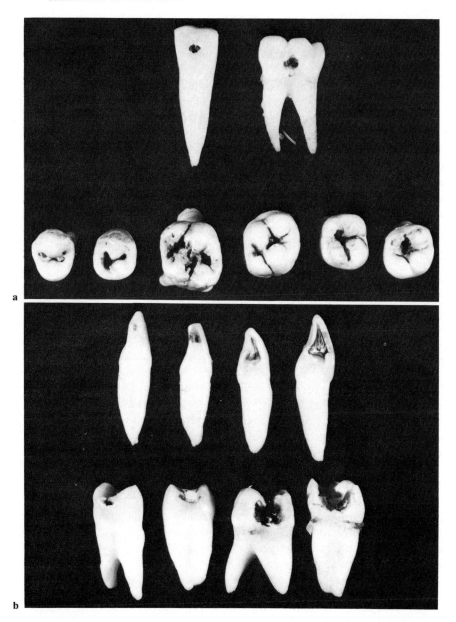

Fig. 1/1. a Extracted teeth showing type I carious lesions in pits and fissures including buccal pits of molars and lingual pits of maxillary incisors (top). **b** Type II lesions on interproximal and labial, buccal or lingual smooth surfaces.

most frequently on the buccal and lingual surfaces of roots; in ancient populations root lesions predominated on proximal surfaces (discussed further in chapter 2). Figure 1/2a, b depicts severe root caries in elderly patients with plaque (organic coating on teeth populated by specific oral bacteria) formation and root caries undermining the enamel.

Linear Enamel Caries (Odontoclasia). An atypical form of dental caries, called linear enamel caries, has been observed in the primary dentition of children, in Latin America and Asian countries (fig. 1/3a, b). The lesions predominate on the labial surfaces of the anterior maxillary teeth, in the region of the neonatal line (more correctly the neonatal zone). The neonatal zone represents the demarcation between pre- and postnatal enamel and is a histological feature of all primary teeth. It is thought to result from the metabolic disturbances associated with the trauma of birth. More recent evidence indicates that the specific metabolic disturbance causing the neonatal line is transient hypocalcemia (low serum calcium concentration) associated with transient hypoparathyroidism – a normal feature of the neonatal period (more on this subject in chapter 7). The position of the neonatal line at the enamel surface of anterior primary teeth results in the carious lesions assuming a crescent shape. Children with linear enamel hypoplasia have an increased predisposition to caries in the posterior primary teeth even though these teeth do not show visible signs of hypoplasia [*Infante and Gillespie,* 1977] (more on this topic later in chapters 2 and 7).
     A variant of the linear enamel form of caries in the primary teeth of children in the Far East has been named odontoclasia (fig. 1/4). The morphological aspects of this type of caries is atypical and results in gross destruction of the labial surfaces of incisor teeth. This may be due to an inherent structural defect in teeth resulting in a rapid carious process.

Classification Based on Severity and Rate of Caries Progression
     Dental caries may be classified according to the severity and rapidity of attack as shown in table 1/I. The severity may be very mild to very severe or rampant. Different teeth and surfaces are involved depending upon the severity of the caries challenge. In mild caries only the most vulnerable teeth and surfaces are attacked such as the occlusal surface of first permanent molars. In moderate caries the occlusal surfaces of other posterior teeth are involved as well as interproximal surfaces. In rampant caries sur-

---

Fig. 1/2. a Caries localized to the dentinal-root portion of teeth in an elderly patient (arrows). **b** Note the heavy plaque and calcareous deposits (arrows), on the lingual of the mandibular incisors (courtesy Drs. *D.W. Banting* and *R.P. Ellen*).

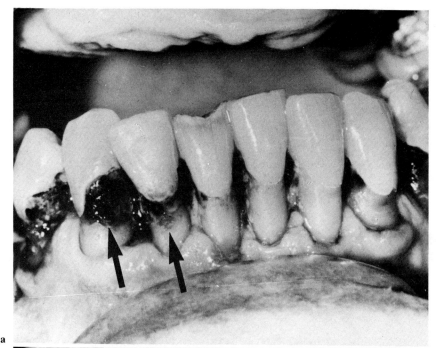

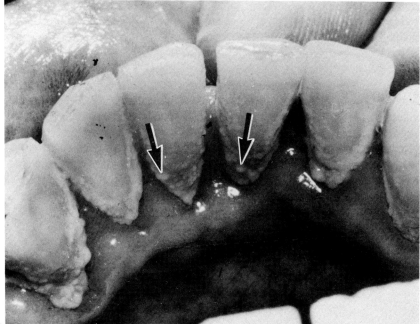

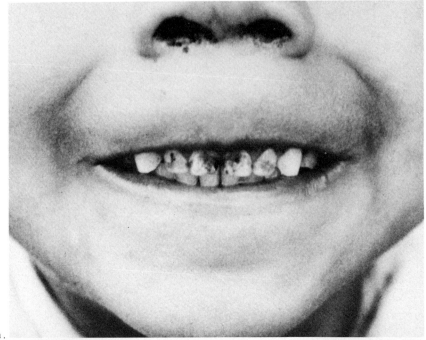

a

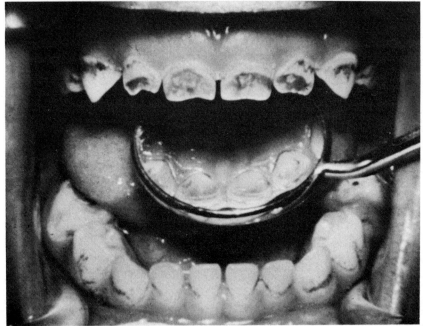

b

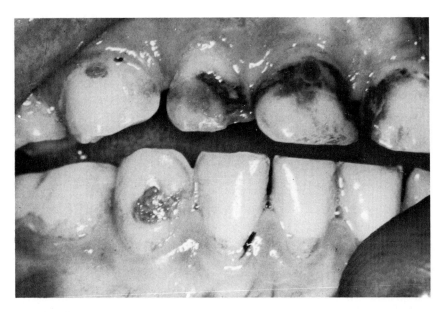

Fig. 1/4. A child with odontoclasia. Note the gross destruction of the labial surfaces of the primary anterior teeth. (Courtesy Dr. *R.G. Schamschula*).

faces of anterior teeth which are relatively less frequently attacked become carious. Rampant caries is a common and important manifestation of the disease in children and some adults and merits a further discussion.

Rampant Caries. One of the most distressful clinical conditions for both patient and practitioner is rampant caries in which there occurs a sudden, rapid and almost uncontrollable destruction of teeth. Rampant caries also involves surfaces of teeth that are ordinarily relatively caries-free. A caries increment of 10 or more new carious lesions over a period of about a year is characteristic of a rampant caries attack. Proximal and cervical surfaces of anterior teeth, including the mandibular incisors which are relatively caries-free, may be affected (fig. 1/5).

Fig. 1/3a, b. Enamel caries superimposed over linear enamel hypoplasia in 2 young children. Note the lesions involving the maxillary primary incisors. These lesions are common in children in some Latin American countries.

Table 1/I. Classification of dental caries based on severity

Classification[1]	Teeth affected	Surfaces affected
Class 1: Very mild caries	6 7	occlusal pits and fissures (in lower molars only)
Class 2: Mild caries (ordinary caries)	6 7 6 7	occlusal pits and proximal contact areas
Class 3: Moderate caries	5 6 7 5 6 7	occlusal and proximal buccal and lingual pits proximals of 1 2 (lingual pits of 2)
Class 4: Severe caries (extensive caries)	1 2 3 4 5 6 7 4 5 6 7	proximal and occlusal and/or occasional cervical areas of 1 2 3 5 6 7 5 6 7
Class 5: Very severe caries (rampant caries)	1 2 3 4 5 6 7 1 2 3 4 5 6 7	proximal of 1 2 3 and/or cervical areas of 1 2 3 4 5 6 7 1 2 3 4 5 6 7

The usual order of susceptibility of the teeth to caries is: $\overline{6}, \overline{7}, \underline{6}, \underline{7}, \underline{5}, \overline{5}, \underline{2}, \underline{1}, 4, \underline{3}, \overline{4}, \overline{1}, \overline{2}, \overline{3}$.
[1] After *Klein and Palmer* [1941].

In North American populations living in non-fluoridated communities about 5% of the child population is affected by rampant caries. Rampant caries is most often observed in the primary dentition of young children and the permanent dentition of teenagers, 11–19 years. Dietary factors affecting oral substrate and oral flora and physiological factors affecting saliva are often significant in the development of rampant caries. Several clinical types of rampant caries that are most common are 'infancy or soother caries' and 'adolescent caries' (see classification of caries according to chronology). All are characterized by a rapid development of numerous carious lesions in teeth and surfaces that are usually relatively caries-free.

In addition to the above classification several other clinical patterns have been described which relate to the degree and rate of progression of caries. The most common clinical forms are incipient, arrested and recurrent caries and caries induced by a marked reduction in salivary flow (xerostomia).

Incipient Caries. The early carious lesion on visible smooth surfaces of teeth is clinically manifested as a white, opaque region, which is best demonstrated when the area is air-dried (fig. 1/6a). At this stage some demineralization of enamel has occurred but there is no cavity and no major histological change of the organic matrix of enamel [*Darling*, 1958].

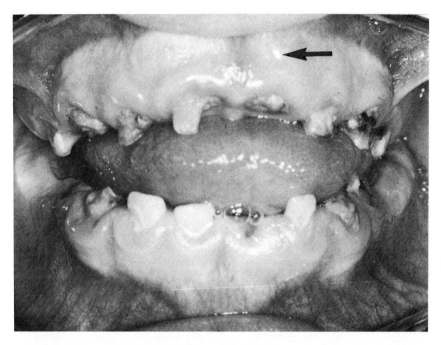

Fig. 1/5. Rampant caries in a child, 2 years old. All primary teeth are carious, the crowns of the anterior incisors have been destroyed leaving only root stumps. Draining fistula is marked by arrow.

An important feature of the early lesion is the apparently intact surface layer overlying subsurface demineralization. Sometimes the relatively intact surface may become pigmented by absorption of extrinsic stain, such an area is called a 'brown spot' and may represent arrested tooth decay.

If a radiographic (bite-wing) examination of a suspected early white-spot lesion shows a small radiolucent area in the outer enamel (fig. 1/6b, I), then histologically it can be demonstrated that the lesion has penetrated into dentin. However, at this stage it is important to recognize that only chemical damage (loss of mineral salts) has occurred in the tissue and that usually there is no significant penetration of the bacteria associated with the dentinal lesion and no cavitation of the enamel surface. Lesions depicted in figure 1/6b, II and III, are more advanced and are characterized by bacterial penetration and cavitation. A white-spot lesion, per se, is not an indication for restoration of the carious lesion. Many incipient lesions undergo remineralization thereby reversing the carious process. If the pa-

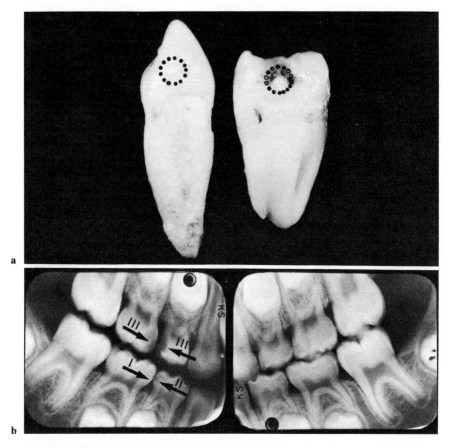

Fig. 1/6. a An incipient white-spot lesion on the interproximal smooth surface of two isolated teeth. **b** (I) Radiographic image of an incipient lesion involving the enamel only, (II) more advanced lesion with dentin involvement and (III) gross lesion with deep dentinal penetration.

tient is not highly susceptible to dental caries an effective preventive procedure is the preferred course of action. A more detailed discussion of the histological and chemical features of an incipient carious lesion is to be found in chapter 10.

Arrested Caries. There is clinical evidence that incipient and even more advanced carious lesions may become arrested if there is a significant shift in oral environmental conditions from those that predispose to those

Table 1/II. Caries progression from age 8 to age 15 on the buccal surface of 184 maxillary first molars [*Backer Dirks*, 1966]

	Age	
	8	15

Sound	93	74 \ 37 } 111
White-spot lesions	72	15 \ 26 } 41
Cavitation	19	4 \ 9 } 32 \ 19

that tend to slow the caries process. Clinical longitudinal data on dental caries in children [*Backer Dirks*, 1966], involving the buccal surfaces of maxillary first molars, indicated that at an age of 8 years about 39% of the surfaces had white-spot, opaque lesions, and about 10% exhibited cavitation. Seven years later, the same surfaces with intial white-spot lesions were reexamined and it was found that about 36% of the original surfaces with white-spot lesions were unchanged and that over 50% had remineralized and regressed to such an extent that the surfaces were considered normal (table 1/II). This suggests that incipient enamel caries can remain dormant for long periods of time and that some lesions may reverse by remineralizing. A case of arrested caries is shown in figure 1/7. A clinical feature of arrested caries involving dentin is the marked brown pigmentation and induration of the lesion (more on the subject of remineralization of incipient lesions later.)

Recurrent Caries. A carious lesion that develops at the interface of a restoration and the cavosurface of the enamel is called recurrent caries. Recurrent lesions may indicate an unusual susceptibility to caries attack, a poor cavity preparation, a defective restoration or a combination of these factors (fig. 1/8).

Xerostomia-Induced Caries (Radiation Caries). A common complication of radiotherapy of oral cancer lesions is radiation-induced xerostomia (from the Greek, xeros = dry; stoma = mouth). Such patients develop rampant dental caries and confirm the important role of salivary secretion in the maintenance of the integrity of the teeth (fig. 1/9). Xerostomia is

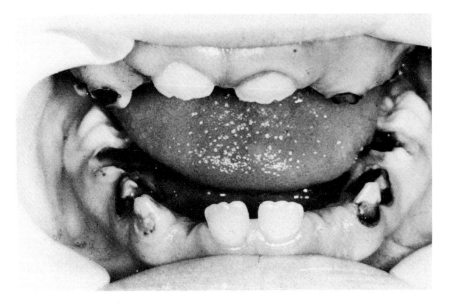

Fig. 1/7. Arrested carious lesions in the primary teeth. The pigmented areas are indurated and glossy.

accompanied by major changes in the salivary flow, salivary composition (electrolytes), salivary and serum proteins and a shift towards a more caries-producing microflora. Collectively, the oral changes following irradiation-induced xerostomia create an overwhelming caries-conducive environment capable of rapidly destroying enamel and root surfaces unless interrupted by intensive preventive measures. Carious lesions appear as early as 3 months after the onset of xerostomia and all patients may be affected irrespective of their past caries history. Xerostomia may be caused by other factors than radiation. Tumors of salivary glands, autoimmune diseases, antisialagogue drugs and prolonged illness may also lead to a reduced state of salivary secretion (for a more detailed discussion of caries due to xerostomia see chapter 9).

Fig. 1/8. Recurrent caries in a child. The lesion is at the junction of the restoration and the enamel surface (courtesy Dr. *N. Levine*).
Fig. 1/9. Radiation caries due to radiation-induced xerostomia in a patient with oral carcinoma (courtesy Dr. *C. Munroe*).

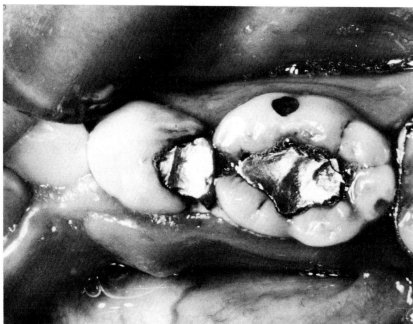

1/8

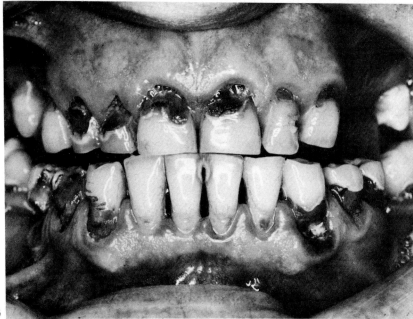

1/9

Classification Based on Chronology

Caries is primarily a disease of children and young adults. As the susceptible surfaces of teeth decay, the new caries increment decreases. Caries experience and age is discussed in detail in chapter 2. The exacerbation of caries at certain age groups has resulted in a descriptive categorization of caries according to age. Again, it is emphasized that these classifications are a convenience in describing clinical features of caries; they do not imply different etiologies.

Infancy (Soother or Nursing Bottle) Caries. Numerous reports by pediatricians and pedodontists describe a rapidly progressing type of dental caries that affects the primary teeth of children, usually during the first 2 years of life and as early as the first year. In children with infancy caries there is a unique distribution of dental decay. The 4 maxillary anterior incisors are affected first (fig. 1/10a, b), these teeth are anatomically so positioned in the mouth as to be most frequently bathed by a feeding formula. If unchecked the decay may extend to the maxillary and mandibular molars. Initially, the lower anterior teeth may not be involved because of the protective environment of the mandibular salivary secretions and the cleansing action of the tongue muscles.

Infancy caries is most often seen in children with an unusual dietary history such as the addition of syrup, honey or sucrose to the formula or the use of a pacifier dipped in honey or other sweeteners [*Ripa*, 1978; *Derkson and Ponti*, 1982]. Rampant caries in young children was very common after the introduction of vitamin syrups in the United Kingdom. A favorite trick to ensure long feeding from the contents of a single bottle was to thicken the formula with a syrup, thereby increasing the viscosity of the fluid and the time required to draw the formula through the nipple [*Winter* et al., 1966]. The use of sweetened apple and other fruit juices as a fluid supplement in infants has also contributed towards development of rampant caries because of the high concentration of 'sweet' fluids bathing the maxillary teeth.

In addition to an increase in caries rates due to use of improper formula in bottle-feeding, it has been reported that prolonged and unrestricted nighttime breast-feeding can result in increased caries rates [*Preston* et al., 1977]. The stagnation of the milk about the neck of anterior teeth and the fermentation of the disaccharide lactose, found in milk, contribute to the carious process. Under usual feeding regimens neither bottle nor breast milk predisposes to caries. Only a prolonged and unrestrictive bottle- or breast milk-feeding regimen may play a role in caries production. Of more significance is the addition of caloric sweeteners to formulas.

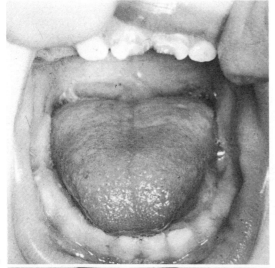

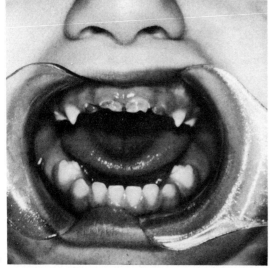

Fig. 1/10. a An 8-month-old child with infancy or nursing bottle caries. In this case corn syrup was added to milk formula at each feeding. **b** An 18-month-old child with nursing bottle caries. Note the destruction of the maxillary, primary anterior teeth.

Adolescent Caries. There are two chronological periods when acute, rapidly progressing caries is commonly observed. Acute exacerbations in caries rates are usually seen at 4–8 years of age and at 11–18 years of age (see chapter 2). The acute caries attack in the latter period is usually characterized as adolescent caries (fig. 1/11a). The characteristic features of this type of caries are:

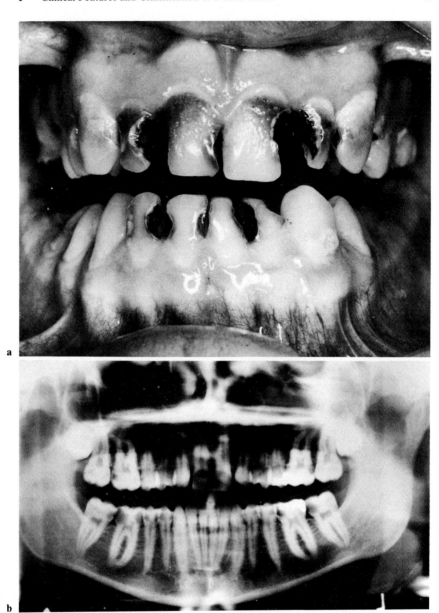

Fig. 1/11. a Rampant caries in an adolescent patient. Note the destruction of surfaces of lower anterior teeth which are normally caries-free. **b** A Panorex view of caries in an adolescent. Note the gross destruction of the interproximal surfaces of posterior teeth.

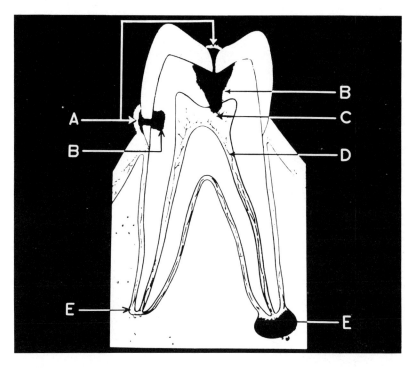

Fig. 1/12. A diagrammatic representation of the clinical progression of an unchecked carious lesion from an incipient lesion, progressing through the enamel, dentin and extending into the pulp and ultimately resulting in a periapical abscess. A = Beginning decay. B = Penetrating decay abscess. C = Diseased pulp. D = Infected root canal. E = Root end abscess.

- Lesions in teeth and surfaces that are relatively immune to caries.
- Relatively small opening in enamel with extensive undermining of enamel.
- Rapid penetration of enamel and extensive involvement of dentin.
- The rapid progression of the lesion which does not permit an effective pulpal response with little or no secondary dentin.

In advanced stages of adolescent caries, as shown in a Panorex radiographic survey (fig. 1/11b), restorative work may be difficult due to undermining and extensive destruction of enamel. It is important to detect cases of rampant caries in the adolescent at an early stage so that preventive procedures may be rigorously applied.

An untreated, unchecked, carious lesion progresses through the enamel and then the dentin and ultimately the pulp (fig. 1/12), leading to a

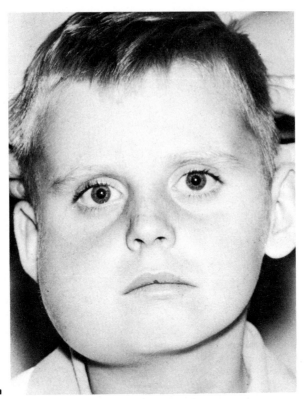

a

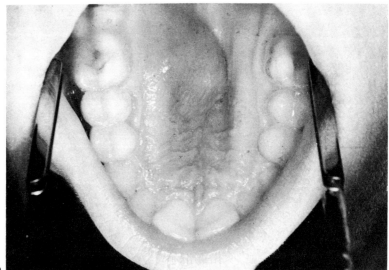

b

periapical abscess. Unsuccessful tissue localization of a periapical infection frequently gives rise to a cellulitis (inflammation of the soft tissues). Acute facial cellulitis of odontogenic origin is shown in figure 1/13a, b.

Rate at which Caries Forms–Clinical Significance

An early diagnosis of the size and location of a carious lesion is important because it helps in evaluating caries activity in an individual. Equally important information is the speed at which the lesion develops once it is established. These two stages, initiation and development, are not necessarily interrelated but for an assessment of caries activity both are relevant.

A carious lesion starts at the enamel surface by a demineralization which clinically appears to be a white spot. Morphologically an initial lesion has an intact surface but a subsurface demineralization (more on subsurface demineralization in chapter 10). The rate at which a cavity grows in size varies between individuals and is a function of several factors like frequency of carbohydrate intake, oral hygiene, and microbial and salivary conditions. A rapid development occurs in patients with an unfavorable combination of caries-initiating and defense factors, as in those individuals whose salivary flow has been significantly reduced by radiation therapy. In normal populations, a cavity develops very slowly and intermittently [*Boyd* et al., 1952]. Each period of demineralization is followed by a period of rest or even remineralization. *Parfitt* [1956] made similar observations, reporting that it may be 3 to over 48 months for occlusal caries to progress through the incipient stage. The progress of a caries lesion in a buccal surface is generally slower, and if no cavity is formed 1.5 years after eruption it is unlikely that a cavity will form before 15 years of age [*Backer Dirks*, 1966]. The progression of lesions is significantly slower in fluoride areas. These general estimations, however, cannot be uncritically used in the treatment of individual lesions. It is clinically important to recognize that large individual variations occur in the rate of caries development.

Occlusal surface lesions develop earlier and often faster than on other surfaces. Further, they are not readily reversible because pits and fissures form highly susceptible surfaces. On the other hand, smooth surface lesions develop later than occlusal cavities and in some individuals may re-

---

Fig. 1/13. a Cellulitis involving the submandibular structures due to a carious mandibular second primary molar. **b** Cellulitis spreading to the palatal area due to a carious maxillary permanent molar.

verse, particularly if dietary conditions change and less cariogenic foods are consumed.

A general practitioner of dentistry has, on a daily basis, to make a decision whether an incipient caries lesion should be treated prophylactically to prevent further progress or if a combined restorative and prophylactic treatment is required. Such an individualized treatment plan must be based on clinical observations and on a proper consideration of the history of the patient. To assist in making an individualized decision, radiographs are often used as an important diagnostic aid for detecting carious lesions. Many radiographic investigations indicate that when a radiolucent area has reached the dentin a cavity is a common finding. Extension of radiolucency through the dentin surface has often been the criterion that a restoration is needed. However, more recent studies [*Gröndahl*, 1979; *Bille and Thylstrup*, 1982] indicate that there is a relative lack of agreement between the radiographic image and the clinical status of an advancing carious lesion. These workers find that overtreatment may result in populations with a low prevalence of dental caries if the decision to treat is based on radiographic interpretations alone. *Bille and Thylstrup* [1982] found that more than half of carious lesions slated for restorations on the basis of radiographic interpretations were found to have no macroscopic cavitation. In the study by *Gröndahl* [1979] it was found that over a third of the lesions diagnosed as enamel caries did not progress beyond the amelodentinal junction over a 6-year period. Further, it was determined that the probability of a radiographically discernable lesion progressing to a clinical cavity is lower the lower the caries prevalence. On the basis of these observations it is essential that decisions to treat or not to treat incipient lesions should be based on combined radiographic and clinical assessments.

References

Backer Dirks, O: Posteruptive changes in dental enamel. J. dent. Res. *45:* suppl. 3, p. 503 (1966).

Banting, D.W.; Ellen, R.P.: Carious lesions on the roots of teeth: a review for the general practitioner. J. Can. dent. Ass. *10:* 496 (1976).

Bille, J.; Thylstrup, A.: Radiographic diagnosis and clinical tissue changes in relation to treatment of approximal carious lesions. Caries Res. *16:* 1 (1982).

Boyd, J.D.; Cannon, J.J.; Leighton, R.E.: Epidemiologic studies in dental caries. V. Placement of fillings as a source of statistical error of estimate as to dental caries progression rates. J. dent. Res. *31:* 354 (1952).

Darling, A.I.: Studies of the early lesion of enamel caries with transmitted light, polarized light and microradiography. Its nature, mode of spread, points of entry and its relation to enamel structure. Br. dent. J. *105:* 119 (1958).

Derkson, G.D.; Ponti, P.: Nursing bottle syndrome; prevalence and etiology in a non-fluoridated city. J. Can. dent. Ass. *48:* 389 (1982).

Gröndahl, H.-G.: Radiographic caries diagnosis and treatment decisions. Swed. dent. J. *3:* 109 (1979).

Infante, P.F.; Gillespie, G.M.: Enamel hypoplasia in relation to caries in Guatemalan children. J. dent. Res. *56:* 493 (1977).

Klein, H.; Palmer, C.F.: Studies on dental caries. XII. Comparison susceptibility of the various morphological types of permanent teeth. Publ. Hlth Rep., Wash. *20:* 203 (1941).

Parfitt, G.J.: The speed of development of the carious cavity. Br. dent. J. *100:* 204 (1956).

Preston, G.S.; Berkowitz, R.J.; Forrester, D.J.: Nursing bottle caries. Pediatrics, Springfield *59:* 777 (1977).

Ripa, L.W.: Nursing habits and dental decay in infants: 'nursing bottle caries'. J. Dent. Child. *45:* 274 (1978).

Winter, G.B.; Hamilton, M.C.; James, P.M.C.: Role of the comforter as an aetiological factor in rampant caries of the deciduous dentition. Archs Dis. Childh. *41:* 207 (1966).

2 Epidemiology of Dental Caries

The word epidemiology is of Greek origin, derived from *epi*, meaning on or upon, *demos*, meaning people and *logos* denoting study. Epidemiology is the study of health and disease states and the effect of ecological or extrinsic factors (nutrition, climate, life-style) and intrinsic factors (age, sex, biological parameters) on these states. Examples of epidemiological research include studies of mortality rates, causes of death and morbidity, and the effects of treatment and prevention. The epidemiologist defines the frequency and severity of health problems in relation to age, sex, geography, race, economic status, nutrition and diet. The epidemiologist can often study parameters of a disease that do not yield to a laboratory approach. He, more often than other investigators, has the panoramic approach to studying disease and health.

Some quantitative measure of the tendency of populations to develop dental caries is essential in delineating the magnitude of the problem, in recognizing the pattern of the disease, in studying underlying causative factors, and in assessing the effectiveness of preventive measures. In addition, epidemiological studies of caries have made it possible to test hypotheses, to evaluate concepts and to assess the effectiveness of health care services.

A single example will illustrate the importance of epidemiology in the study of dental caries. The most significant dental discovery during the current century is that populations consuming water containing approximately 1 ppm of fluoride demonstrate 50–65% less caries than comparable nonfluoride populations. The initial clues to this discovery came about from careful observational studies which linked mottled enamel with lower caries levels. Subsequent research on the microanalysis of fluoride in water led to further discoveries which demonstrated the precise relationship of water fluoride concentrations to dental caries levels among children. Thus, the dramatic story of the link between fluoride and dental health was developed largely by the application of the epidemiological method.

The purpose of this chapter is to provide the reader with an overview of the changing pattern of caries through the ages. The methods of measuring the prevalence of caries is discussed. Use of standardized epidemiological surveys permits a global comparison of dental caries prevalence among contemporary populations. In addition, the effects of environmental and demographic factors on caries prevalence are discussed. The distribution of caries in the permanent and primary dentitions provides clinicians with information about the relative susceptibility of different teeth and surfaces of teeth. There are many sequelae of untreated caries of which the most important is the loss of teeth leading to edentulism. Edentulism is all too common in many parts of the world. Evidence is presented suggesting that edentulism may be more related to the value that individuals place on teeth than to disease states.

Quantitating Caries Activity – DMF and def Index

Before the prevalence and pattern of a disease can be studied it is essential to devise a quantitative measure that will accurately reflect the extent of the disease in a population. Fortunately this is not difficult in the case of dental caries since a carious lesion is, generally, nonreversible and indelible. Thus, permanent stigmata appear in the dentition where surfaces of teeth have open carious lesions, where tooth surfaces have been restored or where teeth have been extracted because of extensive and irreparable damage from tooth decay. It is relatively simple to quantitate the extent of previous damage to the permanent dentition by a measure known as the DMF index, where D represents the number of decayed teeth (surfaces), M the number missing and F the number of filled teeth (surfaces). The DMF index is the sum of these components. It is an arithmetic index of the cumulative caries attack in a population. The designation DMF(T) is used to denote decayed, missing, filled teeth; DMF(S) denotes decayed, missing and filled surfaces in permanent teeth and therefore takes into account the number of surfaces attacked on each tooth. A similar index for primary dentitions is the def(t) or def(s) index, denoting the number of decayed, indicated for extraction or extracted due to caries (to differentiate from loss due to natural exfoliation) and filled teeth or surfaces, respectively.

The DMF/def index can be used to quantitate both the caries prevalence and caries incidence in a given population. Prevalence refers to the number of persons or the proportion of a population afflicted by a disease or condition at a given moment of examination. In the case of dental caries, prevalence refers to the proportion of the population with caries experience, past or current. The incidence of disease refers to the numbers or proportion of persons developing disease in a specified interval of time, usually a year. In the case of dental caries, this would mean the proportion of people developing 1 or more carious lesions during the given time period. In dentistry, however, it is more common to employ a modified form of this index called the caries increment. This latter measure refers to the number of new caries lesions occurring in a specified time interval, either for an individual or averaged over a population. The assessment of the caries increment involves at least two examinations – one at the beginning and one at the end of the period in question. Figure 2/1a, b illustrates the manner in which the DMF(T) index may be applied to a specific case and readily enables the reader to grasp the essential meaning of the index.

The reader will discern practical problems that arise in using the DMF/def index both in children and adults. In children, primary teeth may be lost due to natural exfoliation and, for the purpose of the def index, it is essential that the examiner designate as missing only those teeth that are lost due to caries. In older populations many teeth may be lost for reasons that are not related to dental caries, such as periodontal disease, or removal of teeth for construction of dentures. Such teeth should ordinarily not enter the DMF index calculation. There is, also, the question of whether third permanent molars should be included since these teeth are often removed for reasons other than caries. In many studies missing teeth are scored as equivalent to 4 or 5 carious surfaces. This has been shown to be incorrect; a closer approximation suggested is around 2.25 [*Wagg*, 1974]. Comparisons between surveys are fraught with difficulties since criteria for a carious lesion may be different, e.g. radiographic versus visual criteria. It is often difficult to clinically detect an initial lesion in the proximal surface and the criteria for identifying very early interproximal lesions may vary with different observers. The filled (F) count does not always reflect an accurate indication of past decay since a normal tooth may have been fitted with a metal filling to support an adjoining artificial tooth. In spite of shortcomings of the DMF index it is currently the most widely used measure of caries experience, and efforts are continuing to arrive at international standards in its use and application.

Using the above and other quantitative indices, we shall now discuss the epidemiology of dental caries. First to be considered is the prevalence and pattern of distribution of dental caries in ancient populations and in modern man living in highly industrialized countries, as well as in some isolated populations that still live under primitive conditions. Detailed interpretation of the epidemiological studies will be delayed until later sections of the book, when we consider the current concepts of the etiology of dental caries and discuss the primary causal and the secondary or predisposing factors in caries. The important epidemiological studies which have led to water fluoridation, and the use of topical and systemic fluorides in the prevention of dental caries are considered in volume 2, dealing with prevention.

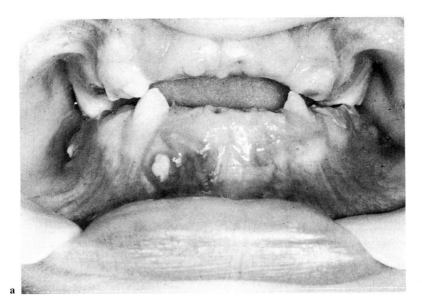

a

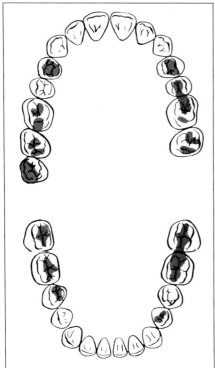

b

Fig. 2/1. a Rampant caries in a 2-year-old child. The decayed, extracted, filled teeth, def(t) index, in this case is 19 since all primary teeth are carious except the right mandibular cuspid. **b** Diagrammatic representation of caries in the permanent dentition. The DMF(T) index and DMF(S) index is readily calculated by counting the number of carious teeth and the number of surfaces affected. The DMF(T) index is 14; the DMF(S) index is 25–26 depending upon the score assigned to a missing tooth. Note that a missing tooth is usually scored as equivalent to 4 or 5 surfaces. A more realistic approximation is about 2.25. Only the maxillary third molar is missing due to caries; the mandibular third molars were extracted due to impaction.

Table 2/I. Percentage of carious teeth found in prehistoric crania of man [*Patrick*, 1914]

Race	Number of teeth examined	Percentage of carious teeth
Asiatics (including Malays, Chinese, Japanese, Armenians, Hindoos, and Burmese)	2,180	2.0
Egyptians and Africans	3,306	3.4
Polynesians and Australians	2,738	4.3
Central Americans	930	4.8
North Americans (including Eskimo)	27,362	5.0
South Americans (including Tierra del Feugians and Guanches)	6,719	5.8
Europeans (including 'a few modern soldiers')	3,422	7.0

Caries in Prehistoric Man (3000–750 BC)

Archaeological and anthropological studies attest to the relative inde-structibility of teeth, postmortem. Enamel is particularly resistant to the physicochemical and microbial agents normally present in soils. This is in sharp contrast to the great vulnerability of teeth to carious attack in living individuals. Since teeth may survive in dry burial sites for thousands of years and since no caries-like lesions have been produced in cadavers, reli-able data on the occurrence of dental caries in ancient populations are available.

With a few recent exceptions, dental caries is to a great extent a dis-ease accompanying advances in civilization. The prevalence of the disease is 'proportionate to the state of civilization to which a particular race has attained' [*Pickerill*, 1914]. There is no evidence of dental caries in the re-latively few teeth found in skull fragments of our earliest known direct ancestors, the Pithecanthropus. Evidence of fairly extensive decay was found in at least one skull of a Rhodesian man from the Neanderthal age. Evidence of caries was found in about one half of the 24 skulls of the prehistoric Ofnet race which lived in central Europe about 15,000 years ago. An examination of prehistoric crania found in the various museums in America indicated that the percentage of carious teeth ranged from 2 to 7% (table 2/I). There is no doubt that prehistoric man suffered from dental caries, although the prevalence and severity of the disease were dramatically less than in modern populations.

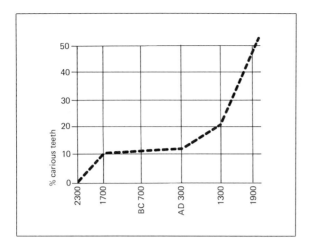

Fig. 2/2. The progress of dental caries in Greece [*Sognnaes*, 1949].

In Greece, which has a long and continuous recorded history, it is possible to compare the caries rates in skulls of individuals living thousands of years ago with those of more recent times. On the basis of such observations *Krikos* [1935] reported a steady deterioration of the teeth of ancient Greek adults and, alarmingly so, during the last few hundred years. Whereas no carious lesions were found in skulls of ancient Greeks before 2300 BC, about 10% of the teeth examined were carious during the period 1700 BC to 300 AD. More recently, fully 48% of teeth examined were found to be carious. Figure 2/2 portrays the progress of dental caries in Greece from 2300 BC to 1900 AD.

Caries in Ancient British Populations

In a survey of the prevalence of dental caries according to tooth type and period of history, *Moore and Corbett* [1971, 1973, 1976] studied the dentitions of ancient populations in the British Isles, spanning the period from the Iron Age (550 BC to 43 AD) to the 19th century. This study indicates that prevalence and pattern of dental caries did not change significantly during the 2,000 years or more from the beginning of the Iron Age to the Medieval period (1066–1500 AD).

During this period the overall caries level was very low, and the most frequent site of caries attack in the younger population was the occlusal surface. Interestingly, the observed frequency of lesions on this surface disappeared with age due to attrition of the teeth resulting from the abra-

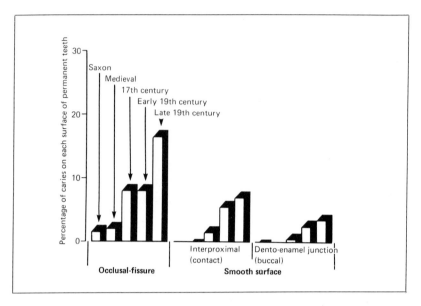

Fig. 2/3. Mean percentage of carious lesions located on specific surfaces of permanent teeth observed in jaws from ancient British populations from the Anglo-Saxon era to the 19th century. The data for each surface is represented by columns in the sequence Saxon, Medieval, 17th century, early and late 19th century, respectively [modified from *Moore and Corbett*, 1971, 1973, 1975, 1976].

sive characteristics of the diet. As occlusal lesions declined with age, the frequency of caries at the cemento-enamel junction of the interproximal surface increased. Unlike the pattern in modern man, carious lesions at or just below the interproximal contact areas or in the buccal fissures were infrequent in the early periods, but were observed more frequently in skulls from the medieval period. By about the 17th century there was a significant increase in the total caries experience and a smaller increase in the number of carious lesions involving the interproximal contact areas of teeth – thus signalling a trend that is more characteristic of the pattern and occurrence of caries in modern populations. The change in the prevalence rates and the pattern of caries involving individual teeth and occlusal-fissure and smooth surfaces is graphically depicted in figures 2/3 and 2/4. The population sample upon which the study of 17th century subjects was based came entirely from burial sites at the time of the 1665 Great Plague of London. Conditions of life in 17th century London were more urbanized than in other cities where a country life-style still prevailed.

The English of this epoch were known to be avid flesh, cheese and

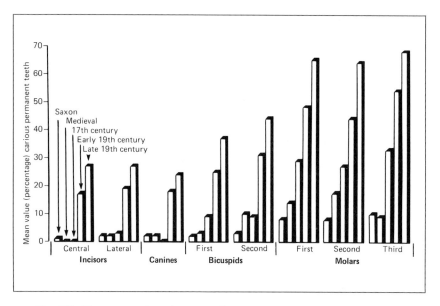

Fig. 2/4. The mean values (percentage) for caries for individual permanent teeth observed in skulls and jaws obtained from ancient British populations from the Anglo-Saxon era to the 19th century. For each tooth group the column sequence is Saxon, Medieval, 17th century, early and late 19th century [modified from the studies by *Moore and Corbett*, 1971, 1973, 1975, 1976].

butter eaters. Poultry, game and a variety of fish were eaten by the wealthy, while the poor had to be satisfied with less expensive salted and pickled fish. Market gardening developed, and corn markets were established during this century. Cane sugar industries were developing rapidly in the New World since the 16th century, and increasing quantities of sugar were also being imported from the East. In 1641, the first sugar factory was built in the British West Indies. Initially sweetmeats, syrup, sweetened puddings and tarts were luxuries of the rich. However, by the year 1850 there were changes in the laws governing wheat and sugar imports which resulted in a rapid dietary change in the direction of increasing consumption of sugar and milled wheat products by all segments of the population.

In the 19th century, caries experience in England increased rapidly after 1850 as shown by studies of dentitions from pre- and post-1850 burial sites. The occurrence of cavities at interproximal contact areas and on occlusal surfaces also increased dramatically. Carious lesions at the cemento-enamel junction, which were not common up to and including the 17th century, increased during the 19th century but to a lesser degree than inter-

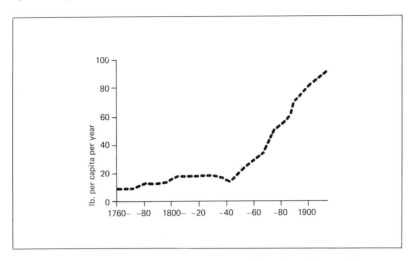

Fig. 2/5. Per capita sugar consumption in Britian during the 18th and 19th century [*Deerr*, 1950].

proximally. Similar trends were also detected in the primary dentition. *Moore and Corbett* [1976] concluded that caries pattern and the increase in prevalence during the 18th and 19th centuries were associated with dietary changes and particularly the increasing consumption of refined carbohydrates. The per capita consumption of sugar in Britain during the 18th and 19th centuries is shown in figure 2/5. A 3-fold increase in sugar consumption occurred between 1830 and 1880.

While the increase in consumption of sucrose parallels the increase in caries activity, it should be noted that other significant changes in dietary patterns occurred during the 18th and 19th centuries. There was a decrease in bread consumption, and an increase in the preparation of foods of fine texture requiring less vigorous mastication and lacking natural cleansing action. The nutritional factors in bread were reduced with the advent of milled, purified flour [*Hardwick*, 1960] (more on diet and caries in chapters 7 and 8).

Caries Rates in Contemporary Isolated Populations

Isolated populations that have not acquired the dietary habits of modern, industrialized man retain a relative freedom from dental caries. Interesting studies have been conducted in several parts of the world on isolated population groups, with varying degrees of exposure to the life-style of man living in the modern technological era. The data on the occurrence

Table 2/II. Increase in the caries experience, between comparable age groups, in the Canadian Inuit population between 1969 and 1973 [*Mayhall*, 1975]

Age, years	n	1969	n	1973	% change
Males					
0–5	88	3.10	53	6.58	+112.5
6–10	44	4.39	66	5.35	+ 21.8
11–15	28	2.68	37	4.54	+ 69.4
16–20	29	3.93	15	5.46	+ 38.9
21–25	29	4.31	19	10.37	+140.6
26–30	21	4.86	10	6.50	+ 33.7
31–40	31	2.96	23	5.74	+ 93.9
41–50	16	4.06	13	4.45	+ 9.7
51–60	11	7.00	8	12.38	+ 76.8
≥61	8	17.13	7	14.86	− 13.2
Females					
0–5	98	2.62	45	7.62	+190.9
6–10	32	4.78	73	6.17	+ 29.1
11–15	31	3.5	40	6.02	+ 71.5
16–20	19	3.15	27	6.63	+110.6
21–25	24	4.25	21	10.14	+138.7
26–30	20	3.90	17	6.82	+ 74.9
31–40	26	7.15	34	8.17	+ 13.5
41–50	14	7.93	13	13.00	+ 63.9
51–60	12	11.17	10	15.00	+ 34.3
≥61	2	12.50	1	2.00	− 84.0

Average DMFT and dft per individual. Exfoliated deciduous teeth and permanent teeth that were congenitally missing were excluded.

of dental caries in the Eskimo population in the North West Territories of Canada, Alaska and Greenland are particularly informative.

In East Greenland, where native food prevailed except at trading posts where imported food was available, *Pedersen* [1938, 1967] reported that 4.3% of males living in isolated settlements of Angmegssalik had caries, as compared to 43.2% of a comparable Eskimo population living at a trading post. On the west part of Greenland, where contact with European technology was greatest, the percentage of male Eskimos with caries was 31.8% for those living in native settlements and 83.3% for those who lived in the proximity of trading posts. In West Greenland, the percent of total caloric intake from flour, sugar and imported foods increased from 17% in 1901 to 63% at the time of the study.

The effect of a rapidly changing culture on the caries experience of an isolated population is dramatically depicted by the study of 425 Canadian

Inuit (Eskimo) by *Mayhall* [1975] in 2 communities in the Foxe Basin (69 North latitude, 82 West longitude) called Igloolik and Hall Beach. The study commenced in 1969. Initially the communities were hard to reach and most people lived off the land. Four years later Igloolic became an administrative center for the area, a landing strip was available for aircraft, and the portion of the population that became wage-earners increased. At this time Hall Beach, already, had a radar site from which many families derived their food and income. During this short period major changes occurred in transportation, wage employment and in consumption of processed foods.

The dental caries experience of the Inuit during 1969–1973 is summarized in table 2/II. The overall increase in the caries experience was 66% in the 4-year period, and was most significant in the younger age groups. Further, in 1969, the diet of most of the population consisted of caribou, seal, fish, flour and tea. By 1973, there was a major shift from a natural diet to one consisting of refined carbohydrates including large amounts of snack food, confectionery and canned soft drinks. These changes were most evident in the younger age groups. There were no significant changes in the timing and frequency (a factor that is significant in caries) of food consumption as Inuit eat when thcy are hungry and do not have rigid meal times.

The significant role of diet in determining caries prevalence over a short period is thus dramatically demonstrated in the Eskimo population. That changes in a diet from one that is essentially primitive to one that is characteristic of a highly industrialized society should result in such rapid changes in the DMF and dft suggests that the determinants of the caries process are essentially local and limited to the oral cavity. It is inconceivable that dietary changes over the short span of 4 years could have systemically affected the structure of teeth. The oral microbiota which is known to be rapidly effected by oral environmental conditions were not studied.

Global Comparison of Dental Caries Prevalence in Contemporary Populations

Dental caries is ubiquitous in modern man living in highly industrialized societies; nevertheless, the caries experience varies greatly among countries, and even within countries. Variations in examination techniques and criteria for caries assessment may account for some of the differences reported in various studies. The more recent investigations by examiners from the National Institute for Dental Research Epidemiology Branch (USA), the World Health Organization (WHO) and the Interdepartmental Committee on Nutrition for National Defense (ICNND), using highly standardized procedures with negligible between-examiner disagreements, cor-roborated that the previously observed differences throughout the world [*Russell*, 1966] are real. The differences in caries rates noted in different parts of the world are extreme, from rates fewer than 1 DMF tooth per person at all ages up to 39 years in Ethiopia [*Littleton*, 1963] to 60 times greater in Alaska-Aleuts [*Russell* et al., 1961].

Findings from the ICNND and recent WHO studies [*Barmes*, 1981] indicate that caries prevalence follows definite regional patterns. Figure 2/6a designates populations and regions with relatively high, intermediate and low prevalence caries rates in persons aged 20–24 years [*Russell*, 1966]. Caries prevalence is generally lowest (0.5–1.7 DMF) for Asian and African countries and highest (12–18 DMF) for the Americas and other Western countries. The caries experience for people of Uruguay, Chile, British West Indies, and Colombia are comparable to those found in Caucasian populations in the USA. Consistently low to moderate caries rates were found in populations of the Indo-Chinese peninsula, in Malaysia, central and southern Thailand, Burma, South Vietnam, Main-land China, Taiwan, India, and New Guinea. Only those populations in the Western hemisphere who live in areas where water supplies contain significant levels of fluoride have a caries prevalence comparable to those living in the Far East. The lowest caries prevalence in the USA was found in the populations living in Colorado Springs where water fluoride levels of 1.5 ppm and over were found (see chapters on Fluorides in volume 2). A recent WHO study [*Barmes*, 1981] of caries prevalence in 35- to 44-year-old adults indicates that variation in DMF according to geographic regions is still the rule (fig. 2/6b).

An approximation of relative prevalence of dental caries (DMFT) among children 10–12 years of age in select regions of the world, derived from a recent, standardized WHO study, is shown in figure 2/7. Generally, highly industrialized countries have the highest caries indices, with a DMFT of approximately 4.5. However, within this large group of countries a very high caries pattern of over 5.6 DMFT occurs in New Zealand, Aus-tralia, Brazil, and Argentina. Populations in Canada, USA, USSR, and in less industrialized countries in western South America and in Mexico have a high (>4.5) to a moderate (2.7–4.4) DMFT caries index. Low caries experience of less than 2.6 DMFT are found among 10- to 12-year-old children in some countries in Africa, and in countries of the Far East such as China and Malaysia. These studies were conducted on small, selected populations and actual figures should not be interpreted literally; however, the relative caries experience among the regions is likely to be meaningful.

Dental caries are not uniform even within large countries as indicated by a major caries study in the USA. In broad agreement with earlier sur-

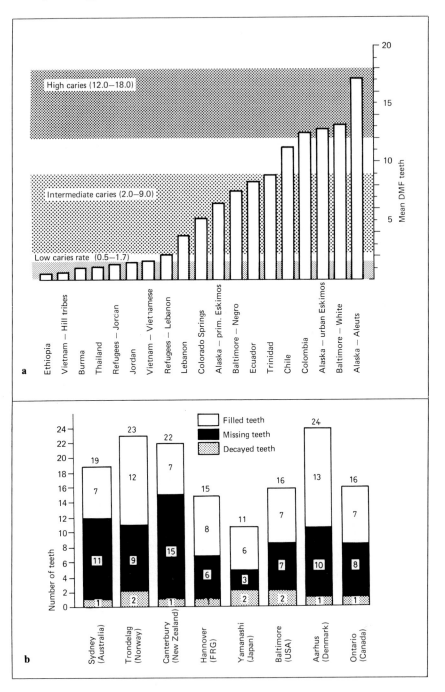

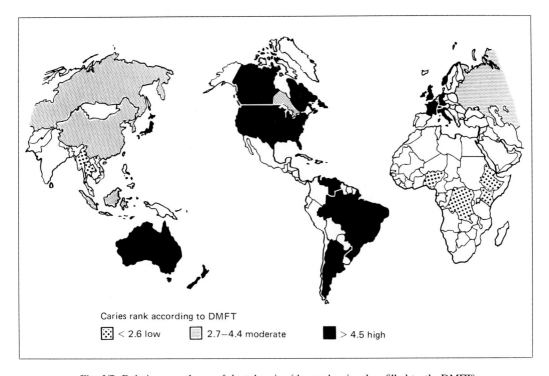

Caries rank according to DMFT

⬚ < 2.6 low   ▨ 2.7–4.4 moderate   ■ > 4.5 high

Fig. 2/7. Relative prevalence of dental caries (decayed, missed or filled teeth, DMFT) among children, 10–12 years of age, in various parts of the world. Blank areas denote inadequate data. These figures are apt to change rapidly as caries prevalence in industrialized countries declines while in some economically underdeveloped countries it increases [*Barmes*, 1979; *Infirri and Barmes*, 1979].

veys [*Britten and Perrott*, 1941; *Nizel and Bibby*, 1944] data on DMFS scores in 1979–1980 among children aged 5–17 in 8 subdivisions of the USA (fig. 2/8) show a high average DMF in the Northeast (about 6), moderate in the Great Lakes States, Midwest and Southeast (about 4.6) and lowest in the Southwest (3.4). The significance of the regional differences are not known. They probably reflect several important variables that affect caries such as diet, trace element composition of soils including fluorides, latitude (discussed later), and racial mix of the population.

Fig. 2/6. a Mean DMF teeth in civilian groups, aged 20–24 years, from different geographical regions [adapted from *Russell*, 1966]. **b** Caries prevalence in adults, 35–44 years old, in different study areas as conducted by WHO [*Barmes*, 1981].

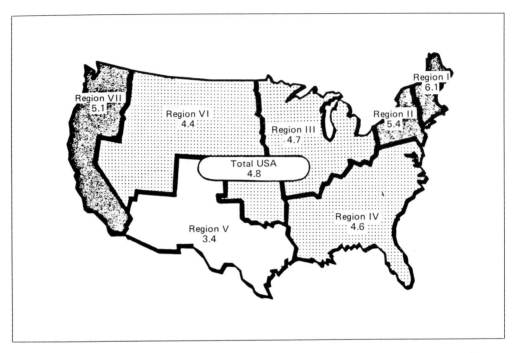

Fig. 2/8. The mean DMFS for US children, aged 5–17 years, according to geographic region [*Brunelle and Carlos*, 1982].

The Recent Decline in Caries Prevalence

The most significant recent epidemiological event has been the dramatic decline in caries prevalence in the nations of the western world. During the last 15 years surveys among schoolchildren in many western countries have unanimously shown a fall in caries prevalence of up to 50% [*Barmes*, 1979; Conference on the Declining Prevalence of Dental Caries, 1982].

Magnitude of the Decline
During 1979–1980 a nationwide survey of the prevalence of caries in US children was conducted. A total of 38,000 children randomly selected from fluoridated and nonfluoridated communities were examined, and this sample was statistically representative of approximately 48 million children aged 5–17 years. The results of this survey and the mean caries prevalence (DMFT) in four national surveys, covering the period 1963–1980, are

Table 2/III. The mean DMFT in children in the USA in four national surveys for the period 1963–1980 [*Brunelle and Carlos*, 1982]

Age, years	NCHS 1963[1]–1970[2]	NCHS 1971–1974	NIDR 1979–1980
6–11	1.4	1.7	1.1
12–17	6.2	6.2	4.6

NCHS = National Centre for Health Statistic;
NIDR = National Institute for Dental Research.
[1] 1963–1965 children aged 6–11 years.
[2] 1966–1970 youths aged 12–17 years.

summarized in table 2/III. The mean DMFS for children in the age group 5–17 years declined from 7.06 to 4.77 (fig. 2/9a).

In a dental survey of 9,000 schoolchildren, from kindergarten through grade 11, in Massachusetts, USA, the DMFT by age obtained in 1979–1981 was compared to a similar survey performed in 1951 (fig. 2/9b) [*DePaola* et al., 1982]. The results indicate a 50% decline in the prevalence of caries. Of significance is the finding that the decline is similar in areas with and without water fluoridation. In a separate study, *Glass* [1982] reported a similar decrease in decayed and filled surfaces, a decrease in extractions of 70%, and a virtual absence of secondary caries in nonfluoridated areas. These observations have been corroborated by reports from countries where water fluoridation programs are absent such as Norway [*von der Fehr*, 1982], Sweden [*Koch*, 1982], The Netherlands [*Kalsbeek* 1982]; Denmark [*Fejerskov* et al., 1982], and in some parts of England [*Anderson* et al., 1982]. Representative studies from four countries showing the decline in caries prevalence are summarized in figure 2/9a. The most dramatic results are shown by the increase in the number of caries-free children as shown in figure 2/9c.

These cumulative studies indicate that the pattern of caries is reversing, resulting in fewer decayed surfaces (particularly smooth surfaces), fewer decayed teeth, and more caries-free individuals. While the present data pertain to the child population and young adults, there is every reason to expect that future studies will demonstrate similar reductions extending into adult life. It is reasonable to conclude that the decline of the past 10 years is significant and real, that it is not a cyclical but a permanent phenomenon, and that it is apt to continue and involve all age groups. A vir-

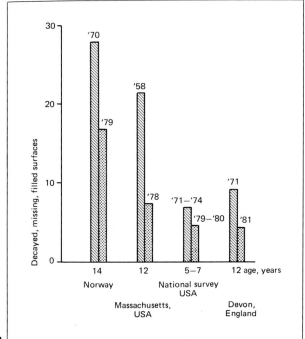

2/9a

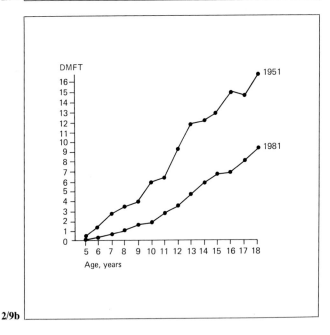

2/9b

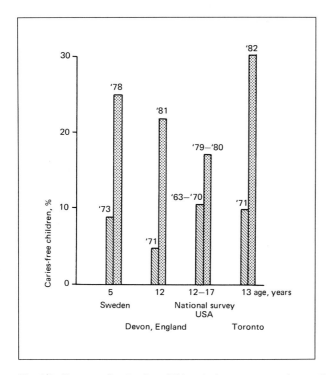

Fig. 2/9c. Percent of caries-free children in four representative studies in nonfluoridated (Sweden and Devon, England) and in fluoridated areas (USA and Toronto, Canada). [Data from *Koch*, 1982; *Anderson* et al., 1982; US Department of Public Health, City of Toronto, 1982.]

tual elimination of smooth surface lesions, in which environmental factors are dominant, is predicted. The inherently susceptible occlusal pits and fissures will be reduced to a lesser extent. The rise in caries prevalence over the ages, the current decline, and the projected prevalence are diagrammatically depicted in figure 2/10.

Fig. 2/9a. Decline in caries prevalence in schoolchildren from three different countries, living in nonfluoridated communities: Norway; Norwood, Mass., USA; and Devon, England. The 5- to 17-year-old children in the US National Caries Program are from fluoridated and nonfluoridated regions; in some schools fluoride rinsing and tablets were introduced. Note the significant caries reduction in each country during the past decade. [Data from *von der Fehr*, 1982; *Glass*, 1982; *Anderson* et al., 1982; US Department of Health and Human Services, 1981.]

Fig. 2/9b. The DMFT by age in Massachusetts children in the 1951 and 1981 surveys. Note a decline of about 50% in the prevalence of dental caries [*DePaola* et al., 1982].

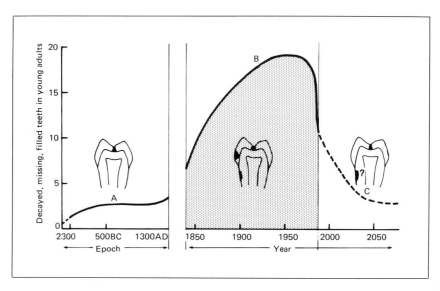

Fig. 2/10. Diagrammatic representation of the rise and fall in the prevalence of dental caries during different epochs. **A** Low level of caries prevalence in prehistoric men. Note that, until the last two centuries, carious lesions were limited to the inherently highly susceptible occlusal surfaces. The later onset of smooth surface (interproximal) and root caries coincided with major dietary changes. The decline in caries due to reduced sugar intake during the war years, 1940–1945, was transient and is not shown on the diagram. **B** The more recent rise and decline of caries prevalence after 1960. The decline is related to the cumulative effects of the widespread use of different fluoride regimens. **C** Projected caries prevalence beyond 1984 when additional preventive measures may become available. Note that the predominant site of lesions may be anticipated to occur on the occlusal and dentinal root surfaces as observed during ancient times.

Factors Contributing to the Decline

A discussion of the reasons for the current decline in caries prevalence must remain cautionary since data that would permit an estimate of the contribution of many factors (improved level of oral health care, sugar substitutes, changing pattern of sugar consumption, improved nutrition, and important preventive methods) are not available. On the other hand, evidence that the widespread use of fluorides substantially reduces caries is incontrovertible. Is fluoride the paramount factor in the current decline?

In regions where the water supply is fluoridated it is reasonable to conclude that this measure is the major factor in the reduction in caries. However, in the Massachusetts and the European studies, water fluoridation was not a factor. During the period under investigation, fluoride rinsing and brushing programs were expanded to cover about 90% of the children in countries such as Norway and Sweden. The use of fluoride dentifrices, dietary fluoride supplements, and topical fluoride regimens (professionally or self-applied) has become widespread and each is known to exert a significant cariostatic action. Of the above measures, the use of fluoride dentifrices has increased most rapidly during the time period of most of these studies, 1965–1980. Fluoride dentifrice sales comprise about 80–90% of the annual dentifrice market in the United States and in Europe. A reasonable conclusion is that the use of fluorides, and especially fluoride dentifrices, provides the most plausible explanation for the impressive and significant decline in caries prevalence in the industrialized nations. (More on this subject in volume 2, chapters 3, 4, and 5.)

Unlike the sharp decline in caries experienced in Western Europe and North America, caries occurrence is increasing rapidly in children in developing countries. When one considers that 36% of the world's population are children, and that there are about 1,500 million children in the world under 15 years, and that about 81% or 1,220 million of this age group resides in underdeveloped countries, then it becomes obvious that prevention is the only hope for improved oral health in the future.

Effect of Environmental Factors on Dental Caries

Diet
Of the many factors that affect caries prevalence none has been studied more exhaustively than the role of diet. The variation in caries prevalence in modern man is thought to be largely determined by diet, especially sucrose consumption. The dramatic changes in caries prevalence during World War II are also explained on this basis. Because of the importance of dietary factors and the significant role of sucrose in caries, chapters 7 and 8 are devoted to this subject.

Latitude
An interesting example of an extrinsic factor that affects caries prevalence is latitude. About 15 more decayed, missing or filled teeth per 100, 12- to 14-year-old children has been reported for each additional degree of latitude north from the Gulf of Mexico to the Canadian border, a total increase of over 200%. In the USSR, where large land masses lie in the northern latitude, the association between this factor and dental caries is strikingly depicted in the study by *Bazijan* [1972]. There are also signs of this effect in the results of the dental survey in the USA in 1979–1980, although the areas included in each of the 8 regions (fig. 2/8) makes it difficult to compare north with south (e.g. the whole of the West Coast of the USA is included in one region).

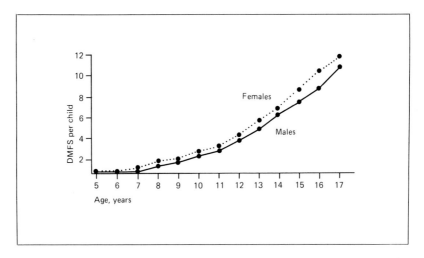

Fig. 2/11. Age- and sex-specific caries prevalence in permanent teeth in the USA [*Brunelle and Carlos*, 1982].

The hypothesis originally suggested to explain the effect of latitude on caries is that hours of sunshine are greater in the south, leading to a greater synthesis of vitamin D in the skin. This in turn influences the mineralization of the hard tissues including enamel, and thus increases the resistance of the teeth to caries. The question of vitamin D and teeth is discussed later (chapter 7) where it is concluded that its influence on caries in westernized countries is probably relatively small but detectable. Although many environmental differences exist between north and south of the USA a possible effect of vitamin D cannot be dismissed. If this is the true explanation, the use throughout the USA of foods fortified with vitamin D would be expected to have reduced the effect of latitude in recent years.

Effect of Demographic Factors on the Prevalence of Caries

Sex

Several epidemiological studies have shown a consistent, albeit small, higher caries experience in permanent teeth of females as compared to males of the same chronological age in spite of a higher average level of oral hygiene in girls. This is shown by the results of the Survey of the US Department of Health and Human Services [*Brunelle and Carlos*, 1982] (fig. 2/11).

The small but consistent difference can be explained, at least up to the age of 15 years, by the earlier eruption of permanent teeth in girls, and

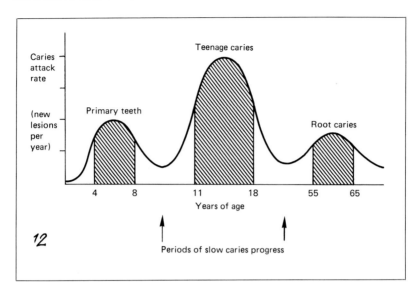

Fig. 2/12. Age periods of high and low caries attack [Preventive Dental Services, 1979; *Massler*, 1969].

hence by the longer exposure of such teeth to the carious environment. This hypothesis has been challenged by some [*Sloman*, 1941; *Backer Dirks*, 1961]. However, a more recent observation by *Carlos and Gittelsohn* [1965] supports the observation that eruption time explains most, but not all, of the age-specific prevalence differences between boys and girls. Even after an adjustment for eruption times the caries rates for the first and second molars were consistently higher in females.

Several careful studies have repudiated the impression created by earlier literature that pregnancy potentiates dental caries. The aphorism 'a tooth for every child' has no scientific basis. Teeth, unlike bones, do not serve as a reservoir of calcium. Further, under normal dietary intake and with increased retention of calcium during pregnancy the stores of calcium are ample for the needs of the developing fetus.

Age

Carious lesions that result in cavitation are irreversible and therefore cumulative with age. There is a strong positive correlation between age and DMF indices. Over a lifetime, caries incidence (new lesions per year) shows three peaks – at ages 4–8, 11–19 and between 55 and 65 years (fig. 2/12). Figure 2/13a, b from a Canadian survey graphically depicts the relationship between prevalence of caries experience, measured as percent of persons with 1 or more DMF teeth (fig. 2/13a), and as the number of DMF teeth per person and chronological age (fig. 2/13b). The trend in figure 2/13b is for older persons to have a high DMFS, a great increase in missing teeth but fewer untreated cavities. At age 65 years, the average Canadian has over 20 decayed, missing or filled teeth; of this figure, over 15 teeth are missing. It should be recognized that in older populations teeth may be lost for reasons other than caries. Nor should one ignore the growing occurrence of root caries in older populations. About 70% of persons older than 60 years have developed root surface lesions. These data, which are characteristic of many industrialized countries, indicate that dental caries affects almost every man, woman or child.

Race

Race or ethnic background is a significant factor in caries prevalence to the extent that it implies cultural, social, economic and possibly genetic differences, and therefore differences in the diet, oral hygiene, and education. The low caries scores of African, Asian and Aboriginal people as compared to the industrialized countries of Europe and North America have been discussed. These differences do not indicate a direct effect due to race since environmental factors were not analyzed.

The relationship between race and caries prevalence is a consistent epidemiological finding in societies characterized by multiculturalism. For example, in Hawaii, caries is more prevalent in children of Korean, Japanese or Hawaiian parentage than in descendants of Chinese, European, Filipino or Puerto Rican parents [*Chung* et al., 1970].

Marked differences in DMF scores between black and white adults of the same age were found in a US survey [1965]. These differences could not be eliminated by standardizing income and education. Other studies do not corroborate this finding. The DMF scores of 14- to 17-year-old blacks in Detroit were found to be only slightly lower than for whites and, in Columbia, South Carolina, the differences were not significant [*Bagramian and Russell*, 1971]. In the National Dental Caries Prevalence Survey [1981] the mean DMFS for white children aged 5 17 years was 4.89 and for black and other colored groups was 4.15 (table 2/IV).

It remains to be determined whether differences in caries scores among races are real, reflecting varying susceptibility to caries or whether the differences reflect culturally related dietary and social factors.

Familial Factors

A familial pattern of caries experience has been detected in several studies. Children of parents with low caries experience also tend to have a low caries experience; the converse is true for children whose parents have

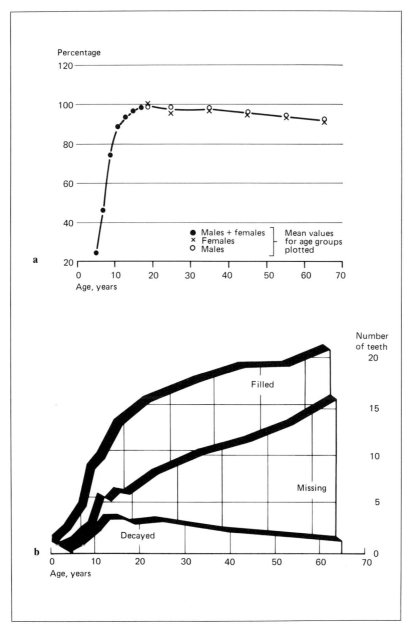

Fig. 2/13. a Percentage of persons with natural dentitions having 1 or more carious teeth [Nutrition Canada, 1977]. **b** Mean number of decayed, missing and filled permanent teeth per person [Nutrition Canada, 1977].

Table 2/IV. DMFS teeth in US children according to race and geographic region [US Department of Health and Human Services, 1981]

Region[1]	Whites		Blacks and all others	
	number in thousands	mean DMFS	number in thousands	mean DMFS
I	2,427	6.09	76	4.79
II	6,179	5.58	1,159	4.40
III	9,970	4.81	1,389	3.68
IV	8,309	4.78	3,274	4.15
V	3,606	3.34	594	3.85
VI	2,460	4.48	142	3.55
VII	5,037	5.15	694	4.93
Total in USA	37,987	4.89	7,327	4.15

[1] Regions correspond to those shown in figure 2/8.

a high caries rate. Siblings of individuals that are caries-free exhibit a low caries rate [*Garn* et al., 1976].

Studies have been made of the dental caries experience in monozygotic and dizygotic twins [*Finn*, 1965]. In a study of identical twins the dominance of hereditary factors should reveal a more closely related caries pattern than would be found in fraternal twins. Such studies indicate that concordance for carious sites in monozygotic twins is much higher than in dizygotic twin pairs. The studies suggest that genetically determined factors, such as tooth morphology and occlusion, may play a significant role in determining caries rates. Nevertheless, environmental factors, such as diet and dental care, are more significant than hereditary factors and are even more responsible for the observed caries pattern in families.

Time Factors for Caries Development after Eruption

Longitudinal studies (studies on the same population over several years) of enamel caries in the permanent teeth indicate that after a tooth erupts there is a rapid rise and then an equally sharp decrease in caries susceptibility. In general the period of peak susceptibility occurs at about 4 years after eruption of the tooth (fig. 2/14) [*Carlos and Gittelsohn*, 1965]. In the second permanent molar the probability of a carious lesion is greatest during the second posteruptive year; for other teeth the period of maximum carious attack is reached about 2 years later. This observation is

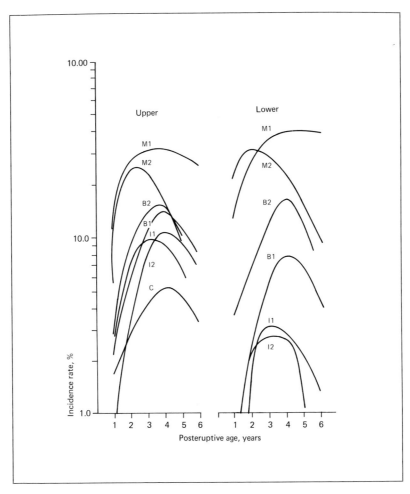

Fig. 2/14. Probability of annual caries attack in permanent teeth, male children in Kingston, New York. Semilogarithmic scale [*Carlos and Gittelsohn*, 1965].

compatible with the idea that 'age confers an increased resistance' to caries upon teeth. This phenomenon is related to the maturation of teeth, whereby the surface composition of enamel is changed by the gradual increase in the concentration of fluoride, decrease in the concentration of carbonate as well as changes in other constituents. Tooth age rather than chronological age is significant in explaining the maturation phenomenon (see section on Maturation of Enamel, chapter 4).

Order Rank in Caries Prevalence in Permanent Teeth

Individual teeth and surfaces have vastly different susceptibilities to dental caries. The most frequent site of caries attack is the occlusal surface of first and second permanent molars. This is the reason why occlusal fillings and sealants, to obliterate pits and fissures, are used predominantly on those surfaces.

In general, susceptibility of teeth increases posteriorly in the oral cavity. Molars are more susceptible than incisors not only because of their posterior location but also because of the anatomy of molar teeth. The pits and fissures and the wider interproximal contact areas are not easily accessible to cleansing action.

On the basis of overall caries patterns permanent teeth can be grouped according to their susceptibility, from the most to the least susceptible, as follows:

Lower first and second molars, upper first molars	Upper incisors
Upper second molars	Upper canine, lower first premolar
Upper first premolar, upper and lower second premolars	Lower incisors, lower canine

Carlos and Gittelsohn [1965]

Occlusal and Pit Caries

The greater inherent caries susceptibility of occlusal, pit and fissure as compared to smooth surfaces is striking and has been studied in detail. The distribution of occlusal lesions does not fit any known analyses of chance distributions, suggesting an inherited predisposition of this surface. The presence of a deep pit or fissure predisposes this surface to dental caries. Caries is prone to develop in a morphologically imperfect area soon after tooth eruption even if the surface is located in a relatively caries-free region of the mouth; examples are deep lingual pits in the maxillary permanent incisor teeth. Not surprisingly, when such pits do not decay they are usually found in mouths that are relatively caries-free.

Smooth Surface Caries

Reid and Grainger [1955] and *Bille* [1980] have shown that the occurrence of smooth, proximal, surface carious lesions may be described as a statistical chance phenomenon (approximating the negative binomial probability distribution); no such statistical approximation is possible for occlusal surfaces. Caries data that fit such a frequency distribution are

Table 2/V. Frequency distributions of subjects according to number of decayed proximal surfaces (DS) for each year from ages 9 to 14 [*Bille*, 1980]

Number of DS	Age, years					
	9	10	11	12	13	14
0	249	217	224	233	198	233
1	37	61	64	51	74	48
2	7	22	19	15	23	22
3	5	7	5	9	9	4
4	4	6	0	2	3	2
5	0		1	2	2	2
6	1			0	2	0
7				1	2	0
8						
9						2
10						
11						

shown in table 2/V. The caries attack rate on smooth surfaces, therefore, tends to reflect environmental and not inherent conditions in the mouth as in the case for pit and fissure surfaces. The increased level of decay on the distal surfaces of both maxillary and mandibular first molars upon eruption of the second molar further suggests that the higher rates for interproximal contact surfaces are associated with restriction of salivary flow and accumulation of dental plaque (chapters 5 and 6).

An analysis of interproximal surface caries in permanent teeth from non-fluoridated regions yields data which permit the surfaces to be ranked from most to least susceptible, as follows:

Mesial and distal surfaces of the first permanent molars
Mesial surface of the maxillary second premolar
Mesial surface of the mandibular second molar
Mesial surface of the maxillary central incisor
Mesial surface of the mandibular second premolar
Mesial surface of the maxillary second incisor
Mesial surface of the maxillary first premolar
Mesial surface of the maxillary canine
Remaining surfaces

Reid and Grainger [1955]

Distribution of Caries in Primary Teeth

Many practitioners recommend that children should first visit a dentist at about 2 years of age, when normally all primary teeth have erupted, and when most children still have a caries-free dentition. This is an ideal age for the effective practice of preventive dentistry including family diet counselling and the use of fluorides.

Even during the first year of life 'soother' or infancy caries may occur. This type of caries usually attacks the primary anterior maxillary teeth, and is associated with an unusual pattern of ingestion of refined, soluble carbohydrates brought about by the addition of honey or syrup to an infant formula. More often caries in the primary dentition is first seen on the occlusal surfaces of the molars.

Due to the geographical variation of caries experience specific figures for prevalence should be interpreted with caution. In many western countries, in nonfluoridated areas, about 1–5% of 1-year-old children exhibit dental caries; this rate may double or triple at 2 years of age [*Infante and Owen*, 1975; *Schwarz and Hansen*, 1979]. The number of children affected continues to rise until at the age of 3–4 years about 50% of children are afflicted. The trend continues, and at age 5 about three quarters of preschool-age children have carious primary teeth. In fluoridated areas the caries experience would be significantly less.

The def index for 8- to 9-year-old children from different geographical areas of the world is shown in figure 2/15a. In children living in a nonfluoride, highly industrialized country (e.g. Denmark) the average df (decayed, filled) teeth as a function of age is depicted in figure 2/15b. Generally, it has been observed that at an early age of 2–3 years occlusal caries predominate while interproximal caries account for about one quarter of the carious lesions in primary teeth. However, as a child grows older the number of interproximal lesions increases rapidly (fig. 2/16). The rank order of caries prevalence in primary teeth, from the highest to the lowest, is as follows:

Lower second primary molar
Upper second primary molar
Lower first primary molar
Upper first primary molar
Upper and lower primary canines

Glass et al. [1970]

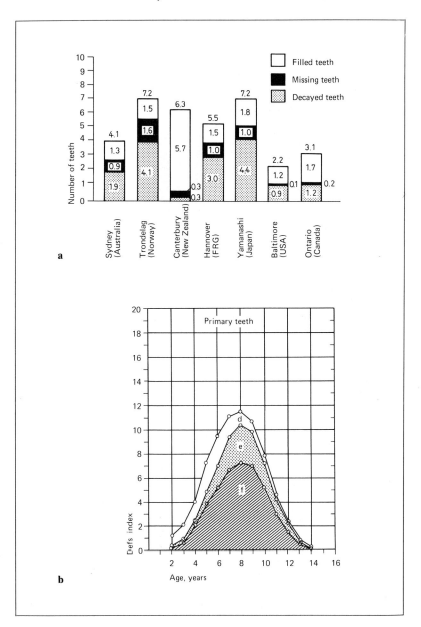

Fig. 2/15. a The def index of children, aged 8–9 years, from different geographical areas [*Barmes*, 1981]. **b** The mean defs for primary teeth in Danish children showing the distribution of decayed, extracted and filled surfaces for the age group 2–14 years [*Schwarz and Hansen*, 1979].

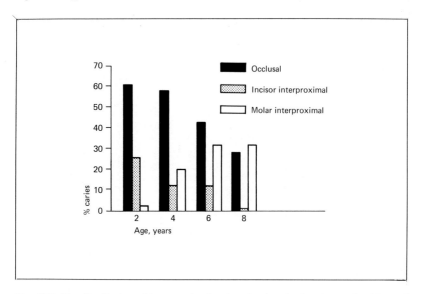

Fig. 2/16. The distribution of interproximal and occlusal caries in primary dentitions of children according to age [*Parfitt*, 1955].

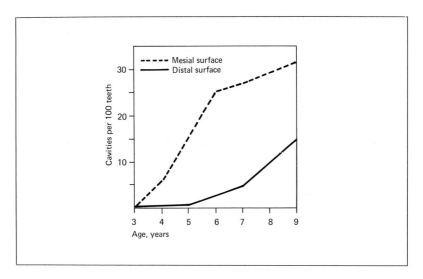

Fig. 2/17. Caries on distal and mesial surfaces of the upper and lower second primary molar in relation to age of children [*Parfitt*, 1956].

Table 2/VI. Percent of persons totally edentulous by location and sex for 33- to 44-year-old adults in study areas of 6 nations [*Bonito*, 1977]

	Australia	FRG	Japan	New Zealand	Norway	USA
Total	13.2	1.6	0.0	35.7	6.4	10.6
Metro (urban) males	5.6	1.9	0.0	24.3	3.0	8.5
Nonmetro (rural) males	21.7	0.4	0.0	33.5	7.1	11.4
Metro (urban) females	5.6	2.5	0.0	29.8	2.3	13.1
Nonmetro (rural) females	26.2	1.6	0.0	52.0	12.6	8.7

Interproximal Surface Caries in Primary Dentition

The distal surface of the first primary molar and the mesial surface of the second primary molar contact each other after completion of eruption of the primary second molars. These are the most susceptible smooth surfaces of primary teeth. The caries attack rates for the two surfaces are about equal indicating that factors affecting caries activity are about the same for the two surfaces.

The distal surface of the second primary molar is interesting from a standpoint of caries susceptibility. This tooth erupts at about 2 years of age, and for 4 years has no approximating tooth on the distal surface until the eruption of the first permanent molar at 6 years. The latter situation is maintained until the natural exfoliation of the second primary molar at about 12 years of age. The interdependence of the proximal contact surfaces on caries activity can be readily studied using the distal surface of the second primary molar as a model. It has been demonstrated that at age 6 years, the occurrence of caries on the mesial surface of the second primary molar is about 10 times greater than for the distal surface of the same tooth; by age 9 the relative decay rate of the mesial surface is only about twice that of the distal surface, thus indicating the significance of contact areas between teeth (fig. 2/17).

Edentulism – a Cultural Trait

Teeth are lost due to diseases of the dental hard tissues (caries), and in later years to a more significant degree due to periodontal disease. The total loss of teeth results in an edentulous state, and, patients, afflicted with the loss of all their teeth are called edentulous.

Edentulism is common in many populations of the world. The prevalence of totally edentulous persons in 6 nations in a WHO study is shown in table 2/VI [*Bonito*, 1977]. In this study New Zealand had the largest

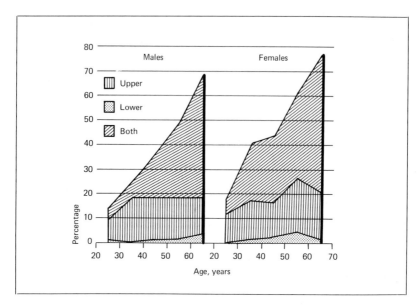

Fig. 2/18. Percentage of persons edentulous in one or both arches [Nutrition Canada, 1977].

proportion of edentulous persons in the 35- to 44-year-old group. Australia, with about one half the proportion of edentulous persons as New Zealand, and the USA with 20% fewer edentulous persons than Australia are second and third behind New Zealand in this statistic. Japan, while experiencing a relatively high caries level, had no edentulous persons in this age group. In persons over 64 years of age in the USA about one half are without natural teeth (60% in 1958; the figure fell to about 51% in 1971). In Canada the figure is equally appalling (fig. 2/18). Over 70% of the female population over 65 years of age are edentulous in one or both arches [Nutrition Canada, 1977]. The loss of function and the high cost of replacing lost teeth impose serious health and economic burdens on the elderly.

An important aspect of edentulism is that the condition is as much a reflection of cultural traits as of disease states. Many people decide to have their teeth removed because of an engrained attitude that loss of teeth is inevitable and, from an economic standpoint, the sooner the better. The attitude of some dentists may also contribute to this situation. This cultural trait was uncovered in a study by *Davis* [1980] in New Zealand. Migrants, who have moved to New Zealand several generations ago from the UK, continue to have edentulous rates which are very similar to their forbears in the UK. This finding is best explained by the perpetuation, from generation to generation, of attitudes and practices that saving teeth is a losing proposition. Health education programs should be sensitive to this fact. Such programs should emphasize that most individuals can have their teeth as long as they wish providing that effective preventive measures are carried out throughout their lifetime. Given the reduced efficiency in mastication and the psychological and physical trauma associated with loss of teeth, the goal of a health service should be the preservation of dentitions for a lifetime. Prevention of oral-dental diseases is the best assurance that a dentition will be retained for the life span of an individual.

References

Anderson, R.J.; Bradnock, G.; Beal, J.F.; James, P.M.C.: The reduction of dental caries prevalence in English schoolchildren. J. dent. Res. 61; spec. issue, p. 1311 (1982).

Backer Dirks, O.: Longitudinal dental caries study of children 9–15 years of age. Archs oral Bio. 6: suppl., p. 94 (1961).

Bagramian, R.A.; Russell, A.L.: An epidemiologic study of dental caries in race and geographic area. J. dent. Res. 50: 1553 (1971).

Barmes, D.E.: Oral health status of children – an international perspective. J. Can. Dent. Ass. 45: 651 (1979).

Barmes, D.E.: International comparative analysis of the findings in Yamanashi; in Onisi, Dental health care in Japan. Progressive report on Yamanashi survey of WHO/ICS (Ishiyaku, Tokyo 1981).

Bazijan, G.V.: Report on the research programme carried out in 1971 under WHO auspices by the Central Institute of Stomatological Research. Paper prepared for WHO, Moscow (1972).

Bille, J.: Development and distribution of proximal caries in 303 9- to 20-year-old individuals in a Copenhagen suburb. Scand J. dent. Res. 88: 291 (1980).

Bonito, A.J.: The oral health and treatment needs of 35- to 44-year-old adults in the Baltimore Metropolitan area in International Perspective; in The United States Study of Dental Manpower Systems in Relation to Oral Health Status: The Private Practice System. Final Report, Contract No. NO 1-DH-34051 (DHEW, Washington 1977).

Britten, R.H.; Perrott, G.S.T.J.: Summary of physical findings on men drafted in the World War. Publ. Hlth Rep. 56: 41 (1941).

Brunelle, J.A.; Carlos, J.P.: Changes in the prevalence of dental caries in US schoolchildren, 1961–1980. J. dent. Res. 61: spec. issue, p. 1346 (1982).

Carlos, J.P.; Gittelsohn, A.M.: Longitudinal studies of the natural history of caries. II. A life-table study of caries incidence in the permanent teeth. Archs oral Biol. 10: 739 (1965).

Chung, C.S.; Runck, D.W.; Niswander, J.D.; Bilben, S.E.; Kau, M.C.: Genetic and epidemiological studies of oral characteristics in Hawaii's schoolchildren. I. Caries and periodontal disease. J. dent. Res. 49: 1374 (1970).

Conference on the Declining Prevalence of Dental Caries. J. dent. Res. 61: spec. issue (1982).

Davis, P.: Tooth loss, the culture of dentistry and the delivery of dental care in New Zealand; in The social context of dentistry (Croom Helm, London 1980).

Deerr, N.: The history of sugar (Chapman & Hall, London 1950).

DePaola, P.F.; Soparkar, P.M.; Tavares, M.; Allukian, M., Jr.; Peterson, H.: A dental survey of Massachusetts schoolchildren. J. dent. Res. *61:* spec. issue, p. 1356 (1982).

Department of Public Health, City of Toronto: Report of the Medical Officer of Health (1982).

Fejerskov, O.; Antoft, P.; Gagegaard, E.: Decrease in caries experience in Danish children and young adults in the 1970's. J. dent. Res. *61:* spec. issue, p. 1305 (1982).

Finn, S.B.: Heredity in relation to caries resistance; in Caries resistant teeth. Ciba Fdn Symp., p. 41 (Churchill, London 1965).

Garn, S.M.; Rowe, N.H.; Clark, D.C.: Parent-child similarities in dental caries rates. J. dent. Res. *55:* 1129 (1976).

Glass, R.L.: Secular changes in caries prevalence in two Massachusetts towns. J. dent. Res. *61:* spec. issue, p. 1352 (1982).

Glass, R.L.; Becker, H.M.; Shiere, F.R.: Caries incidence in human primary teeth during the period of the mixed dentition. Archs oral Biol. *15:* 1007 (1970).

Hardwick, J.L.: The incidence and distribution of caries throughout the ages in relation to the Englishman's diet. Br. dent. J. *108:* 9 (1960).

Infante, P.F.; Owen, G.M.: Dental caries and levels of treatment for schoolchildren by geographical region, socioeconomic status, race, and size of community, J. Publ. Hlth Dent. *35:* 19 (1975).

Infirri, J.S.; Barmes, D.E.: Epidemiology of oral diseases-differences in national problems. Int. dent. J., Lond. *29:* 183 (1979).

Kalsbeek, H.: Evidence of decrease in prevalence of dental caries in The Netherlands: an evaluation of epidemiological cares surveys on 4–6- and 11–15-year-old children, performed between 1965 and 1980. J. dent. Res. *61:* spec. issue, p. 1321 (1982).

Koch, G.: Evidence for declining caries prevalence in Sweden. J. dent. Res. *61:* spec. issue, p. 1340 (1982).

Krikos, A.: The progress of decay in Greece from the most ancient times down to the present. Trans. Am. dent. Soc. Eur. (1935).

Littleton, N.W.: Dental caries and periodontal diseases among Ethiopian civilians. Publ. Hlth Rep. *78:* 631 (1963).

Massler, M.: Teenage cariology. Dent. Clin. N. Am. *13:* 405 (1969).

Mayhall, J.: Canadian Inuit caries experience, 1969–1973. J. dent. Res. *54:* 1245 (1975).

Mills, C.A.: Factors affecting the incidence of dental caries in population groups. J. dent. Res. *16:* 417 (1937).

Moore, W.J.; Corbett, M.E.: The distribution of dental caries in ancient British populations. I. Anglo-Saxon period. Caries Res. *5:* 151 (1971).

Moore, W.J.; Corbett, M.E.: The distribution of dental caries in ancient British populations. II. Iron Age, Romano-British and Medieval Periods. Caries Res. *7:* 139 (1973).

Moore, W.J.; Corbett, M.E.: The distribution of dental caries in ancient British populations. III. The 17th Century. Caries Res. *9:* 163 (1975).

Moore, W.J.; Corbett, M.E.: The distribution of dental caries in ancient British populations. IV. The 19th century. Caries Res. *10:* 401 (1976).

National Dental Caries Prevalence Survey: The prevalence of dental caries in United States Children – 1979–1980. National Caries Program, National Institute of Dental Research, NIH Publ. No. 82-2245 (US Department of Health and Human Services, Washington 1981).

Nizel, A.E.; Bibby, B.G.: Geographic variations in caries prevalence in soldiers. J. Am. dent. Ass. *31:* 1619 (1944).

Nutrition Canada, Dental Report: Bureau of Nutritional Sciences, Food Directorate, Health

Protection Branch (Dept. of National Health & Welfare, Minister of National Health & Welfare, Ottawa 1977).

Parfitt, G.J.: The distribution of caries on different sites of the teeth in English children from age of 2–15 years. Br. dent. J. *99:* 423 (1955).

Parfitt, G.J.: Conditions influencing the incidence of occlusal and interstitial caries in children. J. Dent. Child *23:* 31 (1956).

Patrick, J.J.: Examination of the teeth and mouth; in Marshall, Operative dentistry, p. 121 (Lippincott, Philadelphia 1914).

Pedersen, P.O.: Investigations into dental conditions of about 3,000 ancient and modern Greenlanders. Preliminary report. Dent. Rec. *58:* 191 (1938).

Pedersen, P.O.: Nutritional aspects of dental caries. Odont, Revy *17:* suppl. 10, p. 91 (1967).

Pickerill, H.P.: The incidence of dental caries; in The prevention of dental caries and oral sepsis; 2 ed., p. 9 (White Dental Manufacturing, Toronto 1914).

Preventive Dental Services: Practices, guidelines and recommendations (Dept. of National Health and Welfare, Washington 1979).

Reid, D.B.W.; Grainger, R.M.: Variations in the caries susceptibility of children's teeth. Hum. Biol. *27:* 1 (1955).

Russell, A.L.: World epidemiology and oral health; in Kreshover, McClure, Environmental variables in oral disease, p. 21 (Am. Association for the Advancement of Science, Washington 1966).

Russell, A.L.; Consolazio, C.F.; White, C.L.: Dental caries and nutrition in Eskimo scouts of the Alaska National Guard. J. dent. Res. *40:* 594 (1961).

Schwarz, E.; Hansen, E.R.: Caries experience of Danish schoolchildren evaluated by the Child Dental Health recording system. Community dent. oral Epidemiol. *7:* 107 (1979).

Sloman, E.: Sex and age factors in the incidence of dental caries. J. Am. dent. Ass. *28:* 441 (1941).

Sognnaes, R.F.: A survey of dental caries in Greece. N.Y. St. dent. J. *15:* 15 (1949).

US Department of Health, Education and Welfare; Public Health Service: Decayed, missing and filled teeth in adults, ser. 11, No. 23 (National Center for Health Statistics, Washington 1965).

US Department of Health and Human Services: The prevalence of dental caries in United States children, 1979–1980. The National Dental Caries Prevalence Survey. NIH publ. No. 82-2245 (1981).

von der Fehr, F.R.: Evidence of decreasing caries prevalence in Norway. J. dent. Res. *61:* spec. issue, p. 1331 (1982).

Wagg, B.J.: ECSI – a new index for evaluating caries progression. Community dent. oral Epidemiol. *2:* 219 (1974).

3 Etiology of Dental Caries –
A Review of Early Theories and Current Concepts

The previous two chapters have given the reader an understanding of the clinical features and epidemiology of dental caries. It is clear that fossil teeth provide an accurate record of the state of dentitions of man through the ages. Archeologists continue to bring back evidence of the antiquity of dentistry. Evidence for caries has been found in *Homo sapiens* since Paleolithic times. It is probable that the legendary pain associated with toothache was experienced by prehistoric man at the dawn of civilization. Numerous references to dental caries, including early theories attempting to explain its etiology, have been found in recorded history of ancient peoples. A brief review of the history and early theories of the etiology of caries provides an interesting background for the understanding of the current concepts of dental caries. The word caries is derived from the Latin word meaning 'rot' or 'decay'. It is akin to the Greek word Kēr for death. The term is apt in that the clinical picture of a carious lesion is that of decaying tissue.

Early Theories

The Legend of the Worm

Probably the earliest reference to tooth decay and toothache came from the ancient Sumerian text known as the 'Legend of the Worm'. It was discovered on a clay tablet, excavated from an ancient city within the Euphrates Valley of the lower Mesopotamian area, which dates from about 5000 BC (fig. 3/1). The cuneiform text refers to the creation of the Heavens, the Earth, the Marshes and the latter created the Worm.

A remedy for toothache, recorded during this period, reads as follows: 'Mix beer, the plant SA-KIL-BIR and oil together, repeat thereon the incantation thrice (and) put it on his tooth.'

The tooth worm was prominently invoked in Oriental medicine. In Japanese the word for dental caries is 'mush-ha' (mushi-room; ha-tooth),

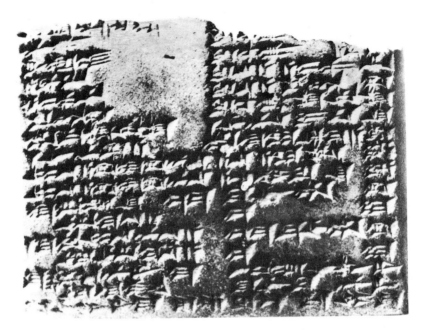

Fig. 3/1. Babylonian tooth worm tablet. This tablet is inscribed in cuneiform writing and contains advice for curing a toothache by medicinal and mechanical treatment along with incantation (British Museum).

meaning hollow tooth. The same terminology is employed by the Chinese; the word for hollow tooth is 'chung choo'.

The early history of India, Egypt, and the writing of *Homer* also make reference to the worm as the cause of toothache. The great surgeon of the Middle Ages, *Guy de Cahuliac* (1300–1368), still espoused the belief that worms cause dental caries. Fumigation devices consisting of burning of leeks and hyocyamus (an alkaloid) were used by the Chinese and Egyptians (fig. 3/2).

An interesting therapeutic method applied by the Chinese about 2700 BC for the treatment of various diseases including those of dental tissues was acupuncture. The treatment consisted of insertion of metal needles into selected points in the body. Acupuncture is used widely today in many parts of the world. The physiological mechanism by which acupuncture reduces pain is unknown. The recent discovery of natural substances called

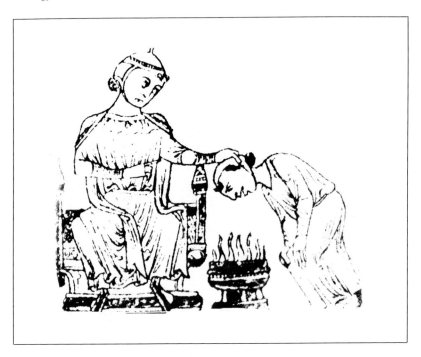

Fig. 3/2. Fumigation for the relief of toothache from a drawing in an Anglo-Saxon manuscript of the 13th century, in Trinity College, Cambridge, England [*Prinz*, 1945].

endorphins which strongly inhibit the pain impulse, and which may be illicited by procedures as acupuncture, may be the basis upon which acupuncture mediates control of pain.

One of the most important medical papyri to be discovered, the Papyrus Ebers, was written about 1500 BC by ancient Egyptians (fig. 3/3). The ideas expressed were copies from older papyri which extend back to many centuries. Of the 50 sections of the Papyrus one is devoted to the diseases of teeth which were treated by incantations and the local application of chemical and vegetable substances in the form of fomentations, masticatories, mouthwashes or plasters. Fumigation devices were used by the Egyptians in early times and in as late as the 19th century in England. The remedies were probably used widely since evidence of calcareous deposits, caries and alveolar abscesses have been found in skulls of the Egyptian aristocrats of the time of the pyramid builders.

Fig 3/3. Part of Ebers' papyrus in the original Egyptian hieroglyphic characters containing 11 dental prescriptions (Courtesy of New York Historical Society) [*Guerini*, 1909].

The first reference to the therapeutic extraction of teeth and to the association of systemic diseases and teeth is probably that obtained from the writings of a court physician of the Assyrian Sargonid dynasty (668–626 BC). The unknown physician wrote to his king: 'The inflammation wherewith his head, his hands (arms), feet (legs) are inflamed is due to his teeth. His teeth must be extracted: it is on this account that he is inflamed ...' It is obvious that such thinking was scientifically considerably advanced from the era that characterized belief in worms as a cause of tooth decay [*Prinz*, 1945].

Endogenous Theories

Humoral Theory. The legend of the worm faded over the early centuries as the Greek physicians advanced the humoral theory of disease. The four elemental humors of the body were blood, phlegm, black bile and yellow bile. According to *Galen*, the ancient Greek physician and philosopher, 'dental caries is produced by internal action of acrid and corroding humors'. An imbalance in these humors resulted in disease. 'The cure must consist in acting upon such vicious humors by means of local or general medicaments according to circumstances and also in strengthening the substance itself of the teeth by the use of astringents and tonic remedies' [*Guerini*, 1909]. *Hippocrates*, the 'Father of Medicine', while favoring the concept of humoral pathology also referred to the accumulated debris around teeth and to their corroding action. He, also, stated that stagnation of juices in the teeth was the cause of toothache. *Aristotle*, who lived during 384–322 BC, referred to elements of the Greek diet, such as figs, which adhered to teeth and thus contributed to decay.

Vital Theory. It was almost certainly apparent to the early Greek physicians, *Hippocrates*, *Celsus*, *Galen*, and *Avicenna*, and to more enlightened physicians of the Middle Ages, that teeth are an integral part of the body, and that they were vitally affected by and in turn affected the body. A vital theory of tooth decay was advanced, towards the end of the 18th century, which postulated that tooth decay originated, like bone gangrene, from within the tooth itself. A forerunner to this theory may have been the observation that internal resorption occurs in some teeth, or from the presence of deep, undermining carious lesions with but pin-point surface involvement of a pit or fissure.

Exogenous Theories
Chemical (Acid) Theory. In the 17th and 18th centuries, paralleling new insights into chemistry, there emerged the concept that teeth are destroyed by acids formed in the oral cavity. The acids implicated were inorganic, an unfortunate choice, since their origin could not be easily accounted for by advocates. One suggestion was that putrefaction of protein gave rise to ammonia which was subsequently oxidized to nitric acid; another was that food in saliva decomposed to form sulfuric, nitric or acetic acids. *Robertson* in 1835 proposed that dental decay was caused by acid formed by fermentation of food particles around teeth. Since fermentation was at this time considered to be a strictly nonvital process, the possibility that microorganisms were involved was not, as yet, recognized.

Parasitic (Septic) Theory. Long before the demonstration of the germ theory of disease, the possibility that microorganisms ('animal culae') can

have toxic and destructive effects on tissue was postulated [*Dubos*, 1954].
These postulations spelled the end of the vital theory and gave rise to
the idea that chemicals can destroy teeth. Early microscopic observations
of scrapings from teeth and of the carious lesions, by *Antoni van
Leeuwenhoek* (1632–1723), maker of the first powerful microscopes, indicated that microorganisms were associated with the carious process. A text
of what he saw is as follows:

'I am in the habit of rubbing my teeth with salt in the morning, and then rinsing my
mouth with water, and often after eating, to clean my back teeth with a toothpick, as well as
rubbing them hard with a cloth, wherefore my teeth back and front remain as clean and white
that only a few people of my age (fifty-one) can compare with me. Also when I rub my gums
with hard salt, they will not bleed. Yet all this does not make my teeth so clean but that I can
see, looking at them with a hollow mirror, that something will stick and grown between some
of the molars and teeth, a little white matter, as batter. Observing it I judged that although I
could not see anything moving in it there were yet living animalcules in it. I then mixed it
several times with purer ain-water, in which there were no animalcules and also with saliva
that I took from my mouth after eliminating the air bubbles lest these should stir the spittle. I
then again and again saw that there were many small living animalcules in the said matter,
which moved very prettily' [Collected Letters of *Antoni van Leeuwenhoek*, 1952].

In 1843, *Erdl* described filamentous parasites in the membrane removed
from teeth. A few years later in 1847 *Ficinus*, a physician, also observed
filamentous organisms in the enamel cuticle (surface protein membrane of
teeth) and in carious lesions. Dental caries was thought to develop as a
result of the infiltration and decomposition of the enamel cuticle, the interprismatic substance of enamel and finally dentin. *Ficinus* may have been
one of the first to recognize the presence of an organic matrix in enamel.
An explanation of the mechanism by which microorganisms caused decay
was not attempted until later.

Miller's Chemicoparasitic Theory. A synthesis of the ideas that acid
and microorganisms were involved in the etiology of dental caries did not
occur until 1889 when *Miller* (fig. 3/4), an American working at the University of Berlin, published a text entitled 'Die Mikroorganismen der Mund-
höhle' [English translation, 1890]. *Miller* was a student of *Koch* and his
extensive studies of the oral microflora and its relationships to caries were
greatly influenced by *Koch* and other scientists of the day. From *Koch* he
learned to isolate, stain and identify bacteria. At this time, *Pasteur* had
discovered that the process of conversion of sucrose to lactic acid is mediated by microorganisms. This enabled *Miller* to assign to oral microorgan-

isms the role of acid formation and thus assigned a chemical role to flora which is the basis of his chemicoparasitic theory of dental caries.

Miller's work at the University of Berlin was crucial to the development of the chemicoparasitic theory, the essential features of which are as follows:

– That the microorganisms of the mouth, by secretion of enzymes or by their own metabolism, degrade the fermentable carbohydrate food material so as to form acids. The chief acids formed are those associated with fermentation, namely lactic, butyric, acetic, formic, succinic and other acids. (The reader will recognize these organic acids as those comprising the glycolytic acids.)
– Carbohydrate food material lodged between and on surfaces of teeth is the source of the acid which demineralizes the lime salts of the tooth. He believed that starchy foods were more effective than soluble sugars – a point which is still somewhat unsettled. Thus, the enamel is destroyed by the acid of fermentation and the disintegrated enamel is subsequently mechanically removed by forces of mastication.
– After penetration of the enamel, the dissolution of dentin is brought about in the same manner with the organisms penetrating along the dentinal tubes.
– The final breakdown of dentin results from the secretion of proteolytic enzymes that digest the organic part of dentin and form a cavity.

The phenomenon of lactic acid fermentation and the role of glycolysis in dental caries is discussed in chapter 5.

The significance of *Miller's* observations is that he assigned an essential role to three factors in the caries process: the oral microorganisms in acid production and in proteolysis; the carbohydrate substrate which microorganisms fermented, and the acid which causes dissolution of tooth minerals. *Miller* used a mixed microbial flora of saliva and carbohydrates in order to demonstrate the destruction of teeth, in vitro. He concluded that caries was caused not by a single species of microorganisms but was related to multiple microbial activity involving acid production and protein degradation. *Miller* summarized his theory as follows: 'Dental decay is a chemoparasitic process consisting of two stages: decalcification or softening of the tissues and dissolution of the softened residue. In the case of enamel, however, the second stage is practically wanting, the decalcification of enamel signifying its total destruction.'

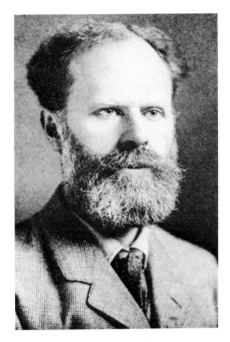

Fig 3/4. *Willoughby D. Miller* (1853 – 1907).

Further support for the role of microorganism in dental caries came from studies by *Underwood and Milles* in 1881. They observed micrococci, oval and rod-shaped bacteria in the dentin of histological sections of carious teeth and concluded that 'caries is absolutely dependent upon the presence and proliferation of organisms; that these organisms attack first the organic material and, feeding upon it, create an acid which removed the lime salt; that the only difference between caries and simple decalcification by acids is due to the presence and operation of germs'.

A very prominent French dental scientist, *Magitot*, demonstrated in 1867 that fermentation of sucrose in vitro led to dissolution of enamel mineral. Also, in 1867, two German physicians, *Leber and Rottenstein*, published a text entitled 'Untersuchungen über die Caries der Zähne'. In it they described the carious mouth as follows:

'In our opinion the progress of caries in enamel is this: By the action of an acid the enamel becomes porous at some point and loses its normal consistency. At the same time there is seen to appear a brown color, in consequence of the change which has taken place in its organic structure. There is formed at the surface a bed of leptothrix, which probably penetrates the dental cuticle, if it still exists, and destroys it. Chinks and fissures are opened in the enamel, which becomes less consistent. Acid liquids and granulations of leptothrix penetrate there, while minute fragments become detached and are promptly enveloped by the elements of leptothrix which, joined to the continued action of acids, hasten the dissolution.'

These workers believed that enamel caries was initiated by acids produced by microorganisms; microorganisms were also implicated in dentinal caries but by an unexplained mechanism. The presence of a specific microorganism, leptothrix buccalis in carious dentinal tubules was noted.

Critique of Chemo-parasitic Theory. *Miller's* chemo-parasitic theory is the backbone of current knowledge and understanding of the etiology of dental caries. Subsequent chapters will deal with recent work that refines *Miller's* theory and adds to our understanding of the complex nature of the carious process and the myriad of factors that influence it. At this point a short critique of *Miller's* theory will assist the reader in placing *Miller's* work in perspective. Of course, the criticism that follows is in the light of present knowledge and should not be interpreted as demerit points for *Miller's* brilliant observations.

–   *Miller's* chemo-parasitic theory was unable to explain the predilection of specific sites on a tooth to dental caries. The initiation of caries on smooth surfaces was not accounted for by this theory. The concept of a dental plaque adhering to teeth and serving to localize bacterial enzymatic activity was not proposed until 1897 by *Williams* and in 1898 by *Black* (see chapter 5 for a detailed discussion of dental plaque).
–   *Miller*, while a disciple of *Koch* who was an avid advocate of specific bacterial etiology of infectious disease, nevertheless worked with mixed cultures from saliva and with techniques that did not attempt to ascertain types of organisms present.
–   *Miller* believed that dental caries was caused by a multiple species of bacteria. This is understandable since many bacterial species possess glycolytic abilities. While current evidence for a specific bacterial infection in dental caries is tantalizing, the concept is not indisputable (more on this point in chapter 6).

– *Miller's* theory does not explain why some populations are caries-free.
– The phenomenon of arrested caries is not explained by the chemico-parasitic theory.
– *Miller* believed that in some systemic conditions the inorganic salts within a tooth could be withdrawn and that the organic-inorganic bonds would be weakened. He did not produce any experimental evidence that the adult tooth is subject to such systemic influences. The concept of tooth resistance while logical did not have any experimental support.

Proteolytic Theory. The surface coverings found on the tooth, in grooves and pits, are organic in nature; also, enamel contains small but significant amounts of organic material. These observations and the fact that carious lesions are characterized histologically by pigmentation, a phenomenon that was interpreted, without evidence, as being indicative of proteolysis, led to the development of the proteolytic theory espoused primarily by *Gottlieb* [1947], *Frisbie and Nuckolls* [1947] and *Pincus* [1950]. They described caries-like lesions that were initiated by proteolytic activity at a slightly alkaline pH, and considered that the process involved depolymerization and liquification of the organic matrix of enamel. *Gottlieb* [1947] proposed that microorganisms invade the organic pathways (lamellae) of enamel and initiate caries by proteolytic action. Subsequently, the inorganic salts are dissolved by acidogenic bacteria. *Pincus* [1950] also maintained that the initial process in dental caries was the proteolytic breakdown of the dental cuticle, the organic membrane found on all teeth.

The above conclusions were made on the basis of early histological observations. An interpretation of a molecular mechanism based on morphological evidence is highly suspect. To date no one has, under physiological conditions, successfully demonstrated significant loss of enamel tissue through proteolytic activity. Enamel is a highly structured tissue and the accessibility of organic material to enzymatic action before decalcification is restricted. Enamel can be dissolved under physiological conditions only by demineralization with acids, chelating or complexing agents.

Proteolysis-Chelation Theory. This theory proposed by *Schatz* et al. [1955] implies a simultaneous microbial degradation of the organic components (hence, proteolysis), and the dissolution of the minerals of the tooth by the process of chelation.

A brief explanation of chelation will permit a clearer understanding of this theory of dental caries. The word 'chelate' is derived from the Greek

word 'chele' meaning claw, and refers to compounds that are able to bind
metallic ions as calcium, iron, copper, zinc and other metals, by the secondary valence bonds. The resulting chelates are nonionic and usually soluble. Biological substances such as amino acids, and other chelators may be
used to remove calcium and other metal ions from a solution. An example
is the reaction between glycine and calcium in which a chelated complex,
calcium glycinate, is formed:

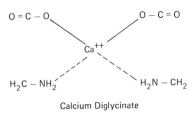

Calcium Diglycinate

There are many other biochemical compounds that form biological
chelates. Citrate forms a soluble, diffusible, anionic calcium citrate complex involving two ionized carboxyl groups and the unshared electrons of
the hydroxyl groups. This complex is most stable at an alkaline pH.

Some formation constants, of organic chelates of calcium, are noted in
table 3/I. Organic acids which contain two or more carboxyl groups and a
hydroxyl group that is sterically available for bonding form the most stable
complex ions with calcium. Lactic acid, a major product of plaque metabolism, can dissolve enamel apatite and, even after neutralization, can do
so as a chelator, but little attention has been paid to this possibility. Chelation, not related to proteolysis, might therefore play some part in caries.

Phosphorus-containing chelators of calcium are abundant in nature,
and indicate the strong attraction of many phosphate compounds for this
cation. Polyphosphates, e.g. hexametaphosphate, strongly complex calcium.

According to the proteolytic-chelation theory, dental caries results
from an initial bacterial and enzymatic proteolytic action on the organic
matter of enamel without preliminary demineralization. Such action, the
theory suggests, produces an initial caries lesion and the release of a variety
of complexing agents, such as amino acids, polyphosphates and organic
acids. The complexing agents then dissolve the crystalline apatite.

Table 3/I. Formation constants[1] of organic and phosphorus-containing chelates of calcium [from *Neuman and Neuman*, 1958]

Calcium chelates	log K_f	Phosphorus-containing chelates	log K_f
Citrate	3.15	orthophosphate	1.79
Malate	2.06	trimetaphosphate	2.02
Oxalacetate	1.6	pyrophosphate	3.17
Malonate	1.36	phytate	3.16
α-Ketoglutarate	1.29	hexametaphosphate	7.62
Succinate	1.0	adenosinetriphosphate	3.58
Carbonate	0.82		
Lactate	0.8		
Glycine	0.		

[1]The higher the formation constant the stronger the calcium complexing. Citrate binds calcium most strongly; some phosophorous-chelates are, also, bound strongly.

Less than 1% of mature enamel is organic in nature and the suggestion that this material upon degradation can give rise to a significant concentration of chelator sufficient to dissolve up to 96% mineral matter has no experimental support. Also, there is no substantial experimental evidence that the initial caries lesion stems from a breakdown of organic matter, i.e. due to proteolytic action. While proteolysis-chelation is an important biological phenomenon, its primary role in the etiology of dental caries has not been corroborated.

Other Theories of Caries Etiology

Sulfatase Theory. Pincus [1950] advanced the sulfatase theory, whereby bacterial sulfatase hydrolyzes the 'mucoitin sulfate' of enamel and the chondroitin sulfate of dentin producing sulfuric acid that in turn causes decalcification of the dental tissues. The concentration of sulfated polysaccharides in enamel is very small and not readily accessible as a substrate for enzymatic degradation. This is a highly unlikely hypothesis for the degradation of tooth enamel.

Complexing and Phosphorylating Theory. It can be readily demonstrated that an uptake of phosphate by plaque bacteria occurs during aerobic and anaerobic glycolysis and the synthesis of polyphosphates. According to the phosphorylating theory of caries [*Lura*, 1967], the high bacterial utilization of phosphate in plaque causes a local disturbance in the phosphate equilibrium in the plaque and the tooth enamel resulting in loss of inorganic phosphate from enamel. Soluble calcium-complexing compounds produced by bacteria cause further tooth disintegration. Saliva is an abundant source of inorganic phosphate for bacterial utilization. Hence, it is highly improbable that depletion of phosphate in plaque by oral microbial metabolism results in phosphate withdrawal from enamel.

The more recent suggestion [*Kreitzman* et al., 1969] that alkaline phosphatase causes a release of enamel phosphate from hypothetical organically bound phosphate is without experimental proof. How alkaline phosphatase which acts on organic phosphates could degrade a solid enamel substrate, in which virtually none of the phosphate is organically bound, remains to be elaborated. Release of phosphate from teeth may be nonspecifically achieved by ammonium sulfate and, since this salt was used in the preparation of the commercial alkaline phosphatase, it may explain this anomalous finding.

Current Concept

Primary (Essential) Factors in the Etiology of Dental Caries
In the epidemiological model, a disease state is due to an interplay of three primary factors: the host, the agent or recruiting factor and environmental influences (fig. 3/5). Obviously, many secondary factors influence the rate of progression of a disease. Many diseases may be viewed as products of the interplay of primary and secondary factors. The term multifactorial is used to denote the interaction between the factors. This model of viewing a disease process is applicable to dental caries.

Interaction between three primary factors is essential for the initiation and progression of caries: a susceptible host tissue, the tooth; microflora with a cariogenic potential; and a suitable local substrate to meet the requirements of the pathodontic flora. A diagrammatic representation of the interaction of the three factors essential for tooth decay is illustrated in figure 3/6. The tooth is the target tissue destroyed in the dental caries process. The cariogenic oral flora which is localized to specific sites on teeth is the agent that produces and secretes the chemical substances (organic acids, chelating agents and proteolytic enzymes) that cause the destruction of the inorganic components and the subsequent breakdown of the organic moities of enamel and dentin. The local substrate provides the nutritional and energy requirement for the oral microflora, thereby permitting them to colonize, grow, and metabolize on selective surfaces of teeth.

Experimental evidence unequivocally supports the concept that bacteria and suitable substrate for the microflora are prerequisites for dental

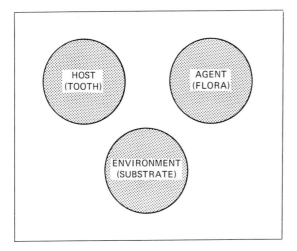

Fig 3/5. Epidemiological model of a disease state as an interplay of the host tissue, the exciting agent and environment influences.

caries. The third factor, the resistance of the tooth, is obviously important since this determines the overall effect of the attack. What is the experimental evidence that bacteria and a suitable substrate are prerequisites for the formation of dental caries?

Essentiality of Oral Bacteria. As early as in 1946 it was demonstrated that penicillin administered in the diet and drinking water to rats significantly reduced experimentally induced caries [*McClure and Hewitt,* 1946]. This study provided concrete evidence for the earlier assumption that bacteria are involved in caries. Also, since the antimicrobial spectrum of penicillin primarily encompasses gram-positive bacteria, this study narrowed the range of species suspected of causing dental caries. The study also provided a direction for studies in caries prevention in humans.

The hypothesis that bacteria are a prerequisite for the initiation and progression of dental caries was clinched by *Orland* et al. [1954] at the University of Chicago, in their classical germ-free animal studies. Germ-free animals obtained by Cesarean delivery and directly transferred to a sterile isolator were fed sterile food. Twenty-two rats which were fed a cariogenic diet, and maintained in a germ-free environment, were caries-free. Of the 39 control rats fed the same diet but maintained in a conven-

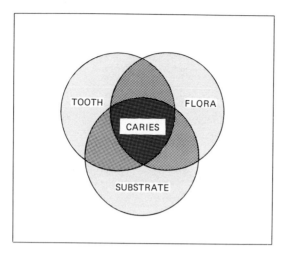

Fig. 3/6. A diagrammatic representation of the primary (essential) factors in dental caries etiology. Concurrent interaction of the three factors over a period of time (overlapping circles) is essential for caries to develop [after *Keyes*, 1960].

tional laboratory environment, and with no interference with their normal microflora, 38 developed carious lesions. This study laid to rest debates extending over a century about the role of bacteria in dental caries. Dental caries is a disease caused by oral bacteria.

The unequivocal demonstration that dental caries did not develop in laboratory rats in the absence of a normal bacterial flora initiated a series of experiments to determine the specificity of microorganisms in the initiation of dental caries. *Orland* et al. [1955] introduced a limited, defined flora in an attempt to produce caries in gnotobiotic animals. The term gnotobiotic (Greek word *gnosis* meaning positive knowledge) refers to laboratory animals with a defined microbiota.

Gnotobiotic animals maintained on a sterile cariogenic diet when infected with an enterococcus and another group inoculated with a combination of an enterococcus and a gram-negative proteolytic bacillus developed dental caries. The control animals that remained germ-free and the animals that were contaminated by pleomorphic bacillus were free of carious lesions. Unfortunately, the metabolic characteristics of these organisms were not stated and interpretations about the mechanisms of caries formation could not be made. This study clearly indicated that dental caries can be produced in laboratory animals with a controlled and limited flora and in the absence of lactobacilli, an organism frequently implicated in caries etiology in the early 1950s. Subsequently, several organisms have been shown to be capable of inducing dental caries in the gnotobiotic animal in pits and fissures, smooth surfaces and on root surfaces. A variety of *Streptococcus mutans* that produce dextrans (an extracellular polysaccharide containing glucose units) from sucrose is cariogenic in gnotobiotic animals. *Streptococcus salivarius* is, also, cariogenic and produces a levan (an extracellular polysaccharide containing fructose units). Also cariogenic are a dextran-producing *Streptococcus salivarius*; a *Streptococcus sanguis*-like organism; *Lactobacillus casei* and *Lactobacillus acidophilus* organisms of which at least one strain produced dextran and *Streptococcus milleri* [*Fitzgerald*, 1968]. Other organisms that have been shown to induce caries in the gnotobiotic rat include *Actinomyces viscosus*, *A. naeslundii* and *Peptostreptococcus intermedius* [*Frank* et al., 1972; *van der Hoeven* et al., 1972; *Rosen and Kolstad*, 1977]. Different types (occlusal vs smooth surface) of caries initiated by different organisms in germ-free rats are illustrated in figure 3/7a-d. Strains of *S. mutans* can initiate caries in pits and fissures as well as on smooth surfaces. In contrast, some strains of *S. sanguis*, *S. salivarius*, *S. mitis*, lactobacilli and actinomyces produce fissure lesions only in the gnotobiotic rat (more on this subject in chapters 5 and 6).

Studies on gnotobiotic animals are important in that they clarify the role of microorganisms in caries. Important summary points are as follows [*Fitzgerald*, 1968]:

– Microorganisms are a prerequisite for caries initiation.
– A single type of organism (for example, enterococcus strain) is capable of inducing caries.
– The ability to produce acid is a prerequisite for caries induction but not all acid–producing (acidogenic) organisms are cariogenic.
– Streptococcus strains that are capable of inducing caries are also able to synthesize extracellular dextrans or levans. Not all strains that produce extracellular polysaccharides are capable of caries induction.
– Organisms vary greatly in their capacity (virulence) to induce caries; comparative virulence cannot be deduced at present with certainty.

Apart from proving that caries cannot occur without the presence of a cariogenic organism, studies on gnotobiotic animals have not succeeded in defining the metabolic characteristics of a cariogenic organism, or of identifying a specific organism. It should be noted that neither the synthesis of dextran or levan, per se, is an absolute determinant of cariogenicity. Strains of dextran-producing *Streptococcus sanguis* and strains of levan-

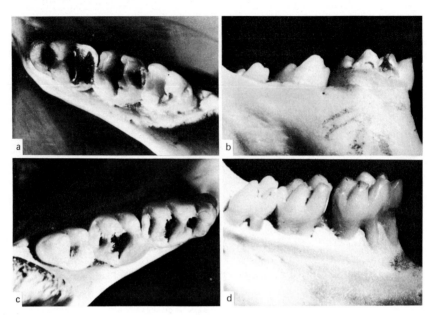

Fig. 3/7. Type of dental caries initiated by various bacteria in the germ-free rat. **a** Sulcal caries produced by *S. mutans*. **b** Typical buccal caries on the first molar produced by *S. mutans*. **c** Sulcal caries produced by lactobacilli. **d** Gingival and root surface caries on the mesial lingual root of the first molar produced by *A. Viscosus* [from *Morhart* et al., 1980, with permission].

producing *Streptococcus salivarius* have been found to be incapable of inducing caries in the gnotobiotic rat. The significance of the synthesis of extracellular polysaccharides, dextran and levan, by cariogenic microorganisms and the question of specificity of microflora in dental caries, the relative virulence of different cariogenic organisms and the interaction of different bacterial species are discussed in chapters 5 and 6.

Even at this early stage of the text one other aspect of microbial activity as it relates to caries should be stressed. Only those members of the bacterial flora of the mouth that are localized to specific sites on teeth are significant in the caries process. Localization of bacterial activity is conferred by adherence of organisms and the formation of a bacterial plaque. The plaque consists of a heterogeneous mass of organisms that implant themselves upon a salivary-derived protein film found on all erupted teeth. This important structure in caries etiology is discussed in detail in chapter 5.

Essentiality of a Local Substrate. The decisive study which indicated that a local substrate is essential for the oral flora to initiate dental caries was the tube-feeding experiment of *Kite* et al. [1950]. Animals that were fed a cariogenic food via a stomach tube, unlike the controls that were fed the same diet ad libitum, did not develop caries. These studies proved that a local food supply for bacteria, ingested ad libitum by the host, is essential for the initiation of dental caries, and that blood plasma constituents cannot mediate this role systematically via salivary secretions or by other mechanisms (more on substrate in chapters 7 and 8).

Secondary Factors that Affect Dental Caries

In a study of disease, primary factors (prerequisites), without which a disease process cannot develop, are often not clearly distinguished from secondary or predisposing factors which control the rate of progress of a disease. Many secondary factors, such as salivary composition and flow rate, oral hygiene and diet influence the caries process. Secondary factors affect one or a combination of the following: increase or reduce the tooth (host) resistance to dental caries; increase or decrease the quantitative and qualitative nature of the oral microflora involved in dental caries; increase or reduce the cariogenicity of the local substrate. The interplay between primary and secondary factors is diagrammatically depicted in figure 3/8 and is summarized in table 3/II.

A question may be asked: 'Is not saliva an essential factor in dental caries etiology?' Indeed rampant caries results when salivation is inhibited (see chapter 9). Saliva has many functions: cleansing effect, buffering capacity, provision of an environment saturated with calcium and phosphate, antibacterial action – these characteristics influence the rapidity at which caries develops. However important a role saliva may play in dental caries it is not a prerequisite for caries initiation in the same sense that organisms, substrate, and the tooth are essential.

Many other factors, in addition to saliva, influence the rate of caries by significantly affecting one of the primary factors. As an example, fluoride is an important trace element that affects the resistance of mineral of enamel to the caries process and enhances remineralization of incipient lesions. Fluoride deficiency potentiates caries since the host factor (tooth) cannot attain its maximum resistance to caries on a suboptimal intake. Other examples of a secondary factors that influence dental caries are oral hygiene and dental plaque control. Scrupulous oral hygiene may completely prevent caries (a perfectly clean tooth does not decay) – but perfect oral hygiene cannot be attained. Oral hygiene affects caries but it is not a primary factor in caries (see volume 2, chapter 10).

Table 3/II. The determinants of dental caries

Primary factors (initiate dental caries)	Secondary factors, environmental and hereditary (control rate of progression of lesion)	Bacterial metabolites important in caries	Mechanism of tooth destruction	Role in caries process
Bacterial plaque	Oral hygiene Oral Flora (quantitative and qualitative) Saliva (pH, composition, buffering capacity, flow rate) Fluoride in plaque Diet and nutrition Transmissibility	Organic acids	Dissolve inorganic phase	Major
Suitable substrate	Carbohydrates, type and concentration Chemical composition of food (fats, proteins) Physical characteristics of food (detergency, etc.) Oral clearance of food Oral hygiene Frequency of eating	Chelators	Bind Ca^{2+} ions	Minor
Tooth	Fluoride concentration Carbonate and citrate level Age of tooth Gross and surface morphology (hypoplasia, fissures) Crystallinity of OH-apatite Trace elements (Zn, Se, Sn, Fe, Mn, Mo) Nutrition (vitamins and minerals, fats, protein, phosphates) Salivary composition and flow rate Surface composition of enamel	Proteolytic enzymes	Breakdown of organic macromolecules after demineralization	Minor in enamel; important in dentin

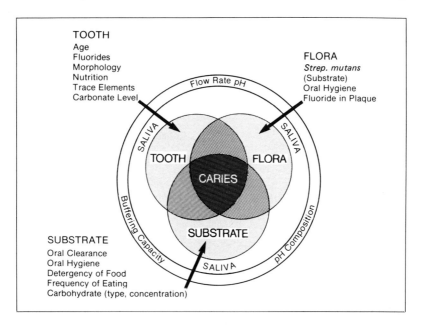

Fig 3/8. Diagrammatic representation of the interplay between primary and secondary factors in caries etiology. The three primary factors, tooth, bacterial flora and substrate are depicted by overlapping circles. Saliva an important secondary, predisposing factor is depicted as a concentric circle surrounding the three primary factors. Other secondary factors (arrows) that influence the tooth, flora and substrate are also, depicted.

Primary Mechanism of Caries Formation

When the three essential parameters for dental caries – cariogenic organisms, susceptible teeth and a suitable local substrate – exist in an individual for a considerable time, then dental caries may develop. What is the primary mechanism by which a carious lesion develops? The mechanism at a molecular level is best understood after considering the nature of tooth substance, substrate and the microbiology of caries, and is presented in the succeeding chapters. In this section, only a gross picture of the mechanism will be sketched.

A detailed picture of the chemical dynamics of enamel dissolution, the factors controlling the chemical reactions involved in a carious process will

Simplified equations depicting the caries progress is as follows (see table 3/II):

Cariogenic bacterial plaque	+	suitable local substrate	→	organic acids
Organic acids (in plaque)	+	tooth mineral	→	loss of enamel
Demineralized tooth (dentin)	+	bacterial proteolytic enzymes	→	cavitation

be delayed until the discussion of the nature of the three primary factors in caries etiology (see chapter 10).

The best available evidence indicates that a carious lesion results from the action of bacterial metabolic endproducts localized to the enamel surface by a dental plaque. In older persons, where gingival recession has occurred, this process may start on the dentin or cementum. Of the metabolic endproducts implicated in the caries process, organic acids are most important in mineral dissolution. The discovery that the pH of dental plaques is rapidly lowered to levels at which the concentrations of calcium and phosphates in the environment no longer saturate it and may therefore cause demineralization following glucose or sucrose rinses is supportive of this view [*Stephan* 1940] (see chapters 5 and 8).

It is obvious from the above summary of the primary and secondary factors that the mechanism of the carious process is relatively complex. The reader quite naturallly must be posing many questions. What members of the oral flora are significant in the etiology of dental caries? Is dental caries due to a specific bacterial infection? What is the metabolic basis for caries pathogenicity of microorganisms? What constituents of our diet contribute to dental caries? Are physical characteristics of diet important? What cultural aspects as they related to customs of eating and selection of food affect caries? What are the characteristics of a noncariogenic diet? Are there caries-resistant teeth? Is the composition and morphology of teeth significant? What is the role of fluoride in caries prevention? What is the role of saliva, oral hygiene in the etiology of caries? These questions will be answered as the chapters unfold. The essentiality of the host tissue, cariogenic flora and substrate in the caries process while experimentally proven is just the beginning of our story and a detailed consideration of each of the three essentials for caries formation is necessary for an understanding of the etiology and mechanism of dental caries.

Additional Reading

Bibby, B.G.; Gustafson, G.; Davies, G.N.: A critique of three theories of caries attack. Int. dent. J. 8: 685 (1958).
Bremner, M.D.K.: The story of dentistry – from the dawn of civilzation to the present ... with special emphasis on the American scene; revised 3 ed. (Dental Items of Interest Publishing, New York 1959).
Jenkins, G.N.: Current concepts concerning the development of dental caries. Int. dent. J. 22: 350 (1972).

References

Dubos, R.J.: Biochemical determinants of microbial diseases, (Harvard University Press, Cambridge 1954).
Fitzgerald, R.J.: Dental caries in gnotobiotic animals. Caries Res. 2: 139 (1968).
Frank, R.M.; Guillo, B.; Llory, H.: Caries dentaires chez le rat gnotobiote inovule avec Actinomyces viscosus et Actinomyces naeslundii. Archs oral Biol. 17: 249 (1972).
Frisbie, H.E.O.; Nuckolls, J.: Caries of the enamel. J. dent. Res. 26: 181 (1947).
Gottlieb, B.: Dental caries (Lea & Febiger, Philadelphia 1947).
Guerini, V.: History of dentistry (Lea & Febiger, Philadelphia 1909).
Hoeven, J.S. van der; Mikx, F.J.M.; Plasschaert, A.M.J.; König, K.G.: Methodological aspects of gnotobiotic caries experimentation. Caries Res. 6: 203 (1972).
Keyes, P.H.: The infectious and transmissible nature of experimental dental caries. Archs oral Biol. 1: 304 (1960).
Kite, O.W.; Shaw, J.H.; Sognnaes, R.F.: The prevention of experimental tooth decay by tube-feeding. J. Nutr. 42: 89 (1950).
Kreitzman, S.N.; Irving, S.; Navia, J.M.; Harris, R.S.: Enzymatic release of phosphate from rat molar enamel by phosphoprotein phosphatase. Nature, Lond. 223: 520 (1969).
Lura, H.E.: The non-acid complexing and phosphorylating theory of dental caries (Holbaek, Ator Tryk 1967).
McClure, F.J.; Hewitt, W.L.: The relation of penicillin to induced rate of dental caries and oral L. acidophilus. J. dent. Res. 25: 441 (1946).
Miller, W.D.: The microorganisms of the human mouth (S.S. White Co., 1890).
Morhart, R.; Cowman, R.; Fitzgerald, R.: Ecologic determinants of the oral microbiota; in Menaker, The biologic basis of dental caries, chapter 12, p. 278 (Harper & Row, Hagerstown 1980).
Neuman, W.F.; Neuman, M.W.: The chemical dynamics of bone mineral (University of Chicago Press, Chicago 1958).

Orland, F.J.; Blayney, J.R.; Harrison, R.W.; Reyniers, J.A.; Trexler, P.C.; Ervin, R.F.;
    Gordon, H.A.; Wagner, M.: Experimental caries in germ-free rats inoculated with en-
    terococci. J. Am. dent. Ass. *50:* 259 (1955).
Orland, F.J.; Blayney, J.R.; Harrison, R.W.; Reyniers, J.A.; Trexler, P.C.; Wagner, M.;
    Gordon, H.A.; Luckey, T.D.: The use of germ-free animal techniques in the study of
    experimental dental caries. I. Basic observations on rats reared free of all microorgan-
    isms. J. dent. Res. *33:* 147 (1954).
Pincus, P.: A new hypothesis of dental caries. J. Calif. St. dent. Soc. *26:* 16 (1950).
Prinz, H.: Dental chronology – a record of the more important historic events in the evolution
    of dentistry (Lea & Febiger, Philadelphia 1945).
Rosen, S.; Kolstad, R.A.: Dental caries in gnotobiotic rats inoculated with strain of *Peptos-
    treptococcus intermedius.* J. dent. Res. *56:* 187 (1977).
Schatz, A.; Karlson, K.E.; Martin, J.J.: Speculation on lactobacilli and acid as possible anti-
    caries factor. N.Y. dent. J. *21:* 367, 438; *22:* 161 (1954, 1955).
Stephan, R.M.: Changes in the hydrogen ion concentration on tooth surfaces and in carious
    lesions. J. Am. dent. Ass. *27:* 718 (1940).

4 The Nature of Tooth Substance

Dental caries leads to a localized destruction of teeth by end products of bacterial metabolism. Carious lesions usually start in a pit, fissure or the smooth surface of enamel. As has already been noted, enamel is avascular and acellular and, therefore, is incapable of vitally resisting the carious process. The cellular events triggered by an infectious process in soft tissues cannot occur in enamel. Destruction of dental tissues by the carious process does not fit into the usual classification of pathological processes. In order to understand the mechanism by which bacterial end products initiate dental caries and the subsequent progression of the carious lesion we must first consider the nature of the hard tissues of the tooth. Because initiation of caries usually involves enamel (some lesions may start in exposed dentin or cementum) this tissue will be discussed in detail.

Dental Enamel

The hard part of a tooth is composed of three mineralized tissues: enamel, dentin, and cementum. Enamel is a secretory product of cells derived from the stratified epithelium of the oral cavity and has some unique biologic characteristics. Dentin and cementum, on the other hand, are of mesodermal origin and possess chemical characteristics similar to bone.

Dental enamel is the most dense biologic substance known. In its adult state enamel has a specific gravity of approximately 3.0, denoting a tissue very high in mineral and low in nitrogen content. Adult enamel contains only about 0.5% protein by weight, as compared with about 20% in bone and dentin, although enamel is very heterogeneous in this respect and reported values for protein content vary enormously. Developing, partially mineralized enamel has an initial protein content similar to that found in bone or dentin.

Developing Enamel

Developing enamel matrix contains about 5–15% calcium (mature enamel contains about 96% mineral) and is composed of an electrophoretically heterogeneous protein with unique features such as amino acid composition, structural configuration and temperature-dependent aggregation [*Eastoe*, 1979]. Two types of protein have been isolated from developing bovine enamel tissue [*Termine* et al., 1979]. About 85% of the enamel matrix consists of a proline-rich protein called amelogenin. In addition, a high molecular weight phosphoprotein, 46,000–72,000 daltons, rich in aspartic and glutamic acids and tightly bound to apatite crystals has been isolated. This protein, called enamelin, is also found in mature enamel. It is not known whether the ameloblasts synthesize a single protein which is subsequently degraded into smaller subunits or whether amelogenin and enamelin constitute distinct protein species. Figure 4/1 describes the laboratory extraction procedure yielding these 2 proteins from developing bovine teeth. Some of the enamel protein is glycosylated as evidenced by the presence of amino sugars fucose, glucose and mannose in hydrolysates [*Burgess and MacLaren*, 1965].

The amino acid composition of amelogenin is characterized by the highest level of proline thus far reported for any protein (200–250 residues per 1,000 amino acid residues) and high concentrations of glutamic acid, histidine and leucine. Biochemical and physical studies using polyacrylamide electrophoresis gels, Sephadex gel molecular sieve filtration have characterized amelogenin as a multicomponent system [*Seyer and Glimcher*, 1977]. However, immunological studies indicate that enamel protein behaves as a single antigen suggesting that the secretion of enamel protein by the ameloblasts is under the control of a single gene [*Nikiforuk and Gruca*, 1969]. An electrophoretic pattern of soluble amelogenin on acrylamide gel showing approximately 12 zones is shown in figure 4/2a. Figure 4/2b shows that the different electrophoretic amelogenin fractions that react with antisera are antigenically identical.

One of the most interesting biological aspects of protein of developing enamel relates to the marked and rapid displacement of amelogenin as enamel calcifies and matures. Over 90% of the amelogenin present in the matrix is removed, probably by hydrolysis of peptide bonds during the mineralization process. Proteolytic activity has been detected in the developing matrix and this may be the mechanism of protein removal. The gross chemical changes and the relation of chemical stages which occur at different stages of enamel maturation is shown in figures 4/3 and 4/4.

The organic matrix which remains in the mature enamel tissue has a composition markedly similar to enamelin, the protein in developing enamel that is tightly bound to crystals. The amino acid composition of mature enamel matrix reveals a high concentration of glycine, glutamic and aspartic aids and serine phosphate. Organically bound phosphate (serine phosphate) has been suggested as playing a key role in the nucleation of hydroxyapatite thus initiating calcification of this tissue. Phosphoproteins

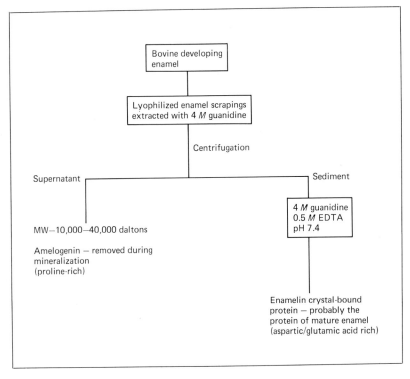

Fig. 4/1. Laboratory procedure for isolation of 2 protein fractions from developing bovine enamel. The proline-rich fraction is called amelogenin. The aspartic-glutamic acid-rich phosphoprotein protein fraction called enamelin is the protein of mature enamel.

are known to inhibit collagen fibrillogenesis. Phosphoproteins from rat dentin have been shown to bind about 40 times as much calcium as collagen in dentin matrix, suggesting that these compounds may play a regulatory role in mineralization of dentin and perhaps in enamel [*Li and Katz*, 1980].

Even the earliest stage of organic matrix formation by ameloblasts has significance from a dental caries standpoint. The ameloblasts are sensitive to some metabolic disorders which result in enamel hypocalcification or enamel hypoplasia. Hypocalcification of enamel denotes a qualitative disturbance in amelogenesis and is clinically recognized as a white area in an otherwise normal surface. Enamel hypoplasia represents a quantitative disturbance in tooth development whereby pits and circumferential defects are seen. Enamel hypoplasia is often associated with a number of childhood diseases such as hypoparathyroidism and vitamin D deficiency. A

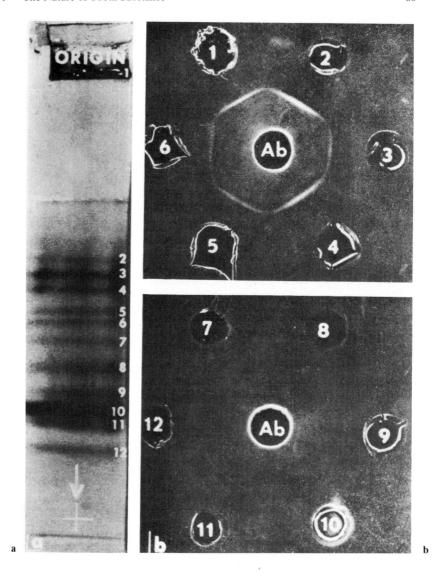

Fig. 4/2. a An electrophoretic pattern of the soluble amelogenin in a vertical, discontinuous acrylamide gel (7%) system; electrode buffer tris-glycine, 0.04 M, pH 8.3; protein loading 2.5 mg. A series of 12 closely spaced bands is shown. **b** Bands from the acrylamide electrophoretic pattern, identified 1–12, were cut from the gel and imbedded in agar plates and then reacted against the purified antisera (Ab). The Ouchterlony plate demonstrates that only the 6 bands most proximal to, and including, the origin formed precipitin lines and that these fractions were antigenically identical [from *Nikiforuk and Gruca*, 1969].

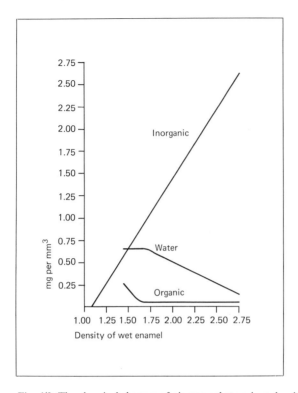

Fig. 4/3. The chemical changes of pig enamel at various densities [*Deakins*, 1942].

common denominator of many metabolic disorders that interfere with ameloblast function is hypocalcemia (low plasma calcium levels). This may be explained by the finding that even the earliest amelogenin secreted contains about 5–10% calcium suggesting a calcium requirement for synthesis of the enamel matrix. Recent evidence suggests that hypocalcemia is a much more specific determinant of enamel hypoplasia than has previously been suspected [*Nikiforuk and Fraser*, 1979]. The subject of enamel hypoplasia and caries is discussed in chapter 7.

Development of Enamel Crystallites
The first evidence of mineral salt deposition in the enamel appears almost simultaneously with the formation of the enamel matrix. The initial crystallites deposited next to the dentin are apparently in juxtaposition to collagen fibrils. Under the electron microscope the initially discernible

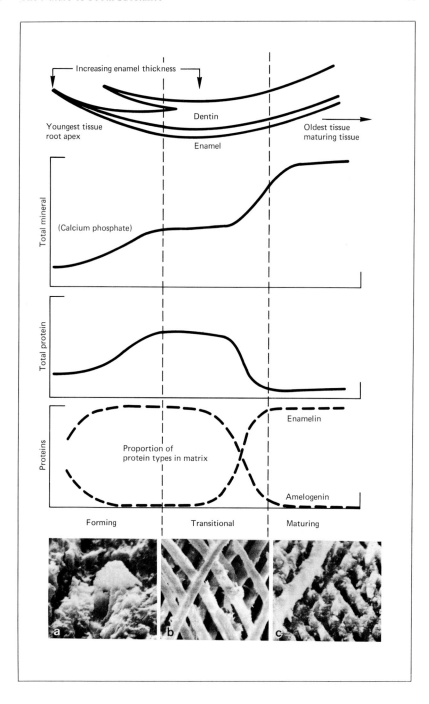

crystallites appear as long plates or ribbons about 15 Å in thickness (fig. 4/5a). It is probable that desiccation required in preparing this highly hydrated tissue for the electron microscope introduces some degree of artifact in these early manifestations of mineral crystallites. The crystallites mature rapidly in width and slowly in thickness. Subsequent growth of the crystallites is primarily limited to a gradual increase in thickness. Figure 4/5c, d) relative to those in the mesenchymal tissues, namely, bone, dentin must occur, since the number of enamel crystallites in mature enamel is about 50% less than in developing enamel.

A unique feature of the mature enamel crystals is their large size (fig. 4/5c, d) relative to those in the mesenchymal tissues, namely, bone, dentin and cementum. Mature enamel crystals are about 1,600 Å in length, 680 Å in width and 260 Å in thickness [*Ronnholm*, 1962; *Daculsi* and *Kerebel*, 1978]. The shape and size of the mature crystal varies with the degree of mineralization and the location within the enamel tissue.

Human enamel crystallites are organized into a basic structural unit called the prism. One enamel prism arises from several ameloblasts [*Ronnholm*, 1962]; therefore, the so-called prism sheath cannot represent a cell boundary, as proposed by earlier morphologists. When cut in cross-sections the prisms are seen as being locked together and resemble a keyhole structure (fig. 4/6a, b). The emphasis on the keyhole structure is misleading and the preferred terminology is to describe circular prisms which are separated by interprismatic regions. What should be stressed is that human enamel prism bodies are continuous with the interprismatic structures cervically. The crystallite orientation within the head of an enamel rod is shown in figure 4/6c.

Crystallinity of a substance refers to the size of the crystal and the strain and stresses within the crystal. There has been a recent suggestion that the alignment of enamel crystallites may be significant in caries resistance [*Cevc* et al., 1980]. The crystallinity of tooth enamel is known to be affected by fluoride. There is experimental evidence that a deficiency of vitamin D retards crystal maturity of bone mineral in rats [*Muller* et al., 1966] and a similar effect may operate in enamel, although the latter tissue has not been investigated from this standpoint. The important point is that

---

Fig. 4/4. Summary of chemical stages at different stages of enamel mineralization. The SEM pictures shows enamel at different stages of maturation on (**a**) relatively structureless enamel, (**b**) prismatic structures in an open arrangement (may be due to shrinkage or absence of interprismatic material) corresponding to the stage of matrix withdrawal, and (**c**) later maturation stage with more mineral acquisition [from *Robinson* et al., 1981, with permission].

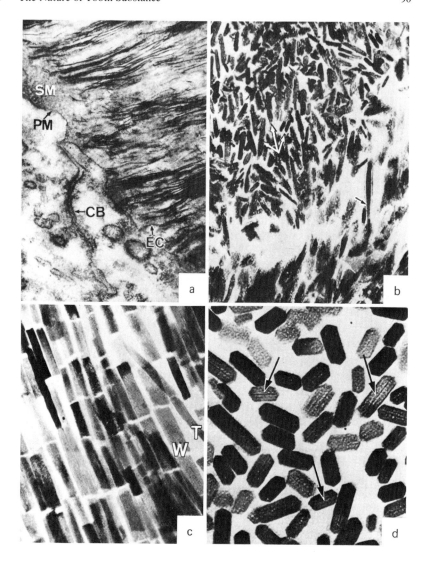

Fig. 4/5 a. Earliest observable human enamel crystallites (EC) formed very close to the plasma membrane (PM). The crystallities are ribbon-shaped and orientated approximately to the long axis of the prism but perpendicular to the cell boundary (CB). Some matrix appears as a stippled material (SM) between the cell surface and the very young crystallites. ×180,000. **b** More mature human enamel crystallites (arrows) than those shown in **a**. Maturation of crystals is accomplished primarily by growth in thickness. ×170,000. **c** Mature rat enamel crystallites sectioned parallel with their long axis. ×150,000. The thickness (T) and the width

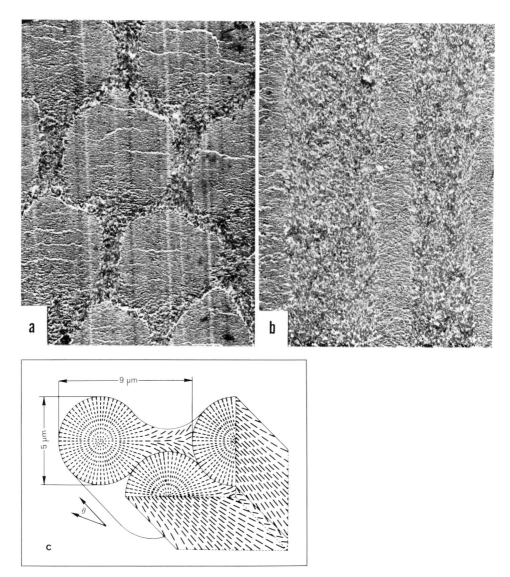

(W) of the ribbons is 200 and 400 Å, respectively. ×150,000. **d** Cross-section of enamel crystallites, showing hexagonal forms (arrows). ×300,000 [4/5a, b from *Ronnholm*, 1962; 4/5c, d from *Nylen* et al., 1963].

Fig. 4/6. a Electron micrograph of sections of human adult teeth depicting the enamel prisms. a Cross-section of enamel prisms. ×5,000. Note the keyhole structure of the prisms. **b** Section cut parallel with the long axis of the prisms. ×5,000 [*Meckel* et al., 1965]. **c** Crystallite orientation in the keyhole-shaped enamel prism [*Cevc* et al., 1980].

Table-4/I. Properties and composition of mature enamel, dentin, cementum and bone

	Embryologic origin	Cell progenitor	Density	Inorganic		Organic		Water		Hydroxyapatite crystal size, Å
				wt%	vol%	wt%	vol%	wt%	vol%	
Enamel	ectodermal	ameloblast (secretes amelogenin and enamelin)	2.9 –3.0	95	87	1	2	3.0	11	l = 250–10,000[1] w = 600– 1,000 t = 263– 350
Dentin	mesenchymal	odontoblast (secretes collagen, phosphoprotein, and glycoproteins)	2.05–2.35	70	47	20	33	10	21	w = 296 t = 32
Cementum	mesenchymal	cementoblast	2.02–2.05	(similar to dentin)						
Bone	mesenchymal	osteoblast	2.1 –2.2	65	36	24	36	15	28	l = 200 w = 50 t = 20

[1] Size and shape of enamel crystallites vary widely, depending upon its degree of mineralization; in the case of adult enamel, with the region studied. Further, it is difficult to resolve individual crystallites because of overlapping and fusion of crystals. These factors explain the wide discrepancies of the published data relating to size of enamel crystals.
Compiled from *Daculsi and Kerebel* [1978], *Ronnholm* [1962], *Grøn* [1978], *Deakins* [1942], *Brudevold and Söremark* [1967].

crystal size is related to chemical reactivity since smaller crystals have larger surface areas per unit volume. The foundation for caries-resistant teeth inheres in normal synthesis of the organic matrix and in optimal microcrystalline structure and chemical composition of tooth enamel.

Maturation of Young Enamel

The process of progressive preeruptive and, to a lesser extent, post-eruptive mineralization of enamel is known as maturation. During the early phases of maturation of enamel, water and protein are replaced by a highly mineralized crystalline calcium-phosphate-carbonate component with structural characteristics of a mineral called hydroxyapatite. The reader should review the chemical changes occurring in developing enamel as it matures by referring to figure 4/3 and 4/4. The process of maturation continues during the entire preeruptive stage of enamel development and to a significant degree after eruption until a crystalline tissue with an unusual density approaching 3.0 is formed.

Physicochemical ionic exchanges and changes in surface enamel due to dissolution and reprecipitation of ions continue throughout the lifetime of a tooth. An important posteruptive chemical exchange results in an increasing concentration of fluorine, and a reduction of carbonate at the enamel surface. Also, ionic exchanges between saliva, plaque fluid, and the tooth play an important role in caries. Although, advanced carious lesions are irreversible, incipient enamel lesions, without any signs of cavitation, may remineralize – more about this phenomenon later.

Gross Chemical Composition of Mature Enamel, Dentin and Cementum

The gross composition of enamel, dentin, cementum and for comparison bone tissue with respect to organic, inorganic, water components and the size of hydroxyapatite crystallites is summarized in table 4/I. The high concentration of the inorganic phase suggests that the most probable mechanism of enamel destruction is by bacterial metabolites such as organic acids or complexing agents, that readily break down this phase.

Adult human enamel of permanent teeth has an inorganic component of between 95 and 96%, while that of primary teeth is between 92 and 93%. The inorganic components occupy a volume of about 87%. The amount of organic material varies within the range of 0.2–2.0% with higher values for primary teeth. The remaining constituent is water. Figure 4/7 depicts the distribution of inorganic, organic fractions and water in enamel.

Of the small amount of organic material in mature enamel, the main components are proteins (about 58%), lipids (about 40%) with traces of sugars, citrate and lactate ions. Triglycerides, cholesterol and cholesterol

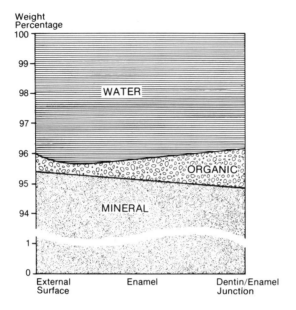

Fig. 4/7. Distribution of inorganic and organic matter and water in human enamel from the dentino-enamel junction to the surface [after *Brudevold and Söremark*, 1967].

esters, lecithins, neutral and complex lipids have been identified in enamel. In addition, adult enamel contains about 3.0% water by weight or 10% by volume. Some of the water is firmly bound to the inorganic phase and is released only after heating enamel to above 250–300 °C for several hours. Water that is firmly bound to the inorganic phase forms the hydration shell of single hydroxyapatite crystals. Water by virtue of space it occupies is important in mediating diffusion of molecules and ions through enamel and in the interaction of enamel with its chemical environment. More will be said about the hydration shell and the surface chemistry of enamel later in this chapter.

Dentin and cementum unlike enamel, are cellular tissues of mesenchymal origin and resemble bone in chemical composition. Dentin contains about 20% organic matter, that is, about 40 times as much as is found in adult enamel; about 79% is inorganic phase. The main organic component is collagen, type I, with its characteristic high content of hydroxyproline, and glycine. A lesser noncollagenous phosphoprotein component, rich in aspartic acid and phosphoserine, that binds to the collagen fibrils in dentin is present [*Butler* et al., 1979]. Also, in common with other connective

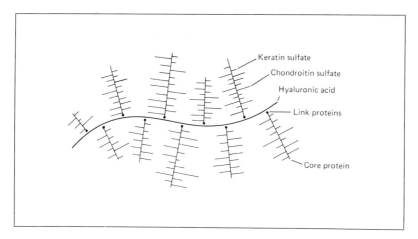

Fig. 4/8. The structure of proteoglycan consisting of an elongated hyaluronic acid backbone to which are attached glycosaminoglycans via a link protein.

tissues, the extracellular spaces of dentin and predentin are filled with macromolecules known as proteoglycans. The structure of proteoglycans consists of an elongated molecule of hyaluronic acid to which is attached a link
protein in a bottle-brush arrangement. The carbohydrate side chains
known as glycosaminoglycans consist of long, nonbranched polysaccharides containing sulfate or carboxylate groups (fig. 4/8). These functional
groups give proteoglycans their strong negatively charged polyanionic
properties. They bind large amounts of water and high concentrations of
Na^+, K^+ and Ca^{2+}. Swelling and turgor of connective tissue is associated
with its proteoglycan content. The role of proteoglycans in dentinogenesis
and mineralization is unknown. The high concentration of organic matter
in dentin relative to enamel suggests that in dentinal caries proteolysis is an
important mechanism of the breakdown of dentin.

Inorganic Constituents of Enamel, Dentin and Cementum

The mineral of enamel, dentin and cementum consists mainly of a
calcium-phosphate-carbonate mineral phase with the inclusion of lower
concentrations of sodium, magnesium, chloride, potassium and a large
number of trace elements, the most significant of which is fluorine. Considerable variation in concentration of minerals in enamel exists because of
different analytical and sampling procedures, and because of the true dif-

Table 4/II. Major inorganic components of mineralized tissues (percent of dry weight)

	Human tooth enamel		Dentin (permenent teeth)	Bone	Calculus	Stoichiometric hydroxyapatite
	permanent	primary				
Ca	36.4	35.0	25.1	39.4	36.1	39.9
P	17.4	18.5	13.9	17.9	19.4	18.5
CO_2	2.7	2.7	4.5	6.1	1.8	–
Mg	0.40	0.31	0.85	0.5	1.8	–
Na	0.66	0.63	0.54	0.9	2.5	–
K	0.03	0.027	0.019	0.2	–	–
Cl	0.23	0.27	0.072	0.2	1.3	–
F	0.01	–	–	–	–	3.77
Ca/P	2.10	1.87	1.80	2.19	1.89	(2.15)
Ca/P molar ratio	(1.61)	–	–	–	–	(1.67)

Compiled from *Patel and Brown* [1975], *Lakomaa and Rytömaa* [1977], *Grøn* [1978].

ferences between persons, between teeth, and even between parts of the same tooth. Since development of the permanent dentition extends over a period of more than 13 years, each permanent tooth takes from 6 to 10 years, and since such a long time span may encompass different metabolic conditions at different ages of an individual, it is not surprising that significant variations in the composition of enamel have been reported.

The concentration of the major elements in enamel in permanent and primary teeth, and the corresponding values for dentin of permanent teeth and for comparison those in bone and calculus is given in table 4/II. The concentration of calcium, the main inorganic elemental constituent of enamel is about 36% by weight, and of phosphorus about 18% by weight, the latter occurs as a phosphate, PO_4^{3-}. About 5% of the total inorganic phosphorus is in the form of HPO_4^2 [*Eanes*, 1979]. The Ca : P ratio (dry weight) in enamel is about 2.0; the molar ratio is 1.62 [*Patel and Brown*, 1975]. Enamel contains about 2.5% by weight of carbonate (CO_3^{-2}); 0.6% Na; 0.3% Cl; 0.35% Mg; and 0.03% K; as well as many other trace elements. Dentin is not as dense a tissue as enamel. It contains about 26% of calcium, 14% phosphorus, and 3.4% carbonate by weight as well as a large number of trace elements.

The crystalline arrangement of the inorganic constituents of dental tissue and the biological significance of the crystalline phase, including its role in dental caries, is discussed next.

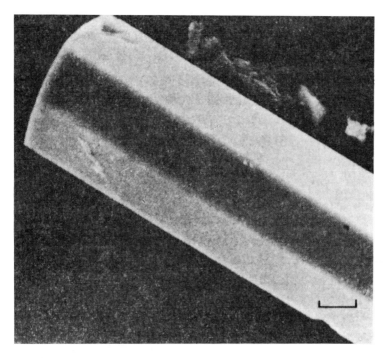

Fig. 4/9. Typical synthetic hydroxyapatite single crystal, carbonate-rich. Bar is 10 μm. The hexagonal cross section is visible in the upper part of the figure [courtesy of *Arends and Jongebloed*, 1979].

Crystalline Phase of Dental Tissues

The major mineral components of enamel, dentin, cementum and bone consist of microcrystals of basic calcium phospate, and the spatial arrangement of the atoms resembles the mineral hydroxyapatite, $Ca_{10}(PO_4)_6(OH)_2$. Enamel consists essentially of apatitic mineral although this is disputed by some researchers; in dentin a part of the mineral phase may be nonapatitic. The formula for hydroxyapatite cannot be used to describe the composition of hard tissues due to substitutions as described later.

High resolution electron microscopy has shown that all biological apatites are composed of very small crystals. Larger synthetic hydroxyapatite crystals in the millimeter range have been prepared [*Arends and Jongebloed*, 1979]. Morphologically, the crystals are rod-like; cross sections may reveal hexagonal forms (fig. 4/9). Much valuable information about the properties of hydroxyapatite has come from studying the atomic arrangements of large single crystals. The analogy with real enamel crystals should be extended with care.

Most of our knowledge about the manner in which atoms are arranged in hydroxyapatite mineral is obtained by a technique known as X-ray diffraction. The apatite nature of the inorganic components of human enamel was first definitely proved by using the X-ray diffraction method. When a parallel beam of X-rays strikes a minute amount of matter, the X-rays are scattered by the electrons of the component atoms. Interference, both additive and subtractive, of the scattered X-rays is a function of the spatial arrangement and the nature of the atomic constituents of the sample of matter. By observing the diffraction effects as spots or lines on a photographic film, or as profiles (diffractograms) of the recorded curves using scintillation detectors it is possible to gain valuable information about the atomic structure of crystals. An X-ray diffraction pattern of enamel and typical diffractogram of dental tissues and mineral apatite is depicted in figure 4/10a, b. Note the similarity of both the positions and the relative intensities of the diffracted X-rays in mineral, biological and synthetic apatite.

Most apatite crystals in nature are very small and poorly developed which in turn results in a poorly defined X-ray diffraction pattern. The exception is fluorapatite which occurs naturally as a macrocrystal that has been extensively studied. Hydroxyapatite crystals in enamel are at least an order of magnitide larger than in other hard tissues and are, therefore also, a good model for studying the crystal structure of biological hydroxyapatite.

The Hydroxyapatite Crystal Structure

The spatial arrangement of the atoms of hydroxyapatite is complex and a detailed, quantitative examination of a 3-dimensional configuration is beyond the scope of this text. Only the basic elements of the structure are presented here. The reader who wishes to gain a better understanding of the apatitic structure is encouraged to consult the selected literature noted at the end of the section and to construct a scale model.

Fig. 4/10. a An X-ray diffraction pattern of enamel. **b** Diffraction patterns of dental hard tissue mineral and synthetic (nonstoichiometric) hydroxyapatite [*Grøn*, 1978]. The patterns are more defined for mineral and synthetic apatite and enamel since the crystals are larger. In dentin and bone the apatite crystals are much smaller and hence the diffraction pattern is less distinct.

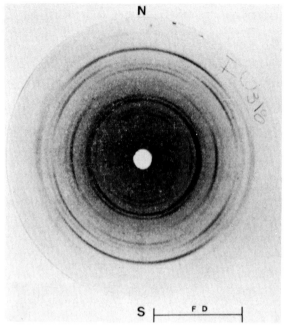

a

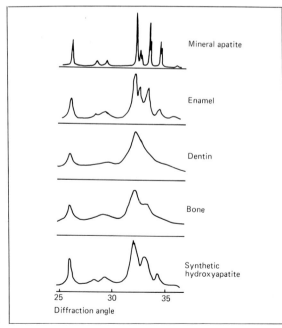

b

The crystal is the true structural unit of apatites. The smallest space unit of the hydroxyapatite crystal is called the unit cell, containing 10 calcium ions, 6 phosphate ions and 2 hydroxyl ions. Isolated unit cells cannot exist and are associated with many repeating units in a crystal. A three dimensional conceptual representation of the unit cell within a crystal is illustrated in figure 4/11. The a- and b-axes lie in the same plane and form the floor and ceiling of a parallelogram with each side 9.42 Å, and with two angles each of 60° and 120°. The height of the unit cell, the c-axis, at right angles to the a-b plane and parallel to the long axis of the crystal, is 6.88 Å.

The location of the hydroxyl ions and calcium ions in a repeating unit cell lattice structure is shown in figure 4/12a. The hydroxyl ions are arranged in columns parallel to the c-axis on a crystallographic symmetry element known as a screw axis at distances of one fourth and three fourths the height of the c-axis. Three calcium ions form an equilateral triangle lying parallel to the a-b plane centered on this column. The oxygen of each hydroxyl ion lies a little (e.g. 0.4 Å) above or a little below one of these Ca triangles. Successive calcium triangles are rotated 180° with respect to each other, in accord with the screw axis symmetry. The stacking of two such triangles of calcium ions, and the hydroxyl ion associated with them along the screw axis is shown in figure 4/12b.

In addition to the location of calcium ions in the triangles, calcium ions are also located in vertical columns, through the structure, inside the unit cell and parallel to the c-axis as shown in figure 4/12 and 4/13. One of the columnar calcium ions is situated just above or below the a-b plane and the other just below or above the halfway point between ends of the cell. Distinction between the two calcium positions occurs because the columnar calcium ions, Ca(1), and the triangle calcium ions, Ca(2), are surrounded by different kinds and numbers of other ions.

The phosphate ions have a tetrahedral structure with the phosphorus at the centre and an oxygen at each apex. . They occupy the bulk of the space within each unit cell as shown in perspective in figure 4/13a. The same structure is projected along the c-axis in figure 4/13b and depicts the position of the calcium, phosphate and hydroxyl ions.

Fluorapatite
Replacement of the dipolar OH⁻ groups by fluoride ions, which are smaller, results in the formation of fluorapatite and causes a decrease in the dimension of the a axis from 9.42 to 9.37 Å. The fluoride ions substituting for the hydroxyl ions go to the centers of the calcium triangles. This substitution exerts several important effects on the physical and chemical properties of the crystal. The fluoride ions in the center of the calcium

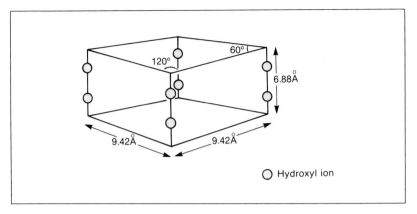

Fig. 4/11. A 3-dimensional representation of a conceptual unit cell of hydroxyapatite. The a-and b-axes form a parallelogram with each side 9.42Å. The height represents the c-axis and is 6.88Å. Only hydroxyl groups are shown; the other ions are omitted for clarity.

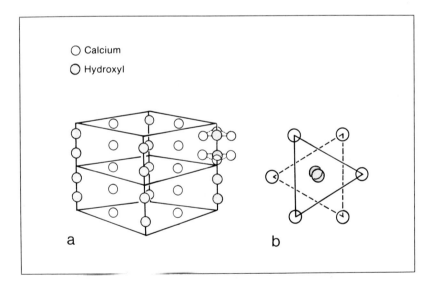

Fig. 4/12. a A diagrammatic representation of a hydroxyapatite unit cell showing the location of hydroxyl ions along the c-axis. Calcium ions are located in two environments: as column-calcium ions located inside the unit cell at the a-b plane and one half the distance between two a-b planes. Calcium ions are also located in the screw-axis position in the form of equilateral triangles around the two hydroxyl groups. **b** Diagrammatic illustration of stacking of calcium ions in the form of equilateral triangles around the hydroxyl groups. Note the adjacent triangles do not lie in the same line but are out of phase by 60° [*Kay* et al., 1964]. Note that when viewing along the c-axis the hydroxyl ions are exactly superimposed.

triangles form strong Coulomb interaction forces with calcium. There is a measurable decrease in calcium to anion and calcium to calcium distances, which is the reason why the a axis is decreased.

In biological tissues fluorides substitution is not entirely isomorphous; some fluoride may be detected in positions other than that occupied by the OH-radical [*Eanes*, 1979]. Spectroscopic studies of enamel indicate that fluoride ions form hydrogen bonds with neighboring OH- ions. The substitution of the OH- ion by fluoride ion and the formation of OH-F bonds stabilizes the lattice structure. The fluoride ions are dispersed so that a small replacement of OH- groups has a large effect on the physicochemical properties of the apatite. Also, a thin layer of fluoridated apatite on the crystal surface will have a disproportionate effect on the crystal's solubility [*Brown* et al., 1977]. This has practical significance since the rate of dissolution of partially fluoridated synthetic hydroxyapatite is less than for pure hydroxyapatite [*Moreno* et al., 1974].

Another effect of fluoride ion is its ability to improve the crystallinity of enamel apatite [*Frazier* et al., 1967]. Improved crystallinity denotes that the apatite structure is more stable, and that there may be fewer imperfections and dislocations within the crystals. The net effect is that even low concentrations of fluoride may result in an increased stability of the substituted lattice structure as demonstrated by lower acid solubilities, increased rates of remineralization and decreased rates of demineralization. All of these effects are significant in the cariostatic activity of fluorides and are discussed further in volume 2, chapter 3.

Carbonate Hydroxyapatite

In addition to the three primary constituents Ca^{2+}, PO_4^{3-} and OH^-, carbonate $(CO_3^=)$ is also present in dental tissues in significant concentrations. Carbonate apatite is less stable than pure hydroxyapatite. The presence of carbonate causes a disruption in the reactions that normally stabilize the apatite structure. Carbonate is an integral part of large apatite crystals in enamel. Carbonate in the mineral probably originates as carbon dioxide and reflects the CO_2 tension of the extracrystalline fluid at the time of crystallite formation. Any factor which alters the rate of metabolism will therefore probably affect mineral carbonate concentrations. Carbonate is present in the lattice as carbonate ions substituting for either 1 phosphate and/or 2 hydroxyl ions [*LeGeros* et al., 1967; *Elliott*, 1965]. Also, in small hydroxyapatite crystals as in bone, in the 100- to 500-Å range, the surface area per unit volume is large enough to accommodate the carbonate on crystal surfaces. It has been reported that as the thin, ribbon-like crystallites of developing enamel thicken [*Hiller* et al., 1975] the carbonate and magnesium content of the tissue falls. Perhaps the carbonate and magne-

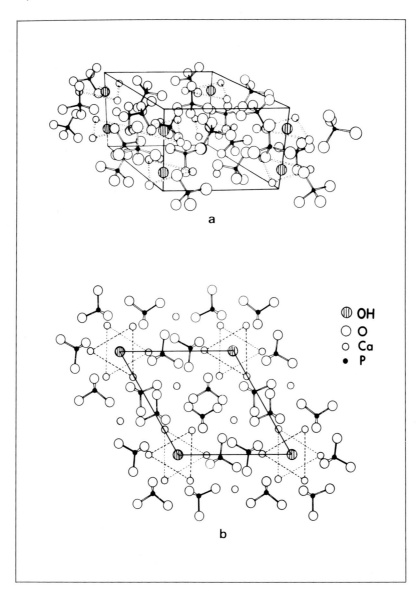

a

b

OH
O
Ca
P

Fig. 4/13. a Hydroxyapatite lattice structure in perspective view. The a and b axis intersecting at 120° are perpendicular to the c-axis. These three axes comprise the unit cell volume which contains the atoms in the formula $Ca_{10}(PO_4)_6(OH)_2$. The position of the OH, O, P and Ca ions are shown. Note the tetrahedral arrangement of the PO_4^{3-} ions. **b** Same structure projected along the c-axis. The columnar, screw axis calcium ions and the tetrahedral arrangement of the PO_4^{3-} ions are more easily visualized in this view [*Young*, 1975].

sium remain in the crystal cores but this suggestion has no experimental support [*Boyde*, 1979].

Carbonates play an important role in enamel maturation and perhaps in the initial phase of dental caries formation. As enamel matures the level of carbonate decreases on the surface of enamel. This may explain the relatively greater caries susceptibility of newly erupted teeth, and the increased resistance of older teeth. Carbonate is more labile than any other component in the apatite crystal and is preferentially lost along with magnesium during chemical erosion and carious destruction of enamel – hence its significance in caries [*Hallsworth* et al., 1973].

Chemical and Physical Characteristics of Hydroxyapatite Crystals

The chemical reactivity of the inorganic components of enamel and dentin is related to the crystalline properties of these tissues. Some important chemical and physical characteristics of hydroxyapatite crystals, relevant in the caries process, are considered here.

Hydration Shell. Solid crystals, such as hydroxyapatite, when exposed to an aqueous solution, take on a definite film of bound water called the hydration layer (fig. 4/14). The exact nature of the bonding of the water is not clear, but is probably related to the strong surface charge [*Neuman and Neuman*, 1958]. The origin of the surface charge may be the electrical asymmetry at the surface and the adsorption of ions, protons in particular. A diagrammatic representation of this concept is given in figure 4/15. As may be deduced from the diagram the isometric distribution of charge at the surface is important in imparting the marked ion-exchange ability of apatite crystals and in explaining the presence of the large number of adsorbed trace elements in dental tissues. Also, this characteristic of hydroxyapatites probably influences the nature of the salivary pellicle on teeth. The salivary pellicle is a proteinaceous structure upon which the bacterial plaque forms. This topic is developed in chapter 9.

Lack of Stoichiometry of Hydroxyapatite Crystals. 'Hydroxyapatite' crystals lack stoichiometry – that is the concentration of the chemical constituents in the crystals is different from that predicted by the formula for hydroxyapatite, $Ca_{10}(PO_4)_6(OH)_2$. A useful exercise for the reader is to calculate the Ca/P and molar ratio of pure apatite and to compare these with enamel (table 4/II). Note that the ratios for enamel are below those of pure apatite. Enamel is nonstoichiometric due to deficiencies of the three primary constituents: Ca^{2+}, PO_4^{3-} and OH^- and due to the presence of CO_3^{2-}, HPO_4^{2-}, trace elements, and possibly H_2O. The concentration of calcium in pure hydroxyapatite is 39.9%, enamel contains only 36.5% cal-

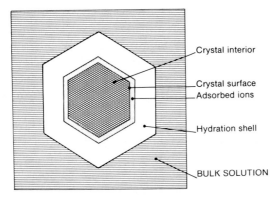

Fig. 4/14. Diagrammatic representation of a hydroxyapatite crystal in an aqueous solution indicating the exchange zones around the crystals.

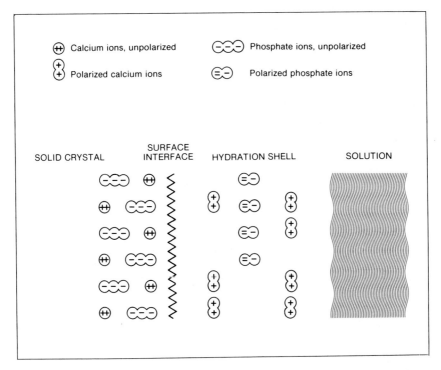

Fig. 4/15. Diagrammatic illustration showing the charge at the surface of crystal due to electrical asymmetry.

cium. Also, enamel is about 20–40% below theoretical value in its OH⁻ content [*Holcomb and Young*, 1980]. The divergence between the stoichiometric and the observed values in biological material may be explained by the large number of internal substitutions that are tolerated by hydroxyapatite crystals, by surface absorption, and by the presence of mineral deficient apatites. Also, some research workers maintain that other chemical phases many exist.

Isomorphous Substitution in Hydroxyapatite Crystals. Cations and anions similar in size and charge to the lattice ions may substitute for them on the surface and the interior of the crystal. This is called isomorphous substitution. For example, Sr^{2+} and Ra^{2+} may substitute for Ca^{2+} in the hydroxyapatite lattice. Magnesium is probably excluded from the crystal structure. Other ions may interact with hydroxyapatite crystals by diffusing into the hydration shell and replacing ions on the crystal surface thus contributing to the neutralization of surface charges. An important substitution in biological hard tissues is the replacement of hydroxyl ions by other anions similar in size and charge such as fluoride and chloride. The substitution of the hydroxyl ion by fluoride results in the formation of a fluoridated apatite (previously discussed). Even though fluoride is a trace element and in whole enamel represents a substitution of about 1 in 40 hydroxyl groups (about 1 to 10–15 in surface enamel) this is sufficient to change the chemical characteristics of enamel with respect to crystallization, dissolution and remineralization. Lattice substitutions are important determinants of properties of enamel (more on this subject in vol. 2, chapter 3).

Surface Area and Reactivity of Hydroxyapatite. The surface area of apatite, particularly the small crystallites of bone and dentin, is enormous, amounting to 10–200 m²/g, thus exposing an enormous area for chemical reactivity involving substitutions, exchanges and absorption. The chemical heterogeneity of apatites is attributed to the large surface reactivity and to the hydration shell of the crystals. Enamel crystals are large, about 30–40 unit cells thick, while bone crystals and many synthetic apatite preparations are two to four unit cells thick. The reactive surface of immature enamel exposed to the oral environment undergoes significant chemical changes. We have already referred to the increase in fluoride concentration and the loss of carbonate in surface enamel following eruption (see Surface Chemistry of Enamel in this chapter).

Dissolution of Hydroxyapatite Crystals
Dissolution of tooth mineral, a primary mechanism in dental caries, is a complex process. The factors controlling dissolution of hydroxyapatite

are also significant in understanding the mechanism of dental caries on a molecular level. There are at least four aspects of the structure and organization of the apatite crystal that are significant in their dissolution. These are lattice impurities, crystal size, crystalline defects (i.e. strains and lattice dislocations) and the rate of diffusion of dissolving ions through intercrystalline spaces [*Eanes*, 1979].

It is known that lattice impurities such as the presence of carbonate increase the solubility of tooth enamel. While impurities may enhance solubility the rate of dissolution is primarily controlled by the surface area of crystals (i.e. size), lattice dislocations and strains in the crystal. Large, perfect crystals with a minimum degree of dislocation dissolve slower than small crystals with poor crystallinity. The rate of mineral dissolution is controlled by surface factors and rate of diffusion of ions into and from the crystal into the dissolving solution. The reader by now will appreciate that dissolution of tooth mineral depends upon the interplay of many contributing factors including the structure and composition of the mineral phase of enamel and dentin. More will be said about dissolution in discussing the mechanism of incipient caries lesions (chapter 10).

When synthetic hydroxyapatite crystallites are subjected to acid etching it can be seen that dissolution starts at an active site located in the basal plane and forms an 'etch pit'. Dissolution continues from the initial 'etch pit' along the central core of the crystal parallel to the 'c'-axis, forming a hollow center (fig. 4/16a). The prism face is the least susceptible to dissolution, the crystal core the most susceptible and the shell in between these two structures is of intermediate susceptibility as diagrammatically noted in figure 4/16b. This pattern of dissolution has also been observed in carious enamel thus providing circumstantial evidence of acid dissolution in caries.

The observed pattern of crystallite dissolution is due to dislocations within the crystal and due to qualitative differences in the core versus the surface of the crystal [*Arends and Jongebloed*, 1979; *Daculsi* et al., 1979]. Dislocations or line defects are common in all materials and crystals. In hydroxyapatite crystals such defects have been observed in the core area. Whether or not carbonate plays an important role in the induction of core dislocations this needs corroboration.

Summary Points – Crystalline Phase of Enamel

The important summary points about the inorganic minerals of hard tissues is that they are structurally similar to a mineral called hydroxyapatite. This mineral has a unique crystal structure. Hydroxyapatites are usually microcrystalline, exhibit a variable stoichiometry with respect to Ca/P ratios, undergo internal substitutions by ions of a similar size and

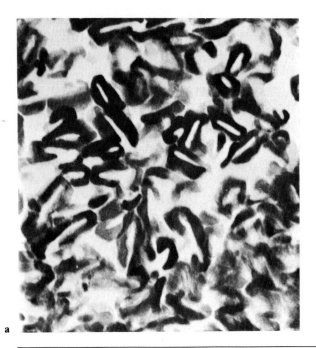

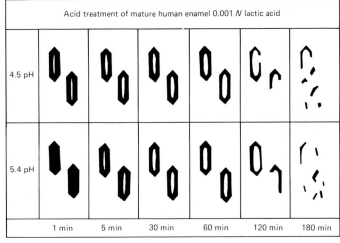

Fig. 4/16. a Pattern of dissolution of human enamel crystals treated with lactate buffer, pH 4.5. Note that centers of crystals show the first sign of dissolution, 170,000 × [from *Scott* et al., 1974, with permission]. **b** Schematic representation of the dissolution sequence of enamel crystals [modified after *Swancar* et al., 1971].

charge, have a large surface area and a high surface reactivity due to the presence of a solvated hydration shell on the crystal. Biological apatite has many defects and is deficient in calcium and hydroxyl ions. It may undergo a maturation whereby the defects and deficiencies are replaced by ions of a similar size and charge. Defects in apatite may also be due to discreet phase changes during apatite crystallization.

Surface Chemistry of Enamel

In the preeruptive stage, the surface crystals of enamel are in a dynamic equilibrium with the adjacent tissue fluid environment. The entry of a large number of ions present in physiological fluids into the hydration shell and the surface of apatite lattice structures of enamel and dentin accounts for the large number of trace elements in these tissues. In the posteruptive stage the enamel surface equilibrates with saliva, crevicular fluid, and ingested fluids in the oral cavity. The continuous physiochemical exchange between the surface of the enamel and the oral fluid and phase changes during dissolution and reprecipitation accounts for the change in the composition of surface enamel (particularly enamel covered by mature plaques) resulting in a gradient concentration of some inorganic elements as one progresses from the outer to inner layers of enamel. Most reactions between surface enamel and ions and molecules of the environment are diffusion-controlled; this contributes to the differences in the composition of surface and inner enamel.

Gradient Concentrations of Elements in Enamel-Surface

Samples of the outer enamel surface may be obtained by microdissection or by using etching techniques [*Brudevold* et al., 1975]. Analyses of such samples of enamel indicate that the surface is more dense and contains a higher concentration of mineral salts than inner enamel. The natural enamel surface has a reduced acid solubility and is also more resistant to the carious process [*Issac* et al., 1958]. Histological and microradiographic studies of the initial carious lesions indicate that marked decalcification is observed in subsurface enamel while the outer surface is relatively intact (see section on Incipient Carious Lesion, chapter 10, for an understanding of this phenomenon). The differential in concentration of elements between surface and subsurface layers increases and stabilizes with age and is part of the process of posteruptive chemical maturation.

The concentration of calcium, fluoride, zinc, silicon, tin, iron and lead in surface enamel is considerably greater than that found in subsurface layers [*Brudevold* et al., 1960]. On the other hand, the concentration of

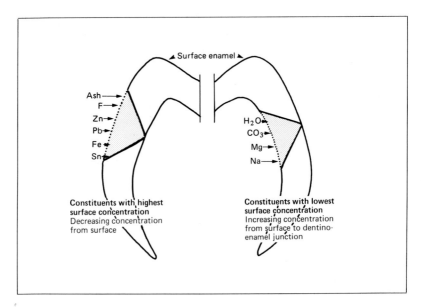

Fig. 4/17. The concentration gradient of chemical constituents of tooth enamel.

carbonate, magnesium and sodium is lowest in the surface layer and increases in layers closer to the dentino-enamel junction. The concentration
of phosphate, and potassium in enamel remains relatively constant after
the completion of mineralization of the tissue, suggesting that chemical
changes on the enamel surface involves primarily the surface of apatite
crystals and that the inner lattice structure is less affected. In addition to
the high concentration of minerals, surface enamel also has a lower concentration of water. The organic fraction is relatively high on the surface of
enamel, decreases slightly in the subsurface and then gradually increases as
the dentino-enamel junction is approached. The major chemical differences between surface enamel and the main bulk of this tissue is depicted
in figure 4/17.

Trace Elements in Enamel

It has been noted that the composition of the hydroxyapatite crystals
reflects the composition of the physiological fluid surrounding the developing tissue. Since physiological fluids contain a host of different ions, it is not

Table 4/III. Trace element concentration in human enamel and dentin [from *Grøn*, 1978]

	Enamel µg/g dry wt (ppm)	Dentin µg/dry wt (ppm)
Aluminum	1.5–700	10–100
Antimony	0.02–0.34	0.7
Barium	0.08–500	10–130
Boron	0.5–39	1–10
Bromine	0.03–35	114
Cadmium	0.03–10	
Chromium	<0.1–100	1–100
Cobalt	<0.02–0.1	0.003–1.1
Copper	0.1–130	0.2–100
Gold	0.02–0.1	0.07
Iron	0.08–200	90–1,000
Lead	1.3–100	10–100
Lithium	0.23–3.40	
Manganese	0.08–20	0.6–1,000
Molybdenum	0.7–39	1–10
Nickel	10–100	10–100
Rubidium	0.2–10	1–10
Selenium	0.1–10	10–100
Silver	0.005–1.3	2.2
Strontium	26–1,000	90–1,000
Sulfur	130–530	
Tin	0.03–0.9	
Titanium	<0.1–100	10–100
Vanadium	0.01–0.03	1–10
Yttrium	0.01–0.2	
Zinc	60–1,800	10–1,000
Zirconium	<0.02–0.6	

surprising that enamel and dentin contain many ions, some of which may be adventitious, such as citrate, sodium and iron. Some 40 trace elements have been found in these tissues. Some of the elements are adsorbed on the surface of the hydroxyapatite crystals; others with appropriate size and charge may substitute for calcium or phosphate in the crystal interior or may fill the voids in the crystal. Others, such as magnesium tend to be excluded from apatitic structures. Some trace elements are also incorporated posteruptively from saliva, food or water. The average concentration of some trace elements found in pulverized enamel is given in table 4/III.

8

Dental Caries and Trace Elements in Human Enamel

Several interesting studies relating to trace element concentrations in enamel obtained from areas high and low in caries prevalence suggest a role for trace elements, other than fluoride. The effect of some trace elements on caries is summarized in table 4/IV.

Trace elements may reduce or potentiate caries rates. Populations ingesting foods and water with a high selenium, copper and cadmium content are more prone to dental caries [Hadjimarkos, 1968]. High molybdenum levels in soils or drinking water have been correlated with reduced caries rates in some studies in humans [Glass et al., 1973].

Higher concentrations of fluoride and strontium in enamel are associated with the lower caries incidence in regions in South Carolina, USA, as compared to the high caries rates found in New England [Curzon and Losee, 1977]. On the other hand, concentrations of barium, aluminum, lithium, copper and zirconium have been related to high caries incidence in the New England population. In areas with a low fluoride water environment the increased strontium levels of surface enamel parallels the increase in fluoride concentrations. The exact role of strontium in the carious process has yet to be evaluated. Current data suggests that the presence of strontium in plaque enhances the resistance of the tissue to dental caries and that strontium and fluoride may have synergistic actions. Several mechanisms have been proposed to explain the reduction of dental caries by fluoride; one of which is related to the ability of the ion to reduce dissolution of hydroxyapatite crystals. Such dissolution is further decreased by the presence of strontium in the apatite crystal lattice [Dedhiya et al., 1974].

An interesting aspect of strontium in teeth deserves mention. The creation of ^{90}Sr as a fission product of atomic explosions and its introduc-

Table 4/IV. The effect of trace elements on caries activity [from Navia, 1972]

Effect	Trace element
Cariostatic	F, P
Mildly cariostatic	Mo, V, Cu, Sr, B, Li, Au
Equivocal effect	Be, Co, Mn, Sn, Zn, Br, I
No effect	Ba, Al, Ni, Fe, Pd, Ti
Caries-potentiating	Se, Mg, Cd, Pt, Pb, Si

tion into the atmosphere and subsequent entry into the food chain as in vegetations and milk has resulted in the incorporation of this radioactive element into bones and teeth. The lack of turnover of minerals of adult enamel, as contrasted with bone tissue, is of particular significance in the utilization of teeth for monitoring the accumulation of ^{90}Sr in the body. The ^{90}Sr : Ca ratio is similar in teeth and bone and therefore the analysis of ^{90}Sr in teeth is of significance in detecting excessive atmospheric amounts of radioactivity during the time the tissue developed and mineralized. A significant correlation between ^{90}Sr in enamel of primary and secondary teeth and its concentration in the atmosphere has been found [*Lindemann*, 1965; *Reiss*, 1961; *Starkey and Fletcher*, 1969].

Tale of Two Cities

Trace elements other than fluoride may account for significant differences in caries prevalence observed between the inhabitants of communities whose diets, living conditions, racial stock, and climate are similar. Two studies in particular deserve emphasis.

In two isolated mountain villages in Columbia, South America, Don Mateas and Heliconia, the level of fluoride in drinking water is approximately 0.1 ppm. The relative DMF in individuals of the same age group was 13.9 in Don Mateas as compared to 5.5 in the population of Heliconia. On the assumption that trace elements in water may reveal clues as to the observed differences in caries rates a study of 21 elements in the fluoride-deficient drinking water of the two communities was undertaken. It was found that levels of copper, iron and manganese were statistically higher in Don Mateas where the dental caries prevalence rate is high. In contrast, the levels of calcium, magnesium, molybdenum, and vanadium were significantly higher in Heliconia [*Mejia* et al., 1969; *Rothman* et al., 1972].

An analogous investigation involved a study of the effects of trace elements on caries rates in residents of two cities in New Zealand. It was observed that children 5–8 years of age had a considerably lower caries experience in the city of Napier than the equivalent age group in Hastings [*Ludwig* et al., 1960]. Both cities have very similar geography, rainfall, hours of sunshine, racial composition, and socioeconomic conditions. The water supplies, with a fluoride level of 0.15 ppm, are drawn from the same artesian strata and the mineral compositions of the water supplies were similar. Differences in soil composition including magnesium and sodium, carbon/nitrogen ratios and phosphorus were minor. However, the pH of the soil was higher in Napier than Hastings, as was the calcium carbonate concentration. The ash of vegetables grown in Napier had higher levels of molybdenum, aluminum and titanium and had lower concentrations of copper, manganese, barium and strontium than ash from vegetables grown in Hastings. High molybdenum levels in soils or in drinking water have also been associated with reduced caries in humans according to other studies in Hungary [review by *Glass* et al., 1973].

Structure and Composition of Teeth and Dental Caries

Caries Immune Teeth – Do They Exist?

From the chapter on 'Epidemiology of Dental Caries' it is apparent that wide variations in the prevalence rates of dental caries exist. The WHO evaluation of dental health in 22 countries indicates that in 12-year-olds the number of carious teeth may vary from a low of about 0.6–1.0 in Sudan, Zimbabwe-Rhodesia and Zaire to as high as about 8 in Australia, Finland and Norway. In the highly industrialized countries of Europe and North America, where the prevalence rates are generally high, about 1–2% of the population is caries-free. Does this denote the existence of teeth that are caries immune in a small segment of the population? The answer to this question is no. The structure and composition of teeth undoubtedly influence the initiation and the rate of a progression of a carious lesion. However, in spite of the obvious effect of the host tissue (the tooth), it seems highly unlikely that any tooth is completely immune from an intensive and prolonged cariogenic challenge. A diet low in cariogenic potential or the absence of a cariogenic flora are more probable explanations for the caries-free status of individuals. In addition, fluoridation of water supplies and the extensive use of fluoride preparations (dentifrices, mouthrinses) has resulted in a significant increase in caries-free individuals (vol. 2, chapters 4 and 5).

Given the nature of the carious mechanism – that is, the initial dissolution of the hydroxyapatite crystal in enamel – it is improbable that enamel would remain intact when subjected to low pH values or complexing agents for prolonged periods. If a caries-resistant tooth is a possibility, given a better understanding of its constituents, this goal has so far eluded research efforts. However, it is not inconceivable that a chemical surface coating which imparts noncorrosive, nonwettable properties to teeth may someday be developed which may reduce the prevalence of dental caries below current levels.

Determinants of Tooth Susceptibility to Caries

What factors relating to tooth composition and tooth morphology tend to resist the initiation of dental caries? A discussion of determinants of tooth susceptibility will synthesize much information in this chapter.

First, the element fluorine imparts a high degree of resistance against caries in many populations of the world. The role of fluorine in caries prevention is so important that several chapters are devoted to the subject (vol. 2, chapters 2–5).

Populations that live closer to the equator are less prone to dental caries (chapter 2), so also are populations living in areas where the mineral content (F⁻, P and Ca) of water is high and where the level of strontium in water is relatively high.

Populations with morphological defects in the form of accentuated pits or fissures are susceptible to dental caries [*Bossert*, 1937]. Also, the child population with linear enamel hypoplasia [*Sweeney* et al., 1971]; populations ingesting foods and water with a high selenium, copper and cadmium content are more prone to dental caries. The buccolingual diameter of carious molar teeth in children tends to be larger than for noncarious teeth [*Paynter and Grainger*, 1961]. The observations are countered by several studies where no specific relationship between tooth size and caries are found. Also, caries prevalence is less in children whose first permanent molars were missing the hypoconulid (four cusped), but greater in children with agenesis of the third molars [*Anderson and Popovich*, 1977].

Carbonates in enamel are a relatively labile component to dissolution. The incorporation of carbonate in synthetic hydroxyapatite increases its solubility [*Grøn* et al., 1963]; hence the probability that the carbonate content of teeth may affect the caries rate. Unfortunately, the earlier studies which reported that low carbonate levels in teeth of experimental animals are associated with caries resistance [*Sobel* et al., 1960] have not been corroborated by subsequent studies [*McClure and McCann*, 1960]. The reduction of the carbonate concentration in surface enamel and the parallel increase in fluoride levels as enamel matures has been suggested as a possible mechanism for the reduction in caries susceptibility of mature teeth [*Nikiforuk*, 1961].

In summary it may be stated that teeth, undoubtedly, vary greatly in their predisposition to caries attack. However, with the exception of the well-demonstrated correlation between ingestion of fluoridated water and caries other factors relating to tooth composition and caries have not been subjected to the same rigorous studies. Recent reports that relate strontium to caries reduction are interesting, as are the preliminary studies with regard to the beneficial effect of vanadium, molybdenum and boron. More definitive data is required about the role of micro- and macronutrients and the manner in which they influence the chemical and crystallographic structure of teeth before any effect they might have on dental caries is established.

Additional Reading

Chemistry and Physiology of Enamel. Symp. University of Michigan, 1971.

Grøn, P.: Inorganic chemical and structural aspects of oral mineralized tissues; in Shaw, Sweeney, Cappuccino, Meller, Textbook of oral biology (Saunders, Philadelphia 1978).

Nylen, M.V.; Termine, J.D. (eds): Tooth enamel. III. Its development, structure and composition. Proc. 3rd Int. Symp. on Tooth Enamel. J. dent. Res. *58:* spec. issue B (1979).

Osborn, J.W.; Ten Cate, A.R.: Advanced dental histology; 4th ed. (Wright, Bristol 1983).

Stack, M.V.; Fearnhead, R.W. (eds): Tooth enamel. I. Its composition, properties and fundamental structure (Wright & Sons, Bristol 1965).

Weatherell, J.A.; Robinson, C.: The inorganic composition of teeth; in Zipkin, Biological mineralization (Wiley & Sons, New York 1973).

References

Anderson, D.L.; Popovich, F: Dental reductions and dental caries. Am. J. phys. Anthrop. *47:* 381 (1977).

Arends. J.; Jongebloed, W.L.: Ultrastructural studies of synthetic apatite crystals. J. dent. Res. *58:* 837 (1979).

Bodecker. J.: The colour of teeth as an index of their resistance to decay. Int. J. Orth. Dent. Child. *XIX:* 386 (1933).

Bossert, W.A.: The relation between the shape of the occlusal surface of molars and the prevalence of decay. J. dent. Res. *16:* 63 (1937).

Boyde, A.: Carbonate concentration, crystal centers, core dissolution, caries, cross striations, circadian rhythms, and compositional contrast in the SEM. J. dent. Res. *58:* spec. issue B, p. 981 (1979).

Brown, W.E.; Gregory, T.M.; Chow, L.C.: Effects of fluoride on enamel solubility and cariostasis. Caries Res. *11:* suppl. 1, p. 118 (1977).

Brudevold, F.; Reda, A.; Aasenden, R.; Bakhos, Y.: Determination of trace elements in surface enamel of human teeth by a new biopsy procedure. Archs oral Biol. *20:* 667 (1975).

Brudevold, F.; Söremark, R.: Chemistry of the mineral phase of enamel; in Miles, Structural and chemical organization of teeth, vol. II, chap. 18, p. 247 (Academic Press, New York 1967).

Brudevold, F.; Steadman, L.T.; Smith, F.A.: Inorganic and organic components of tooth structure. Ann. N.Y. Acad. Sci. *85:* 110 (1960).

Burgess, R.C.; MacLaren, C.M.: Proteins in developing bovine enamel; in Stack, Fearnhead, Tooth enamel, its composition, properties and fundamental structure, p. 74 (Wright & Sons, Bristol 1965).

Butler, W.T.; Munksgaard, E.C.; Richardson, W.S.: Dentin proteins: chemistry, structure and biosynthesis. J. dent. Res. *58:* spec. issue B, p. 817 (1979).

Cevc, G.; Cevc, P.; Schara, M.; Skaleric, U.: The caries resistance of human teeth is determined by the spatial arrangement of hydroxyapatite microcrystals in the enamel. Nature, Lond. *286:* 425 (1980).

Curzon, M.E.J.; Losee, F.L.: Dental caries and trace element composition of whole human enamel: Eastern United States. J. Am. dent. Ass. *94:* 1146 (1977).

Daculsi, G.; Kerebel, B.: High-resolution electron microscope study of human enamel crystallites: size, shape, and growth. J. Ultrastruct. Res. *65:* 163 (1978).

Daculsi, G.; Kerebel, B.; Kerebel, L.M.: Mechanisms of acid dissolution of biological and synthetic apatite crystals at the lattice pattern level. Caries Res. *13:* 277 (1979).

Deakins, M.: Changes in the ash, water and organic content of pig enamel during calcification. J. dent. Res. *21:* 429 (1942).

Dedhiya, M.G.; Young, F.; Hefferen, J.J.; Higuchi, W.I.: Inhibition of hydroxyapatite dissolution by Sr^{++} and Mg^{++} under partial saturation conditions in solutions containing F^-. J. dent. Res. *53:* 105 (1974).

Eanes, E.D.: Enamel apatite: chemistry structure and properties; in Proc. 3rd Int. Symp. on Tooth Enamel. J. dent. Res. *58:* spec. issue B, p. 829 (1979).

Eastoe, J.E.: Enamel protein chemistry – past, present and future. Proc. 3rd Int. Symp. on Tooth Enamel. J. dent. Res. *58:* 753 (1979).

Elliott, J.C.: The interpretation of the infra-red absorption spectra of some carbonate-containing apatites; in Stack, Fearnhead, Tooth enamel, p. 20 (Wright & Sons, Bristol 1965).

Frazier, P.D.; Little, M.F.; Casciani, F.S.: X-Ray diffraction analysis of human enamel containing different amounts of fluoride. Archs oral Biol. *12:* 35 (1967).

Glass, R.L.; Rothman, K.J.; Espinal, F.; Velez, H.; Smith, J.: The prevalence of human dental caries and waterborne trace metals. Archs oral Biol. *18:* 1099 (1973).

Grøn, P.: Inorganic chemical and structural aspects of oral mineralized tissues; in Shaw, Sweeney, Cappuccino, Meller, Textbook of oral biology, p. 484 (Saunders, Philadelphia 1978).

Grøn, P.; Spinelli, M.; Trautz, O.R.; Brudevold, F.: The effect of carbonate on the solubility of hydroxyapatite. Archs oral Biol. *8:* 251 (1963).

Hadjimarkos, D.M.: Effect of trace elements on dental caries; in Staple, Advances in oral biology, p. 253 (Academic Press, New York 1968).

Hallsworth, A.S.; Weatherell, J.A.; Robinson, C.: Loss of carbonate during the first stages of enamel caries. Caries Res. *7:* 345 (1973).

Hiller, C.R.; Robinson, C.; Weatherell, J.A.: Variations in the composition of developing rat incisor enamel. Calcif. Tissue Res. *18:* 1 (1975).

Holcomb, D.W.; Young, R.A.: Thermal decomposition of human tooth enamel. Calcif. Tissue Res., *31:* 189 (1980).

Isaac, S.; Brudevold, F.; Smith, F.A.; Gardner, D.E.: Solubility rate and natural fluoride content of surface and subsurface enamel. J. dent. Res. *37:* 254 (1958).

Kay, M.I.; Young, R.A.; Posner, A.S.: Crystal structure of hydroxyapatite. Nature, Lond, *204:* 1050 (1964).

Lakomaa, E.-L.; Rytömaa, I.: Mineral composition of enamel and dentin of primary and permanent teeth in Finland. Scand. J. dent. Res. *85:* 89 (1977).

LeGeros, R.Z.; Trautz, O.R.; LeGeros, J.P.; Klenin, E.: Colloq. Int. Phosphates Mineraux Solides, 1967, p. 66.

Li, S.-T.; Katz, E.P.: Dentinal phosphoproteins: evidence for a regulatory role (Abstract). IADR 59: spec. issue, p. 901 (1980).

Lindemann, J.: [90]Strontium in teeth. A preliminary report. Saertryk af »Tandlaegebladet« *69:* 297 (1965).

Ludwig, T.G.; Healy, W.B.; Losee, F.L.: An association between dental caries and certain soil conditions in New Zealand. Nature, Lond. *186:* 695 (1960).

McClure, F.J.; McCann, H.G.: Dental caries and composition of bones and teeth of white rats. Effect of dietary mineral supplements. Archs oral Biol. *2:* 151 (1960).

Meckel, A.H.; Griebstein, W.J.; Neal, R.J.: Structure of mature human dental enamel as observed by electron microscopy. Archs oral Biol. *10:* 775 (1965).

Mejia, R.; Espinal, F.; Velez, H.; Velez, A.: Communidad Colombiana con baja prevalencia de caries sin antecedentes de fluor. Boln Of. sanit. pan-amer. *66:* 501 (1969).

Moreno, E.C.; Kresak, M.; Zahradnik, R.T.: Fluoridated hydroxyapatite solubility and caries formation. Nature, Lond. *247:* 64 (1974).

Muller, S.A.; Posner, A.S.; Firschein, H.E.: Effect of vitamin D deficiency on the crystal chemistry of bone mineral. Proc. Soc. exp. Biol. Med. *121:* 844 (1966).

Navia, J.M.: Prevention of dental caries: agents which increase tooth resistance to dental caries. Int. dent. J. *22:* 427 (1972).

Neuman, W.F.; Neuman, M.W.: The chemical dynamics of bone mineral, (University of Chicage Press, Chicago 1958).

Nikiforuk, G.: Carbonates and fluorides as chemical determinants of tooth susceptibility to caries. Symp. Present Status Caries Prevent. Fluorine-Containing Dentifrices, Zürich 1961, p. 62.

Nikiforuk, G.; Fraser, D.: Etiology of enamel hypoplasia and interglobular dentin: the roles of hypocalcemia and hypophosphatemia. Metab. Bone Dis. rel. Res. *2:* 17 (1979).

Nikiforuk, G.; Gruca, M.: Immunological reactions of the organic matrix of developing bovine enamel. Calcif. Tissue Res. *4:* 129 (1969).

Nylen, M.U.; Eanes, E.D.; Omnell K.A.: Crystal growth in rat enamel. J. Cell Biol. *18:* 109 (1963).

Patel, P.R.; Brown, W.E.: Thermodynamic solubility product of human tooth enamel: powdered sample. J. dent. Res. *54:* 728 (1975).

Paynter, K.J.; Grainger, R.M.: Influence of nutrition and genetics on morphology and caries susceptibility. J. Am. med. Ass. *177:* 306 (1961).

Reiss, L.Z.: Strontium-90 absorption by deciduous teeth. Science *134:* 1669 (1961).

Robinson, C.; Fuchs, P.; Weatherell, J.A.: The appearance of developing rat incisor enamel using a freeze fracturing technique. J. Crystal Growth *53:* 160 (1981).

Ronnholm, E.: II. The development of the enamel crystallites. J. Ultrastruct. Res. *6:* 249 (1962).

Rothman, K.J.; Glass, R.L.; Espinal, F.; Velez, H.: Caries-free teeth in the absence of fluoride ion. J. Publ. Hlth Dent. *32:* 225 (1972).

Scott, D.B.; Simmelink, J.W.; Nygaard, V.: Structural aspects of dental caries. J. dent. Res. *53:* 165 (1974).

Seyer, J.M.; Glimcher, M.J.: Evidence for the presence of numerous protein components in immature bovine dental enamel. Calcif. Tissue Res. *24:* 253 (1977).

Sobel, A.E.; Shaw, J.H.; Hanok, A.; Nobel, S.: Calcification. XXVI. Caries susceptibility in relation to composition of teeth and diet. J. dent. Res. *39:* 462 (1960).

Starkey, W.E.; Fletcher, W.: The accumulation and retention of strontium-90 in human teeth in England and Wales 1959–1965. Archs oral Biol. *14:* 169 (1969).

Swancar, J.R.; Scott, D.B.; Simmelink, J.W.; Smith, T.J.: The morphology of enamel crystals; in Stack, Fearnhead, Tooth enamel, vol. 2, p. 233 (Wright & Sons, Bristol 1971).

Sweeney, E.A.; Saffir, A.J.; Leon, R. de: Linear hypoplasia of deciduous incisor teeth in malnourished children. Am. J. clin, Nutr, *24:* 29 (1971).

Termine, J.D.; Torchida, D.A.; Conn, K.M.: Enamel matrix: structural proteins. J. dent. Res. *58:* 773 (1979).

Young, R.A.: Some aspects of crystal structural modeling of biological apatites. Physico-chim. Cristallogr. Apatites Interêt biolog. *230:* 21 (1975).

5 Formation, Structure and Metabolism of Dental Plaque

Introduction

In the previous chapters it is noted that dental caries is a local disease in which destruction of dental tissue is initiated by organic acids produced by oral bacteria as a result of their glycolytic metabolism of readily fermentable dietary carbohydrates. The essentiality of bacteria and local substrate interacting with host tissue in the disease process is discussed in chapter 3. Although the role of microorganisms in caries etiology is indisputable, much is still to be learned about the characteristics of a cariogenic flora. The oral environment and the bacterial flora of the mouth are complex, and many interactions occur involving nutrients from the host, the diet and other bacteria. Also, an individual's state of oral hygiene, frequency of eating, and the amount and composition of oral secretions influence the disease process. Only a small fraction of the total oral flora is involved in caries initiation and these microorganisms colonize in highly localized and specific sites on the teeth. The manner by which bacteria attach themselves to teeth is only now being unraveled, and this fascinating story forms an important part of this chapter.

Teeth, with their unique morphological characteristics for biting and grinding food, also provide protective niches which favor colonization of specific bacteria. Teeth are indispensable habitats for some bacterial species. However, bacteria do not initiate colonization of teeth by attaching themselves to the naked dental enamel but rather to the acquired organic film, termed the pellicle, that forms on teeth from saliva (chapter 9).

The organic deposits on teeth and microbial dental plaques have been the subject of exhaustive studies. Much of the earlier confusion in this field could be eliminated by the recognition that salivary coatings and dental plaques are distinct structures which are not homogeneous and do not possess a well-defined composition. Any efforts in the laboratory to characterize dental plaque as an easily definable entity have not been rewarding. Although a detailed review of the organic deposits on teeth is beyond the scope of a single chapter, the student is directed to several reviews which have synthesized various aspects of the subject [*McHugh*, 1970; *Bowen*, 1976; *Gibbons and van Houte*, 1980]. In this chapter and chapter 6 answers to the following questions will be explored: What is dental plaque? What factors affect bacterial colonization of the teeth and the formation of dental plaques? What are the predominant bacterial species in plaques? What are the metabolic characteristics of plaques and the specific bacteria known to be associated with dental caries initiation?

An appropriate background for an exploration of these questions is to consider first the acquisition and the general distribution of the flora in the mouth. This sequence gives a better perspective for a discussion of the formation, structure and microbiology of plaque and its role in caries etiology. The evidence for bacterial specificity in the etiology of caries and a detailed presentation of the metabolism of the *Streptococcus mutans* group of bacteria implicated in caries is presented in chapter 6.

Acquisition of Oral Flora

Bacteria can be isolated from the oral cavity shortly after birth. The microflora of infants, prior to tooth eruption, consists predominantly of facultative or microaerophilic organisms such as *Streptococcus mitior*, *Streptococcus salivarius*, *Neisseria*, staphylococci, and lactobacilli. Anaerobic organisms such as *Veillonella alcalescens* and fusobacteria are commonly found a few weeks after birth. Major changes occur in the oral flora when teeth erupt into the mouth (table 5/I). Teeth provide unique surfaces for bacterial colonization because they contain retentive sites and they do not desquamate. An increase in anaerobic forms including *Bacteroides* species, fusobacteria and vibrios are found in the gingival crevice. Also, certain organisms such as *S. sanguis*, *S. mutans* and *A. viscosus* may be detected only after the eruption of teeth which appear to constitute their primary habitat. *S. mutans* can be isolated from predentate infants with acrylic resin obturators [*Berkowitz* et al., 1975] which indicates that the

Table 5/I. Qualitative changes in oral flora associated with eruption of teeth [*Gibbons and van Houte*, 1978]

Organism	Predentate Infants	Dentate Infants
Streptococcus sanguis	not detectable	always detected
Streptococcus mutans	not detectable	frequently detected
Bacteroides sp.	infrequently detected	frequently detected
Fusobacterium sp.	infrequently detected	frequently detected
Actinomyces sp.	infrequently detected	frequently detected
A. viscosus	not detectable	frequently detected

organism requires a non-desquamating surface for oral colonization. Loss of the dentition causes a reversion of the microflora to one that is predominantly facultative, but those species dependent on teeth for colonization, such as *S. mutans* and *S. sanguis*, are no longer detectable. Infants are often infected with *S. mutans* by their mothers as shown by the finding that when the numbers of *S. mutans* were reduced below 3×10^{-5} in nursing mothers, the establishment of *S. mutans* in the mouths of the babies was prevented or delayed [*Köhler* et al., 1983].

Distribution of Bacteria in the Mouth

The largest masses of bacteria are found on the surfaces of teeth and on the dorsum of the tongue. Dental plaques contain in the order of 10^8 organisms per milligram wet weight, i.e. 10^9 organisms are present in 10 mg of plaque, which is typically the accumulation on a tooth in one day without tooth-brushing. Epithelial cells scraped from the tongue dorsum average over 100 microorganisms per cell. The bacterial concentrations on cheek and palatal surfaces are considerably lower. Saliva as secreted from the salivary glands contains few, if any, bacteria; but in excess of 10^8 organisms per milliliter are found in whole saliva as a result of their dislodgement from oral surfaces. The tongue and the teeth are the major sources of bacteria found in saliva.

Quantitative surveys indicate that the mouth contains several distinct microcosms, each with a characteristic collection of bacteria. Thus, the flora of coronal dental plaque differs significantly from the flora found in subgingival plaques and these, in turn, differ from the flora found on tongue and buccal mucosa (fig. 5/1). The proportions of various bacteria in plaque also differ significantly from those found in saliva. For example, *S. salivarius* comprises about 50% of the streptococci found on the tongue dorsum and in saliva but it makes up less than 1% of the streptococcal populations of plaque. In contrast, *S. sanguis* comprises only a minor percentage of the salivary flora which bathes the teeth on which it often predominates. Such data make it clear that salivary bacterial populations are not representative of the plaque flora.

As will be discussed later, the selective ability of bacteria to attach to various surfaces of the mouth is thought to be one of the major reasons which account for differences in the host age at which bacteria establish in the mouth and their intraoral distribution patterns. The mouth contains surfaces exposed to the flow of saliva and other oral fluids, and colonization requires that bacteria either attach to a surface or else be able to multiply at a rate which exceeds their removal caused by the flowing fluids,

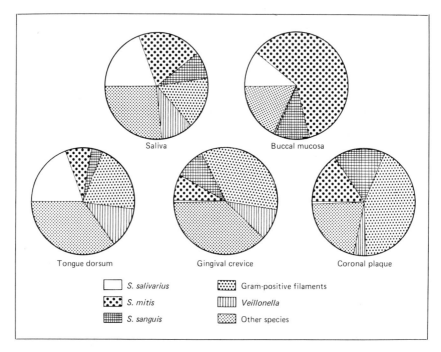

Fig. 5/1. The approximate distribution of selected prominent bacteria on various oral surfaces and in saliva [data from *Gibbons and van Houte*, 1980]. Note the marked differences in their relative proportions at various sites.

mastication and swallowing. It has been estimated that the overall oral flora probably averages only a few divisions per day. Because humans swallow every few minutes, it is obvious that unattached bacteria cannot maintain themselves in the mouth solely by their rates of multiplication. Presumably, some progeny of attached bacteria are able to withstand clearance and reattach, thus maintaining a surface-associated community of slowly proliferating microorganisms.

Dental Plaque

Definition and Composition

Plaques consist of densely packed bacteria which are embedded in an amorphous material called the plaque matrix. A characteristic of plaques is that they resist removal by physiological oral cleansing forces such as saliva and tongue movement but plaques are removable by toothbrushing if the bristles can reach them. Bacterial cells have been estimated to comprise 60–70% of the volume of plaque whereas the matrix makes up the remainder. The matrix is thought to impart structural integrity to the microbial masses. It consists of extracellular carbohydrate polymers synthesized by the bacteria and of macromolecules and other elements derived from saliva and crevicular fluid. By accumulating in greater masses on specific surfaces (e.g. pits, fissures), plaque bacteria localize and concentrate their chemical activities to these areas. If the plaque mass is located interproximally or in fissures it is relatively less affected by salivary secretions.

Plaque must be distinguished from food debris. Insoluble constituents of foods such as meat or plant fibers may become lodged between the teeth or in fissures but the plaque grows around these structures. Masses of starch may also accumulate in these areas during eating but they are superimposed on existing plaque rather than being incorporated within it. This is clinically important because it is often assumed that the aim of toothbrushing is to remove food debris and it is not always realized that it is plaque removal which must be achieved if oral hygiene is to reduce caries and gingivitis. Plaque bacteria are exposed to virtually every substance ingested, and to complex mixtures of microorganisms in foods and our environment. The plaque is also subject to salivary influences and may eventually become mineralized to form dental calculus. Such heterogeneous microbial deposits which are constantly changing would not be expected to have a fixed chemical composition. Therefore, analyses of the chemical composition of plaques must be interpreted with caution.

Plaques are composed of about 80% water and 20% solids. Bacterial and salivary proteins comprise about one half of the dry weight of plaque. Plaque matrix, in addition to its high protein concentration, contains carbohydrates and lipids which account for approximately 25% of the plaque dry weight [Silverman and Kleinberg, 1967]. Much of the carbohydrate in the matrix consists of polymers (glucans, fructans and heteropolysaccharides) synthesized by bacteria. Some of these polymers are thought to play a role in bacterial attachment and cohesion and others are more important as a reservoir of fermentable substrates which are metabolized by bacteria when other more readily utilized carbohydrates in plaque become depleted (more on this subject in chapter 6) [Hotz et al., 1972].

Bacterial cells may also contain carbohydrate in the form of polysaccharides associated with their cell walls and intracellular glycogen-like polymers. The latter polysaccharides are stored as granules observable by electron microscopy [Saxton, 1969]. They are believed to function as a reservoir of fermentable carbohydrate to be used once dietary substrates are depleted in much the same way that glycogen stores are used to fuel glycolysis in muscle cells when glucose is depleted.

Inorganic Components of Plaque

Inorganic components account for approximately 5–10% of the dry weight of plaques. The concentration of calcium and phosphate in dental plaque is several magnitudes higher than in saliva [*Dawes and Jenkins*, 1962]. In addition, potassium, sodium, magnesium, copper, lead, iron, strontium and fluoride are also present. The high concentration of calcium and phosphate in plaques is thought to be due, in part, to the infiltration of salivary proteins containing these constituents in bound form. These probably include statherin (chapter 9), the salivary protein which, by adsorbing onto early crystal nuclei and preventing crystal growth, maintains supersaturation of the fluid phase of plaque with apatite. In addition, bacteria may also accumulate polyphosphates and possess components which bind calcium. Most of the calcium found in plaque is nonionic. Solubilization may occur as the pH drops. Thus, as plaque calcium becomes ionized, it may play a significant role in determining rates of dissolution and in remineralization reactions by serving as a reservoir which helps to satisfy the solubility product of enamel at different pH values.

The fluoride concentration of dental plaque (wet weight) is about 5–10 ppm as compared to about 0.01–0.05 ppm in saliva and is higher in communities with fluoridated water. Most of the fluoride is probably bound on or within bacteria but some may be in the form of calcium fluoride or fluorapatite. The ionic concentration of fluoride has been estimated to be less than 10% of the total [*Jenkins and Edgar*, 1977; *Agus* et al., 1980]. This concentration may increase as the pH of plaque decreases and additional fluoride is released. The concentrations of bound fluoride in plaque are sufficiently high to inhibit bacterial metabolism by its effect on several essential enzymes, especially at pH values below 5.5 when bacteria become more sensitive to fluoride. Plaque fluoride also plays a significant role in the remineralization of enamel (vol. 2, chapter 3).

Table 5/II. The relationship between caries experience and plaque mineral concentration [*Schamschula* et al., 1980–1982]

Element	High DMFS mean	Low DMFS mean
Fluoride, ppm	12.4	36.0
Calcium, %	0.416	2.158
Magnesium, %	0.156	0.185
Phosphorus, %	1.58	2.11

It has been shown that a pH drop associated with a cariogenic challenge results in a reduction of total fluoride and other plaque minerals [*Agus* et al., 1980]. These findings are important in view of the observations that concentrations of calcium and phosphorus [*Ashley*, 1975] and fluoride [*Agus* et al., 1980] are higher in plaque in subjects with lower caries experience. The reverse is true for high caries experience.

It is not known whether the lower average concentration of fluoride, calcium and phosphate ions in plaque of individuals with high caries experience is a cause of their high caries or a result of the higher acid production and lower pH leading to greater outward diffusion or less retention of these ions (table 5/II). Nevertheless, factors leading to an increase in the fluoride, calcium and phosphate concentrations in plaque are significant in cariostasis as well as in reactions that lead to a reversal of incipient carious lesions (chapter 10).

Clinical Features

Plaques are classified as supra- or subgingival, according to the anatomical area in which they form. Subgingival plaque present in a healthy gingival sulcus is generally scanty and thin, but much larger bacterial accumulations are found in diseased periodontal pockets. Supragingival plaque, when not limited by mechanical factors, may develop into a thick film, several hundred micrometers thick, as a result of the proliferation of attached microorganisms and the successive deposition of additional bacteria and salivary material [*Schroeder and de Boever*, 1970]. Plaques obtained from the fissures of teeth differ in their bacterial and chemical composition from those developing on smooth tooth surfaces [*Theilade* et al., 1976]. Fissures represent sites which are protected from normal cleansing, where food can become impacted and weakly adhering bacteria may accumulate. Supragingival plaques play an essential role in the pathogenesis of dental caries while marginal and subgingival plaques are responsible for the initiation of different types of periodontal diseases.

The amount of plaque can be assessed directly by clinical examination or indirectly by examination of dental photographs. Often dye solutions, referred to as disclosing agents, are used to stain plaques to improve visual scoring (fig. 5/2). Erythrocin, basic fuchsin, fast green or fluorescein are frequently used for this purpose. Clinical indices have been developed which permit comparative estimates of the amount of dental plaque to be made between different areas of the mouth or between different individuals. For research purposes the most accurate method of assessing the amount of plaque is by collecting it with a scaler (sometimes from one quadrant of the mouth) and weighting it. Disclosing solutions stain very

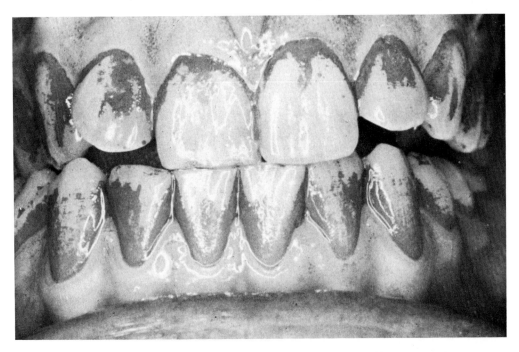

Fig. 5/2. Dental plaque stained with basic fuchsin dye as observed in a young patient.

thin layers of plaque of doubtful clinical significance and therefore give inflated plaque scores.

Plaques accumulate most rapidly on areas of the teeth that are protected from mechanical forces resulting from mastication, movement of the tongue, lips, cheeks, and from oral hygiene procedures. Plaque is usually first detected around defects and irregularities of the teeth and along the gingival margin. More plaque accumulates in interproximal areas near the contact points of teeth than on lingual or labial surfaces. The incisal and occlusal areas of teeth generally have less plaque than the gingival third. More plaque accumulates in posterior than in anterior and more in the mandibular than in the maxillary regions. The lingual surfaces of mandibular molars and the buccal surfaces of the maxillary molars tend to have the heaviest plaque deposits, while the labial and lingual surfaces of the maxillary incisors tend to have the least.

There is great variation among persons with regard to the rapidity and the extent to which plaques form. The reasons for such differences are often not clear and have not been systematically studied but are likely to be attributed to differences in saliva composition and flow, differences in diet composition and the frequency of eating, differences in health status of the gingiva, variations in the anatomical features of teeth, and differences in the composition of the oral flora.

Oral hygiene procedures, including tooth brushing and interdental cleansing, can dramatically reduce the quantity of plaque; these form the basis for plaque control procedures discussed in volume 2, chapter 11. While it is true that a clean tooth never decays, this ideal state is unattainable under normal conditions. Imperfect oral hygiene is the norm for most individuals and carious lesions most often develop in sites which are difficult to keep free of bacterial plaques. Further, the colonization of defined sites on teeth by specific organisms implicated in caries, such as *S. mutans*, suggests that oral hygiene measures alone are not very effective in controlling a specific infection.

Although carious lesions will not develop without plaque, it should be emphasized that plaques can often be relatively innocuous. In fact, salivary pellicles and plaques perform many beneficial functions. They have a high buffering capacity and they exhibit perm-selective properties, protecting the teeth from exposure to acids present in many foods. However, when plaques contain appreciable proportions of highly acidogenic bacteria, such as *S. mutans* and are exposed to readily fermentable dietary sugars, they produce sufficient concentrations of acids to demineralize the enamel. Setting up a dangerous cycle, such acidic conditions may even select for more acid-tolerant bacteria. Therefore, pathogenicity of plaque depends upon its microbial composition in both quantitative and qualitative terms, and upon the availability of dietary sugars.

Ultrastructure of Dental Plaque

Shortly after a tooth is cleaned, clusters of bacteria can be found on the acquired pellicle. Some of these clusters represent remnants of plaque which were not completely removed by oral hygiene procedures; others represent newly deposited bacteria. Initially the clusters tend to be well separated, and they are found in highest concentrations at protected sites, especially near the gingival margin. They gradually increase in size as a result of bacterial proliferation and form microcolonies. Simultaneously, additional bacteria adsorb to the surface, and eventually a continuous bacterial layer is formed (fig. 5/3, 5/4) which progressively increases in thickness. Thick, smooth surface plaques usually have densely arranged, mostly coccoid cells near the pellicle interface and a looser arrangement

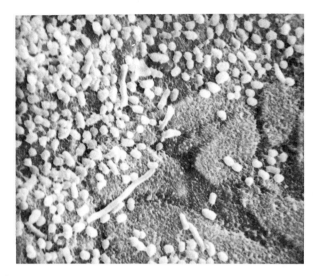

Fig. 5/3. An electron micrograph of early plaque formation (after 24 h) reveals coccoid cells with a few rods in a monolayer growth pattern. ×3,900 [from *Lie*, 1979, with permission]. The monolayer is transient; clusters of bacteria soon predominate.

containing both coccoid and long filamentous forms near the salivary interface (fig. 5/5).

Histologic sections of mature smooth surface plaques formed on epoxy resin crowns demonstrate the presence of columns of similar bacteria extending perpendicularly from the inside towards the plaque periphery (fig. 5/5) [*Listgarten* et al., 1975]. This columnar development is most likely the result of growth of bacterial colonies after a continuous bacterial layer has formed. It is probably due to a much more rapid rate of growth of bacteria at the plaque periphery and to the presence of adjacent organisms which physically impair lateral spreading. A morphological comparison of bacteria near the saliva and pellicle interfaces confirms the abundance of septa resembling bacterial division planes among bacteria near the periphery [*van Houte and Saxton*, 1971]. In contrast, bacteria deep within dental plaques often show morphological evidence of imbalanced growth, such as thickened cell walls and numerous intracellular polysaccharide granules. These granules represent carbohydrate stores which allow the bacteria to extend metabolic activity during periods of relative inaccessibility to the host's dietary carbohydrate intake.

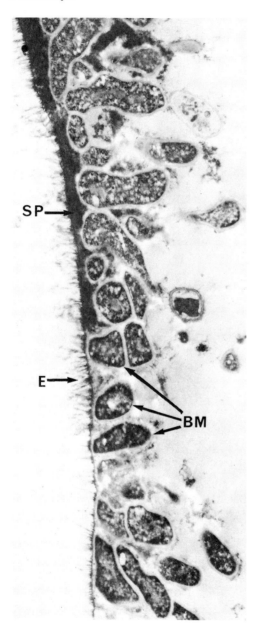

Fig. 5/4. TEM. Early plaque formation showing a bacterial colonization (BM) of salivary pellicle (SP) covering enamel (E) [from *Newman*, 1979, with permission].

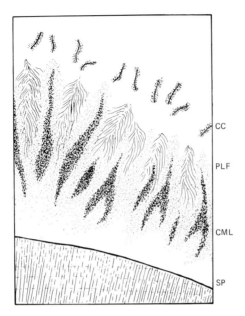

Fig. 5/5. Diagrammatic illustration of the morphological features of the supragingival plaque. Note the characteristic zones consisting of the following: salivary pellicle at the plaque-tooth surface (SP); the microcolonies of the condensed microbial layer (CML); the palisade-like filamentous bacteria in the body of the plaque (PLF); the corn cob-like microbial colonization at the plaque surface (CC).

Because of their proximity, plaque bacteria have evolved diverse surface structures for mutual attachment which impart cohesive properties to the plaque. These range from short tufts of fuzz-like projections to long surface fibrils or fimbriae. Bacteria with differing cell wall structures are often seen in direct contact in photomicrographs which may imply that there is some cohesion specificity in bacterial contact. The salivary interface of supragingival plaques often harbors morphological forms which are called 'corn-cobs' because their central filament totally coated with coccal cells is very suggestive of that morphology (fig. 5/5, 5/6). Another pairing in subgingival plaque has been termed 'bristle brushes' and is composed of rods and filaments radiating out from a central long filamentous bacterial cell.

Most of the aforementioned morphological features have been elucidated by studying dental plaques deposited on smooth enamel or resin surfaces worn in the mouths of volunteers for various time periods but

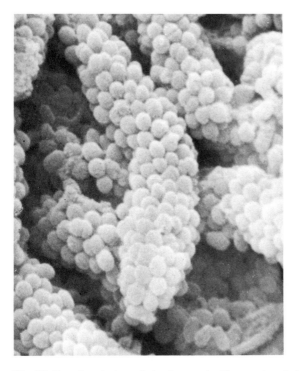

Fig. 5/6. Scanning electron photomicrograph of human dental plaque showing 'corn cob' structures. These arrangements consist of coccoid cells of a type of *S. sanguis* attached to filamentous cells of *Bacterionema matruchotii* (courtesy of Dr. *Z. Skobe*, Forsyth Dental Center).

is presumed to resemble naturally formed plaque. The ultrastructures of cariogenic and noncariogenic plaques have not been adequately compared.

Plaques deep in occlusal fissures differ significantly from those on smooth surfaces. Fissure plaques consist of dense microbial aggregates composed predominantly of gram-positive coccal and filamentous organisms [*Schroeder and de Boever*, 1970; *Frank*, 1973]. The scanty plaque matrix is slightly fibrillar and many ghost-like structures exist, which appear to be dead bacterial cells or remnants of cell walls or vegetable matter. In some cases, bacteria in photomicrographs of plaques may be seen invading the local tooth structure (fig. 5/7) [*Frank*, 1973]. For a more detailed description of plaque ultrastructure, readers should refer to *Ellen* [1980].

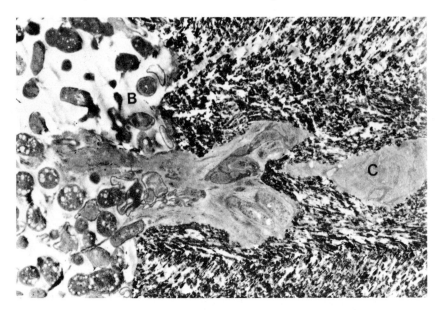

Fig. 5/7. Electron microscopic view of early fissure caries. Coccal cells (B) of the occlusal fissure microflora are shown. There is diffuse destruction of enamel crystals surrounded by an amorphous substance (C) [from *Frank*, 1973 with permission].

Dental Plaque Formation

Formerly, it was considered that plaque formed by the deposition of salivary mucins which entrapped bacteria onto the tooth surface. Further, it was hypothesized that mucin was precipitated from saliva through the action of bacterial acids or enzymes. Though it was known that the bacterial composition of plaques differed from that of saliva, it was assumed that differences in the rates of growth of various bacterial species on the teeth accounted for these differences. These views are no longer tenable. Careful studies of the nutritional requirements of prominent oral bacteria indicate that they possess generally similar and simple nutritional requirements and this does not support the hypothesis that selective growth is responsible for the bacterial population differences between plaques and saliva. Rather, factors affecting adherence of the oral flora to mucous membranes and dental surfaces determine the populations at different sites.

It is now considered that the formation of dental plaques requires two types of specific bacterial adherent interactions. First, bacteria attach selectively to the acquired pellicle and, secondly, bacteria accumulate via specific adhesive and cohesive interactions involving components of the plaque matrix and direct bacterial cell contact. The high specificity of these adherent processes largely accounts for the differences in bacterial composition which exist between dental plaques and other sites within the mouth.

Colonization of Salivary Pellicle

The first step in plaque formation involves the selective adsorption of bacteria from oral fluids to the pellicle surface (fig. 5/4, 5/8). This process is highly selective and involves clumps of bacteria near the gingival margin as well as single cells on other areas [*Saxton*, 1973; *Lie*, 1979]. Some organisms, such as *S. salivarius*, which are prominent on the tongue dorsum and in saliva, do not adsorb well to teeth. Other organisms, such as *S. sanguis* and *A. viscosus*, which are not as numerous in saliva, adsorb avidly to the pellicle surface and are prominent in newly developing plaque. The selectivity of this adsorption process has been documented in experiments in vivo as well as studies in vitro which have used enamel powder or hydroxyapatite coated with experimental salivary pellicles. Evidently, bacterial strains bind to different salivary components, and this accounts for the selectivity of the adsorption process (fig. 5/9). The important point is that organisms are not passively entrapped but rather selectively attached because of specific interactions involving their cell surface constituents and the macromolecules of salivary pellicle.

The number of cells of a given bacterium which attach to a clean tooth surface also depends upon the salivary concentrations of the organism available for adsorption. Only a small percentage of the available bacteria in oral fluids becomes associated with the pellicle surface. For example, approximately 10^4 cells of *S. mutans* per milliliter of saliva must be present before some streptococcal cells can be recovered from an initially clean, smooth tooth surface. In the case of *S. sanguis*, which has a greater avidity for the pellicle surface, approximately 10^3 organisms per milliliter of saliva are required. The available data further suggest that the salivary concentration of *S. mutans* required to initiate colonization of a fissure is probably lower than that required to initiate colonization on a smooth tooth surface. Presumably fissures as well as smooth surfaces are exposed to similar concentrations of *S. mutans* in the mouth, but the higher cleansing action on smooth surfaces prevents organisms with a comparably weak affinity for teeth from becoming firmly attached to a smooth surface. These observations probably explain why *S. mutans* can be isolated more frequently from

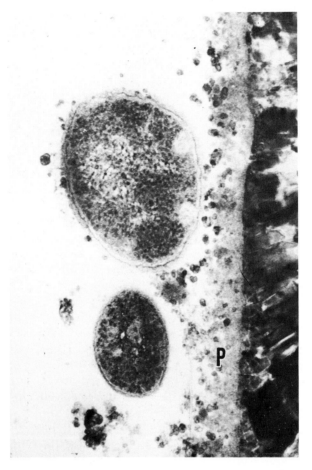

Fig. 5/8. Electron micrograph of a section of an extracted human tooth showing the acquired pellicle (P) and the selective attachment of bacterial cells to the pellicle [from *Frank and Houver*, 1970, with permission].

fissures and contact points of molar teeth than from buccal or lingual smooth surfaces.

Studies of the attachment of several oral bacteria have demonstrated that their relative adherence to teeth or to oral mucosal surfaces correlates with their natural distribution in the mouth (table 5/III). This has led to the realization that adherence per se is a major ecological determinant which influences bacterial colonization of host tissues. The selectivity of bacterial adherence, therefore, accounts for differences in the distribution of various

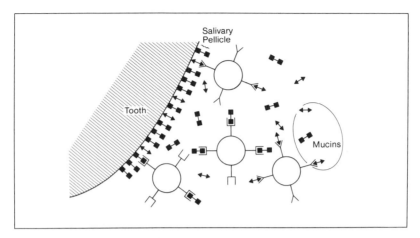

Fig. 5/9. Diagrammatic representation of bacteria interacting with the acquired pellicle covering the enamel. The pellicle is composed of salivary macromolecules (proline-rich proteins) which have become adsorbed to the enamel mineral. Bacterial cells possess lectin-like adhesins on their surface which bind to certain types of molecules present in the pellicle. Mucins and other glycoproteins in saliva can also interact with these adhesins and block attachment of the organisms to teeth [*Gibbons and van Houte*, 1980].

bacterial species within different sites of the mouth and, in part, for the host age at which these species first establish intraorally.

Mechanisms of Bacterial Adherence

Bacteria attach to solid surfaces in many natural environments, but the mechanisms involved have not been thoroughly investigated. Studies of the attachment of marine bacteria have suggested that two phases may be involved. Almost all bacteria and all natural surfaces, including teeth, have a net negative charge. In the first phase of loose association, the organisms are thought to be attracted to the surface by van der Waals forces, but firm contact does not occur because of the repulsive effects of the negative electrostatic charges. The second phase of attachment results in more firm bonding and appears to involve polymeric substances on the surface of the bacterium which link the organism to the target surface (fig. 5/10). The polymeric material may bond to the surface by the formation of hydrogen, hydrophobic, ionic, or other types of bonds, and often calcium ions are involved.

The adsorption of proteins and other materials to hydroxyapatite occurs via electrostatic attractions involving calcium and phosphate groups on the mineral surface. It may be that initial adsorption of bacteria, such as

Table 5/III. Correlation between the experimentally observed adherence of bacteria and their natural distribution on surfaces of the mouth [from Gibbons, 1980]

Organism	Approximate proportions[1] present naturally on oral surfaces					Experimentally observed adherence		
	saliva	gingival plaque	coronal plaque	tongue dorsum	buccal mucosa	coronal surfaces	tongue dorsum	buccal mucosa
Streptococcus salivarius	20	<0.5	<0.5	20	11	low	high	moderate
Streptococcus mitis	20	8	15	8	60	high	moderate	high
Streptococcus sanguis	8	8	15	4	11	high	moderate	moderate
Streptococcus mutans	<1	<1	0–50[2]	<1	<1	low	low	low
Lactobacillus sp.	<1	<1	0–1	<0.1	<0.1	low	low	low
Veillonella sp.	10	10	2	12	1	low	high	low
Neisseria sp.	<1	<0.5	<0.5	<0.5	<0.5	low	low	low
Bacteroides gingivalis	<1	6	<1	<1	<1	low to moderate[3]	low	low

[1] Data expressed as a percentage of total flora cultivable in an anaerobically incubated agar.
[2] Proportions vary with dietary sucrose intake.
[3] Low to clean tooth surfaces; moderate to preformed gingival plaque

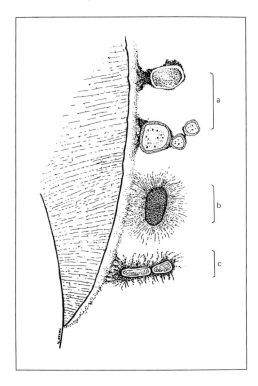

Fig. 5/10. Diagrammatic illustrations of bacterial adherence to the salivary pellicle indicating polymer bridging **(a)** by secretion of a polysaccharide substance, **(b)** by protein fimbriae or pili, **(c)** by fine polysaccharide fibrils.

S. mutans, to pellicle also involves electrostatic interactions. It has been postulated that cell wall teichoic acids which contribute to the net negative charge possessed by bacteria may form bridges with calcium ions to the tooth enamel or pellicle. However, as the only mechanism such a hypothesis does not account for the specificities involved in bacterial attachment because no relationship has been found between the elaboration of teichoic acids by various bacterial species, or their net negative charges, and their relative abilities to attach to the pellicle surface. However, bacteria appear to possess surface components that have recognition potential and which bind to specific receptors on pellicle and other host tissues (fig. 5/9). These surface components are referred to as adhesins. Some adhesins bind to saccharide receptors. Protein adhesins which bind to specific sugars are called 'lectins' (from Latin *legere*, to pick or choose). Other adhesins which contain hydrophobic moieties may interact with hydrophobic residues in specific receptors. Adhesins therefore act like preformed codes that permit bacterial cells to recognize and adhere to complex macromolecules. Often adhesins are present within long surface appendages on the bacterial cell termed 'pili', 'fibrils' or 'fimbriae' (fig. 5/10). Strains of *Actinomyces* and *Bacteroides gingivalis* possess such structures which permit them to attach to erythrocytes and to oral epithelial cells. For example, B-galactosides serve as the erythrocyte, epithelial cell, and streptococcal receptors for the fibril-borne lectin adhesin of *Actinomyces viscosus*. However, *A. viscosus* attachment to pellicle-coated teeth probably involves fibril adhesins which do not contain the galactosyl-binding lectin [for review see *Ellen*, 1982].

The exact chemical nature of the receptors on pellicle or other host tissues to which bacteria attach has not yet been determined; none have yet been isolated and characterized. However, it is clear that bacteria can specifically bind various salivary macromolecules causing bacterial aggregation. Addition of saliva, in vitro, to pure cultures of some oral bacteria leads to their forming aggregates. This aggregation probably occurs in the mouth, and some of the smaller aggregates may become attached to the pellicle. In contrast, other larger aggregates could be cleared more easily and swallowed. Aggregating factors may also favor the attachment of some bacteria to those already bound to the pellicle. Salivary components which are known to bind specifically to bacteria include blood group-reactive mucins, high molecular weight glycoproteins in parotid saliva, lysozyme and salivary immunoglobulins [*Ericson* et al., 1976]. Several of these salivary components have also been shown to be present in the pellicle on teeth.

Bacterial Accumulation on Teeth
Once bacteria have attached to the pellicle and growth occurs, additional adherent interactions must take place to permit the organisms to accumulate. Both bacterially derived polymers and salivary components appear to play important roles in this process.

Role of Bacterial Polymers. Because of the high cariogenic potential of *S. mutans*, considerable information is available concerning the role of bacterial polymers in its accumulation on teeth. This subject has been reviewed by *Hamada and Slade* [1980] and *Gibbons and van Houte* [1980]. Early studies demonstrated that *S. mutans* accumulated on the teeth of rats or hamsters fed diets rich in sucrose but not glucose. It was subsequently found that *S. mutans* synthesized extracellular glucans and fructans from sucrose but not from other common carbohydrates (fig. 5/11), and polymer

---

Fig. 5/11. a Emptied culture vessels of a strain of *S. mutans* grown in broth containing either glucose or sucrose. Note the adherent accumulations of *S. mutans* associated with extracellular polysaccharides specifically synthesized from sucrose (courtesy of *R. Gibbons*).

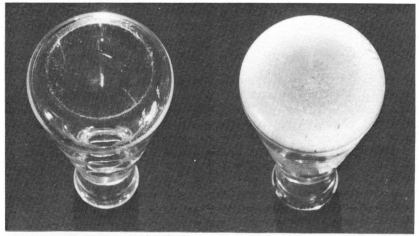

S. mutans 2T6T   S. mutans 2T6T
glucose   sucrose

a

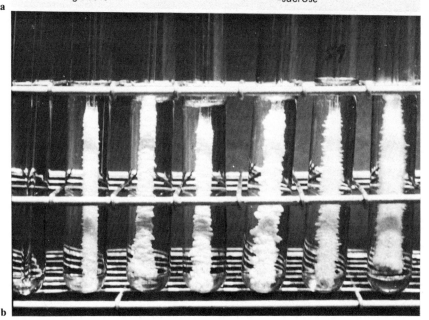

b

b Demonstration of specificity of formation of extracellular polysaccharides by *S. mutans*. On the right are voluminous plaques formed on glass rods by each of 6 strains of *S. mutans* during growth in 5% sucrose broth. No plaque formed in the control tube on the left, inoculated with a *Fusobacterium* species (courtesy *T. Ikeda and J. Sandham*, unpublished).

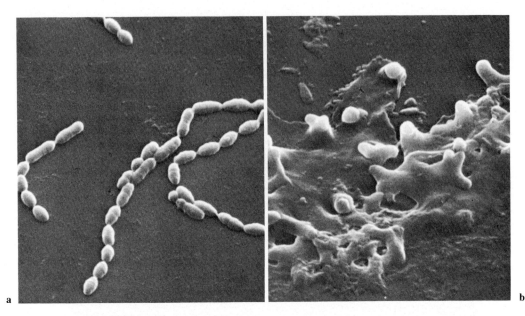

a   b

Fig. 5/12. Scanning electron micrograph of *S. mutans* (serotype d) grown in glucose broth (**a**) and sucrose (**b**). Note the amorphous material covering of colonies grown in sucrose which permitted the organisms to accumulate on a glass surface [from *Hamada* et al., 1975, with permission].

synthesis enabled the organism to accumulate, sometimes in large masses, on a variety of solid surfaces (fig. 5/12). Of the two classes of polysaccharides, the glucans are of more importance in promoting *S. mutans* accumulation. The chemical structure and synthesis of glucans and fructans is discussed in chapter 6.

S. mutans cells are able to bind to high molecular weight glucans and this results in their agglutination (fig. 5/13). Surfaces of streptococci possess several glucan-binding ligands which include the glucosyltransferases (enzymes involved in the synthesis of glucans) and a glucan-binding protein (lectin) devoid of enzymatic activity. The sum of the interactions of these ligands with glucan molecules is thought to promote the accumulation of *S. mutans* cells growing on the teeth.

The importance of glucan-mediated agglutination and glucan-mediated adhesion to dental surfaces in determining smooth surface virulence of *S. mutans* has been examined by studying mutant strains. A common characteristic of the mutants of *S. mutans* studied is their inability to synthesize

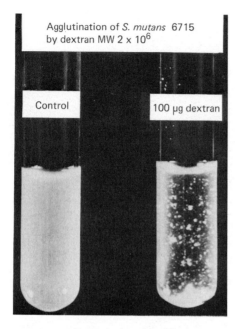

Fig. 5/13. Agglutination of washed glucose-grown *S. mutans* cells in the presence of high molecular weight dextran. The streptococci possess glucan-binding ligands on their surface which interact with glucan molecules.

highly insoluble α(1–3)-linked glucans (fig. 5/14). This metabolic defect greatly reduces their in vitro and in vivo adhesion and virulence but not their agglutination by glucan. This indicates that the α(1–3)-insoluble glucan is essential for cariogenicity on smooth surfaces but it does not necessarily exclude a role for α(1–6) more soluble glucan in virulence (see chapter 6 for a further discussion of the role of bacterial polymers in caries).

Some early data suggested that glucans might also be involved in the initial attachment (as distinguished from accumulation) of *S. mutans* to teeth but subsequent studies have indicated that this organism can colonize the teeth of experimental animals in the absence of glucan synthesis. Similarly, other studies [*van Houte* et al., 1976] have made it clear that *S. mutans* can interact directly with components of salivary pellicles and that the presence of glucan on the organism's surface does not enhance this process. The adsorption of several *S. mutans* strains to experimental salivary pellicles can be inhibited by galactose and by various amines, and this suggests that these moieties comprise part of the pellicle receptors for this organism.

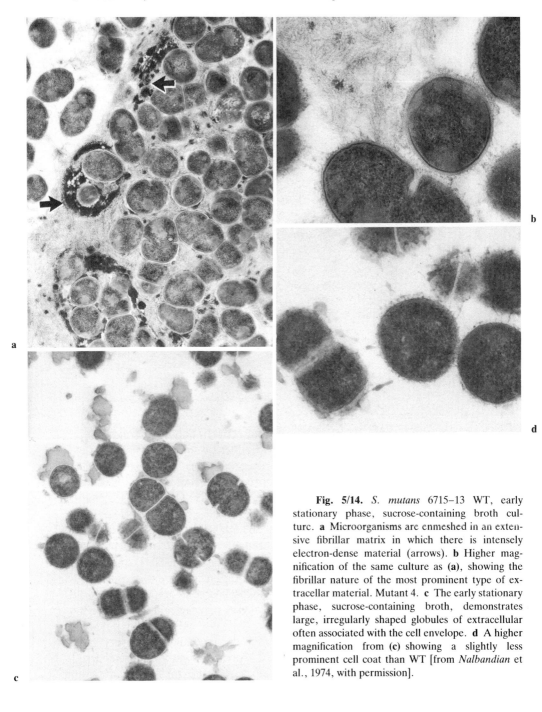

Fig. 5/14. *S. mutans* 6715–13 WT, early stationary phase, sucrose-containing broth culture. **a** Microorganisms are enmeshed in an extensive fibrillar matrix in which there is intensely electron-dense material (arrows). **b** Higher magnification of the same culture as (**a**), showing the fibrillar nature of the most prominent type of extracellar material. Mutant 4. **c** The early stationary phase, sucrose-containing broth, demonstrates large, irregularly shaped globules of extracellular often associated with the cell envelope. **d** A higher magnification from (**c**) showing a slightly less prominent cell coat than WT [from *Nalbandian* et al., 1974, with permission].

Although other bacteria can probably accumulate on teeth by synthesizing extracellular polymers, direct evidence is lacking. *A. viscosus* and *A. naeslundii* cells accumulate on solid surfaces in cultures containing a variety of carbohydrates. Some strains produce fructans from sucrose and others synthesize an extracellular heteropolysaccharide composed largely of *N*-acetyl glucosamine and lesser amounts of glucose and galactose [*Rosan and Hammond*, 1974; *van der Hoeven*, 1974]. However, the role of these polysaccharides in promoting bacterial accumulation remains to be clarified. It is known that human isolates of *Actinomyces* species are not agglutinated by commercially purchased glucans, fructans, galactans, mannans or by polysaccharides synthesized from sucrose by streptococci [*Ellen*, 1982].

Host-Derived Polymers. Many species of bacteria isolated from human dental plaques do not accumulate on solid surfaces in laboratory cultures. This suggests that they are unable to synthesize polymers which promote their accumulation and it raises the likelihood that their accumulation on teeth may be mediated by substances present in the oral environment. Salivary and serum components which are able to bind to bacteria and cause their aggregation would be expected to promote accumulation if they interacted with organisms proliferating on the teeth. This possibility is supported by analyses which indicate that the matrices of plaques contain blood group-reactive and sulfated mucins, immunoglobulins, and albumin. In addition, components which have properties similar to those of salivary mucins and which can aggregate bacteria have been extracted from plaques. These so-called agglutinins do show a high degree of specificity for various bacterial strains and thus may influence colonization selectively. It seems likely that host-derived substances are of considerable importance in promoting the accumulation of bacteria on teeth, but the chemical nature of individual macromolecules with these functions have not yet been elucidated fully.

Bacterial Succession as Plaque Accumulates

Almost everyone has observed a barren piece of land which over a period of time becomes overgrown by a succession of different species of plants. A deforested area is repopulated by a succession of different botanical species indigenous to the area and in most of the Northern hemisphere ends up with stately pines and firs. The same principles are applicable to the flora of dental plaques. In young plaques, streptococci usually predominate, but other organisms such as *Neisseria* and *Actinomyces* species may also play a role in the initial development of plaque. *S. sanguis* is among the more prominent initial colonizers of tooth surfaces. *A. viscosus*,

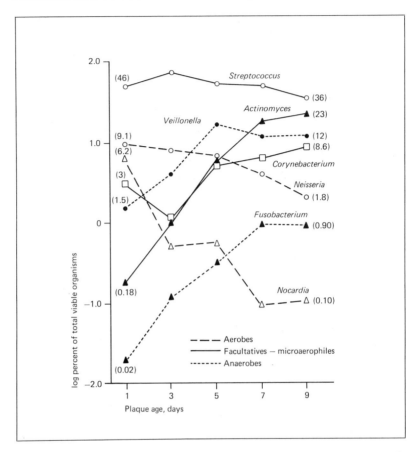

Fig. 5/15. Graph showing the changes in relative proportions of selected organisms in plaque as it thickens and matures [from *Ritz*, 1967, with permission].

S. mitis and *Veillonella* species have also been consistently found in newly developing plaque [*Socransky* et al., 1977].

When a plaque is undisturbed, it will become thicker after a few days and additional bacterial species may be detected. The flora of the plaque changes from its predominantly coccal form to a mixed filamentous flora. The rods and filaments increase proportionally as the plaque thickens and become dominant in a 7- to 14-day-old plaque. The changes in the relative proportions of some organisms in plaque as it thickens is shown in figure 5/15.

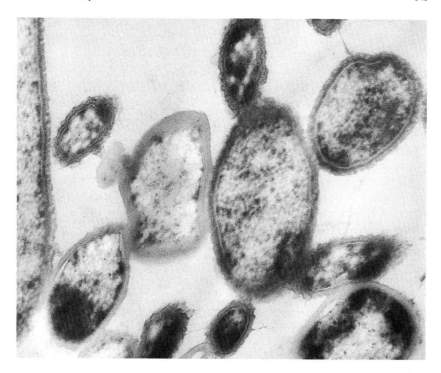

Fig. 5/16. Electron micrograph of a section of human dental plaque showing dissimilar organisms attached to each other. These interactions are thought to promote bacterial accumulation (courtesy of *Z. Skobe*, Forsyth Dental Center).

The changes in the morphological forms of the plaque flora have been attributed to changing metabolic and environmental conditions within the plaque over time. As plaque accumulates and matures it becomes more anaerobic and this may permit the emergence of certain obligate anaerobes. The degree of anerobiosis of plaque is reflected in its redox potential (Eh). The Eh of early developing plaque is about +200 mV, which is similar to that of saliva and of aerobically metabolizing tissue. However, a plaque several days old will have an Eh of about −100 mV and this may decrease still further to about −300 mV for older plaques [*Kenney and Ash*, 1969]. Growth of anaerobes is encouraged at low Eh levels.

The developing flora of dental plaque also provides new surfaces for bacterial colonization. Dissimilar organisms attached to each other are often seen in electron microscopy studies (fig. 5/16). For example, pre-formed plaques have been found to promote the colonization of organisms, such as *B. gingivalis*, which is associated with certain types of periodontal disease. This organism adheres avidly to the surfaces of *Actinomyces* and other gram-positive species present in newly formed plaques.

The interbacterial attachment mechanism which has been studied most thoroughly is that between streptococci (particularly *S. sanguis*) and *A. viscosus* and *A. naeslundii*. Although these interactions involve several mechanisms, a common one studied in vitro consists of the galactosyl-binding lectin of the *Actinomyces* cell surface fibrils interacting with a galactoside-containing receptor on the streptococcal cell surface. Thus, like bacterial attachment to pellicles, these interbacterial interactions are highly specific and may contribute to the sequence in which bacterial types accumulate on the teeth. Adherence to a rapidly plaque-forming bacterium offers an opportunity for tooth colonization to an organism which may otherwise attach very poorly to the salivary pellicle.

Microflora of Established Plaque

An electron microscopic examination of established plaque often shows large masses of organisms, some with identical morphology, sometimes merging or sometimes sharply divided from other forms (fig. 5/5). A bewildering array of species may be cultivated from established plaques as a result of the unique morphology of teeth and the varying microenvironments of the oral cavity. Deficiencies in the precise quantification of bacterial species (sampling, dispersion, recovery, identification of viable organisms and difficulty of growing some organisms in culture) precludes an exact description of microbial composition applicable to a 'typical plaque'. However, a general description of main bacterial groups common to most dental plaques is possible.

The microbial composition of approximal plaque is shown in table 5/IV. The predominant groups of bacteria are gram-positive, consisting mostly of the genera *Actinomyces* and *Streptococcus*. These two groups are found in virtually all plaques. In addition, *Veillonella*, *Neisseria*, and additional genera of gram-positive rods are also present at most sites. This collection of genera may be considered a 'basic plaque' flora which is consistently present along with diverse mixtures of a large number of other less common types of microorganisms.

Because of fluctuations in relative numbers among the basic plaque members and the other species, the bacterial composition of plaque varies significantly at different sites of the oral cavity and even at different surfaces on the same tooth [*Donoghue*, 1974]. For example, samplings from plaque adjacent to the gingival crevice yield a high proportion of anaerobes including many *Bacteroides* and fusobacteria, depending on the state of

Table 5/IV. The microbial flora of dental plaque [from *Bowden, Hardie and Slack*, 1976, unpublished data; reproduced from *Silverstone* et al., 1981, with permission]

Type of organisms	Percent viable count, range	Isolation frequency, %
Streptococcus	17–38	100
Gram-positive rods and filaments	22–52	100
Neisseria	0–2	99
Veillonella	1–13	94
Gram-negative anaerobic rods	0–17	98
Fusobacteria	0–7	55

These figures have been assembled from five independent surveys by different authors, who have used a variety of sampling methods and laboratory procedures.

Table 5/V. Variations of cultivable plaque flora on 3 sites of the same tooth [from *Silverstone* et al., 1981, with permission]

Subject	Site	*Streptococcus*	*Actinomyces*	*Bacteroides*	*Fusobacterium*	*Veillonella*
1	A	11.4	0.04	8.5	0.85	11.4
	B	65.5	5.7	9.0	11.4	0
	C	0.4	0.6	0.08	0.26	73.0
	Mean	25.7	2.1	5.9	4.2	28.2
2	A	8.6	85.3	0.65	0	1.7
	B	71.5	18.7	8.0	0.93	0
	C	14.3	56.6	0	0	16.6
	Mean	31.2	53.5	2.9	0.3	6.1
3	A	30.0	14.0	2.0	0	23.0
	B	65.0	7.0	25.0	3.0	14.0
	C	64.0	25.0	0	0.5	10.0
	Mean	53.0	15.3	9.0	1.2	15.6
	Mean for all sites	36.6	23.6	5.9	1.9	16.6

Figures expressed as percentage of total viable count. Site A = contact area; site B = gingival crevice below contact; site C – buccal surface.

gingival health. Table 5/V indicates the wide variations of cultivable plaque flora from three separate sites of the same tooth.

S. mutans has been implicated as a specific organism associated with caries (chapter 6). For this reason the location of the organism at different tooth sites has been widely studied. This species has been found to localize in retentive areas and to persist at these specific sites; it is not easily transmitted to other similar sites except through deliberate implantation [*Loesche* et al., 1979].

In summary, important aspects of the bacterial composition of dental plaque are as follows:

–   A dominant characteristic of the microflora of plaques is its hetero-geneity.
–   The initial flora of a newly forming plaque consists predominantly of gram-positive streptococci and rods; the predominant flora becomes more complex to include more filamentous and gram-negative species as the plaque becomes established.
–   Each microenvironment within the mouth and on well-defined tooth surfaces harbors its own unique flora.
–   The metabolic features of dental plaque in a specific site must be deter-mined primarily by the particular bacterial composition of the plaque.

Metabolism of Dental Plaques

The heterogeneity and complexity of the chemical and microbial com-position of dental plaques has been emphasized. It is not surprising, there-fore, that a very wide range of metabolic reactions may be detected in plaques. Degradative reactions whereby bacteria convert organic sub-strates to end products (metabolites) and thereby derive energy are readily detectable in plaques. Opposite biochemical processes also occur which entail the synthesis of complex molecules from basic building blocks and which utilize the energy released from the breakdown of substrates. Of the metabolic reactions occurring in plaque, glycolysis is perhaps the most im-portant from the standpoint of dental caries etiology.

Glycolysis
Anaerobic catabolism of carbohydrates (called fermentation or gly-colysis) predominates in plaques which have a reduced oxygen tension. The bacteria in dental plaque are capable of using different carbohydrates such as starch, dissacharides and monosaccharides as substrates. The end products of glycolysis have the same empirical formula as the starting sub-strate as illustrated by the breakdown of 1 molecule of glucose ($C_{12}H_{12}O_6$) to 2 molecules of lactic acid $2(C_3H_6O_3)$. This reaction has a net yield of 2 mol of ATP from each mole of glucose. Some streptococci and many lactobacilli ferment sugars producing 90% or more of lactic acid among their end products; such bacteria are homofermentative. Heterofermen-tors produce a mixture of metabolites including other organic acids, such as

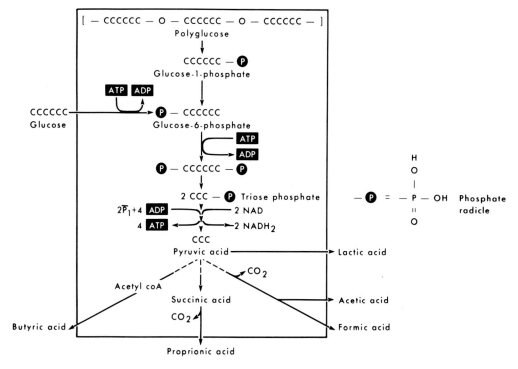

Fig. 5/17. A schematic representation of glycolytic fermentation by plaque bacteria leading to various acidic end products. The formation of phosphorylated sugars as metabolic intermediates, the utilization and synthesis of ATP (adenosine triphosphate) and the production of $NADH_2$ (reduced nicotinamide or adenine dinucleotide) are shown.

propionic, butyric and succinic acids and ethanol. A schematic representation of the breakdown of glucose to various end products in dental plaque is shown in figure 5/17.

Oral bacteria do not all metabolize glucose to the same end products because they utilize divergent metabolic pathways. Pyruvic acid, an intermediate in glycolysis, may be metabolized via several paths. For example, it may be reduced to lactic acid by the enzyme lactic acid dehydrogenase or split into formic acid and acetyl-CoA by the enzyme pyruvate formate lyase. The acetyl-CoA is then converted into acetate and ethanol. The proportion of lactic or other organic acids formed by plaques may be markedly affected by growth conditions and by the bacterial types present.

When the concentration of cariogenic bacteria and sugars in plaque is high, the pathway leading to lactic acid formation is dominant. On the other hand, when carbohydrate is limited the latter reactions are favored [*Yamada and Carlsson*, 1975].

Concept of Critical pH

The loss of tooth mineral during caries formation is caused by the formation of bacterial acids which lower the pH to the point where the hydroxyapatite mineral of enamel dissolves. The concept of critical pH was initially applied to indicate the pH at which saliva was no longer saturated with respect to calcium and phosphate ions, thereby permitting hydroxyapatite to dissolve [*Ericsson*, 1949]. However, it is now realized that the immediate fluid environment involved in demineralization of a tooth is not saliva but the fluid phase of plaque, now known as 'plaque fluid'. It has been shown experimentally that both saliva and plaque fluid cease to be saturated at pH values in the range 5–6 with an average of 5.5. The critical pH varies in different plaques depending mainly on the concentrations of calcium and phosphate ions but is also influenced by the buffering power and ionic strength of the environment so that a simple numerical value is not applicable to all plaques. However, it is unlikely that demineralization would occur above 5.7 and this value has often been accepted as being 'safe for the teeth'. These considerations are especially important in the very early stages of caries when the outer enamel is being dissolved. As a carious lesion develops, the demineralization occurs within the body of the lesion (chapter 10) rather than on the outer surface which retains a high degree of mineralization. This implies that the acids must diffuse into the enamel and dissolve the apatite within the lesion. There is good evidence that unionized lactic acid molecules diffuse more readily into enamel. Being uncharged, the un-ionized molecules are less likely to react with apatite than their constituent hydrogen or lactate ions [*Gray*, 1966]. The proportion of un-ionized molecules increases as the pH falls:

$$H^+ + [lactate]^- \underset{(high\ pH)}{\overset{(low\ pH)}{\rightleftarrows}} H\ lactate.$$

The critical pH may therefore be the pH at which the environment of the enamel becomes unsaturated and in addition that pH at which sufficiently high concentrations of un-ionized acid are present to ensure the inward diffusion of enough acid to extend the inner lesion. As the undissociated acid diffuses it will reach conditions, such as a high pH, at which it will dissociate and be capable of dissolving apatite (see p. 280). The validity of the existence of a critical pH is confirmed by clinical data.

Clinical Data on Plaque pH in Relation to Caries

Bacterial plaques present in protected sites of the teeth subject localized areas of the enamel to high concentrations of metabolic acid end products. Salivary pH does not correlate well with caries activity since it is not markedly affected by acid production within the plaques. Direct measurements of plaque pH in vivo clearly indicate the significance of these deposits in synthesizing, concentrating, and localizing the acid end products of bacterial metabolism.

Stephan [1940], using antimony microelectrodes, recorded the pH values of dental plaques in situ before, during and after a glucose rinse. A typical pH response to plaque following exposure to a glucose rinse is illustrated in figure 5/18. These curves are often referred to as 'Stephan' curves, and they have three main characteristics. Under resting conditions, the pH of plaque is reasonably constant, though differences can be noted between individuals. Following exposure to sugars, the pH drops very rapidly (in a few minutes) to its lowest level and then slowly returns to its original value over a period of approximately 30–60 min. *Stephan* [1944] observed that plaques of caries-free or caries-inactive individuals usually had a resting pH of between 6.5 and 7 and they usually remained above pH 5 following exposure to glucose. In contrast, plaques of highly caries-prone persons had a lower resting pH and attained acidities well below pH 5 after exposure to glucose (fig. 5/18) – values shown experimentally to be low enough to cause enamel demineralization. These early studies also demonstrated that differences could exist in the metabolic properties of plaque which relate to dental caries activity. *Stephan* [1940] postulated that there must be microbial differences between plaques in caries-free and caries-prone subjects, but his efforts to demonstrate these in the 1940s were not successful. In addition to differences in bacterial composition, other factors which may affect the extent and rate of pH changes in plaque are the type and concentration of carbohydrates and other substrates ingested, the frequency of ingestion, salivary composition and flow, and the thickness and age of the plaque.

More recently, miniaturized glass electrodes and fine antimony electrodes, about 5 μm in diameter, have permitted measurement of pH changes in plaques in interproximal areas and in pits and fissures (chapter 8, fig. 8/10). Also, continuous pH measurement is possible by embedding electrodes in partial dentures abutting on plaque-laden proximal surfaces of natural teeth. Using indwelling electrodes, pH values below 4.0 for interproximal plaques have been recorded [*Graf and Mühlemann*, 1966]. This subject will be developed further under cariogenicity of diets in chapter 8 and vol. 2, chapter 8.

The reason that the resting pH of plaques of caries-prone individuals can be considerably below neutrality for extended periods after meals is

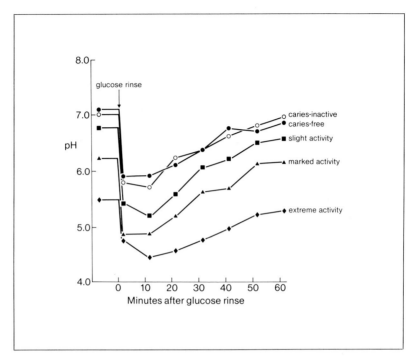

Fig. 5/18. A typical pH response in plaque following a 10% glucose rinse in caries inactive individuals and those with marked caries activity. The pH plotted represents means for individuals in each group. Note the rapid fall in pH, the pH minimum and subsequent return to the resting pH value of plaque. The curve, known as the 'Stephan curve', is the net result of acid production in plaque, its neutralization by salivary and plaque buffers, the diffusion of sugar and by the production of ammonia and amines in plaque, its utilization by bacteria such as *Veillonella*, and the rate of acid diffusion from plaque [after *Stephan*, 1944].

most probably related to the ability of many plaque bacteria to store carbohydrates in the form of polysaccharides. These can be utilized for energy with the production of acidic by-products when dietary carbohydrates become depleted. Plaques in caries-prone individuals contain increased proportions of bacteria capable of synthesizing intracellular polysaccharides (IPS) of the glycogen-amylopectin type. Laboratory studies have shown that the degradation of these polysaccharides occurs in the absence of environmental sugar and leads to the production of lactic acid. Streptococci capable of synthesizing IPS have also been observed to utilize more environmental substrate and to produce acid at higher rates per unit time than mutants defective in IPS synthesis [*van Houte* et al., 1969]. Moreover,

IPS-defective mutants of *S. mutans* have been found to be less cariogenic than their IPS-producing parent strains [*Tanzer*, et al., 1976]. Thus, the higher proportions of glycogen-synthesizing bacteria in caries-active persons not only helps to explain why the resting pH of their plaques is lower, but also why such plaques generate more acid from exogenous carbohydrate.

Some extracellular polysaccharides synthesized by bacteria may also serve as carbohydrate storage compounds. For example, glucans and fructans are synthesized within dental plaque from dietary sucrose and they are subsequently degraded. Fructans are degraded rapidly, and they usually cannot be detected in plaques a few hours after eating. Glucans, however, persist for longer periods. The catabolism of both intra- and extracellular polysaccharides, therefore, extend the time during which plaque pH may be low. The acids produced from stored polysaccharides may be of special significance in the caries process if they are formed when salivary flow is diminished.

Base Production

The pH of plaque is usually highest upon wakening in the morning, and it is often higher than the pH of saliva. This appears to be due to the production of ammonia, amines and other basic components by bacterial degradation of proteins, peptides, urea, and other nitrogenous components [*Kleinberg and Jenkins*, 1964].

Ammonia may be derived from the breakdown of urea or from deamination of amino acids. On the other hand, amines originate from the decarboxylation of amino acids. The net effect of decarboxylation is loss of the carboxyl group of an amino acid due to the production of CO_2. This causes a rise in pH. Amines detected in plaque include α-amino butyric acid, putrescine, histamine, and cadaverine. Most evidence suggests that deamination and decarboxylation reactions have a significant neutralizing effect in plaque under conditions of moderate sugar intake. However, when intake of sugar is frequent and excessive, these reactions are not of sufficient magnitude to neutralize the high concentrations of organic acids produced.

Although base production is not directly involved, some acid-neutralizing activity in plaque may be derived from the metabolic conversion of lactic acid to weaker organic acids. A prime example involves bacteria of the genus *Veillonella* which metabolize lactic acid produced by cariogenic and other bacteria, converting it to propionic and other volatile acids. It is interesting, from an ecological point of view, that strains of *Veillonella* are often found in plaques associated with strong lactic acid producers (chapter 6).

Properties of Cariogenic Plaque

If acid production from readily fermentable substrates by certain plaque bacteria is the mechanism involved in enamel destruction during the formation of a carious lesion, the metabolism and microbial composition of plaque should reflect these properties. These parameters have been studied in samples of plaque derived from carious areas (cariogenic plaques) and plaques obtained from sound enamel surfaces of the same teeth (non-cariogenic plaques) [*Minah and Loesche*, 1977a, b]. This study has provided significant data about the metabolic and bacteriological properties of cariogenic and noncariogenic plaques which may be summarized as follows:

- The rate of sucrose consumption was noticeably higher in cariogenic plaques.
- The rate of lactic acid formation was considerably higher in cariogenic plaques.
- Bacteria in cariogenic plaques synthesized more intracellular glycogen-amylopectin-type polysaccharides.
- Up to 20% of the sucrose consumed within 15 min was converted into intracellular polysaccharides by cariogenic plaques.
- Cariogenic plaques formed more lactic acid from stored intracellular polysaccharides.
- Cariogenic plaques formed approximately twice as much extracellular polysaccharide from sucrose as did non-cariogenic plaques.
- Cariogenic plaques contained higher levels of *S. mutans* than non-cariogenic plaques.
- Noncariogenic plaques harbored higher levels of *S. sanguis* and *Actinomyces* than cariogenic plaques.
- Noncariogenic plaques had significantly higher proportions of dextranase-producing organisms.
- Noncariogenic plaques had higher levels of *Veillonella* and contained slightly lower concentrations of lactic acid and slightly higher concentrations of acetic and propionic acids.

It is apparent that clear differences exist in the metabolic patterns of plaques associated with carious areas as compared to plaques associated with noncarious surfaces. These studies confirm and extend the earlier findings of *Stephan* [1944] concerning the metabolic potential of plaques in caries-free and caries-active individuals as revealed by measurements of plaque pH. The rate of lactic acid formation and depletion of plaque minerals is considerably higher in the latter group. These differences reflect a different microbial composition between cariogenic and noncariogenic plaque. A detailed examination of the microflora associated with caries follows in chapter 6.

References

Agus, H.M.; Un, P.S.H.; Cooper, M.H.; Schamschula, R.G.: Ionized and bound fluoride in resting and fermenting dental plaque and individualized caries experience. Archs oral Biol. 25: 517 (1980).

Ashley, F.P.: Calcium and phosphorus concentrations of dental plaque related to caries in 11- to 12-year-old male subjects. Caries Res. 9: 351 (1975).

Berkowitz, R.J.; Jordan, H.V.; White, G.: The early establishment of Streptococcus mutans in the mouth of infants. Archs oral Biol. 20: 171 (1975).

Bowen, W.M.: Nature of plaque; in Preventive dentistry: nature, pathogenicity and clinical control of plaque. Oral Sci. Rev. 9: 3 (1976).

Dawes, C.; Jenkins, G.N.: Some inorganic constituents of dental plaque and their relationship to early calculus formation and caries. Archs oral Biol. 7: 161 (1962).

Donoghue, H.D.: Composition of dental plaque obtained from eight sites in the mouth of a ten-year-old girl. J. dent. Res. 53: 1289 (1974).

Ellen, R.P.: Surface coatings of the teeth; in Ten Cate, Oral histology. Development, structure and function, chap. 15, p. 290 (Mosby, Toronto 1980).

Ellen, R.P.: Oral colonization by gram-positive bacteria significant to periodontal disease; in Genco, Mergenhagen, Host-parasite interactions in periodontal diseases (Am. Society for Microbiology, Washington 1982).

Ericson T.; Carlen, A.; Dagerskog, E.: Salivary aggregating factors; in Stiles, Loesche, O'Brien, Microbial aspects of dental caries, p. 151 (Information Retrieval, Washington 1976).

Ericsson, Y.: Investigations into the calcium phosphate equilibrium between enamel and saliva and its relation to dental caries. Acta odont. scand. 8: suppl. 3 (1949).

Frank, R.: Microscopic electronique de la carie des sillons chez l'homme. Archs oral Biol. 18: 9 (1973).

Frank, R.M.; Houver, G.: An ultrastructural study of human supragingival dental plaque formation; in McHugh, Dental plaque, p. 85 (Livingstone, Edinburgh 1970).

Gibbons, R.J.: Adhesion of bacteria to surfaces of the mouth; in Berkeley, Lynch, Melling, Rutter, Vincent, Microbial adhesion to surface, p. 351 (Ellis Horwood, 1980).

Gibbons, R.J.; Houte, J. van: Bacteriology of dental caries; in Shaw, Sweeney, Cappuccino, Meller, Textbook of oral biology, p. 975 (Saunders, Toronto 1978).

Gibbons, R.J.; Houte, J. van: Bacterial adherence and the formation of dental plaques; in Beachey, Receptors and recognition, bacterial adherence, series B, vol. 6, P. 60 (Chapman & Hall, London 1980).

Graf, H.; Mühlemann, H.R.: Telemetry of plaque pH from interdental area. Helv. odont Acta 10: 94 (1966).

Gray, J.A.: Kinetics of enamel dissolution during formation of incipient caries-like lesions. Archs oral Biol. 11: 397 (1966).

Hamada, S.; Mizuno, J.; Murayama, Y.; Ooshima, T.; Masuda, N.; Sobue, S.: Effect of dextranase on the extracellular polysaccharide synthesis of Streptococcus mutans: chemical and scanning electron microscopy studies. Infect. Immunity 12: 1415 (1975).

Hamada, S.; Slade, H.D.: Mechanisms of adherence of Streptococcus mutans to smooth surfaces in vitro; in Beachey, Receptors and recognition bacterial adherence, ser. B, vol. 6, p. 105 (Chapman & Hall, London 1980).

Hoeven, J.S. van der: A slime-producing microorganism in dental plaque of rats, selected by glucose feeding. Caries Res. 8: 193 (1974).

Hotz, P.; Guggenheim, B; Schmid, R.: Carbohydrates in pooled dental plaque. Caries Res. 6: 103 (1972).

Houte, J. van; Burgess, R.C.; Onose, H.: Oral implantation of human strains of *Streptococcus mutans* in rats fed sucrose or glucose diets. Archs oral Biol. *21:* 561 (1976).

Houte, J. van; Saxton, C.A.: Cell wall thickening and intracellular polysaccharide in microorganisms of the dental plaque. Caries Res. *5:* 30 (1971).

Houte, J. van; Winkler, K.C.; Jansen, H.M.: Iodophilic polysaccharide synthesis, acid production and growth in oral streptococci. Archs oral Biol. *14:* 45 (1969).

Jenkins, G.N.; Edgar, W.M.: Distribution and forms of fluoride in saliva and plaque. Caries Res. *11:* suppl. 1, p. 226 (1977).

Kenney, E.B.; Ash, M.M.: Oxidation-reduction potential of developing plaque, periodontal pockets and gingival sulci. J. Periodont. *40:* 630 (1969).

Kleinberg, I.; Jenkins, G.N.: Influence of saliva and meals on plaque. Archs oral Biol. *9:* 493 (1964).

Köhler, B.; Bratthall, D.; Krasse, B.: Preventive measures in mothers influence the establishment of the bacterium *Streptococcus mutans* in their infants. Archs oral Biol. *28:* 225 (1983).

Lie, T.: Morphologic studies on dental plaque formation. Acta odont. scand. *37:* 73 (1979).

Listgarten, M.A.; Mayo, H.E.; Tremblay, R.: Development of dental plaque on epoxy resin crowns in man. J. Periodont. *46:* 10 (1975).

Loesche, W.J.; Svanberg, M.L.; Pope, H.R.: Intraoral transmission of *Streptococcus mutans* by a dental explorer. J. dent. Res. *58:* 1765 (1979).

McHugh, W.D. (ed.): Dental plaque (Livingstone, Edinburgh 1970).

Minah, G.E.; Loesche, W.J.: Sucrose metabolism in resting cell suspensions of caries-associated and non-caries-associated dental plaque. Infect. Immunity *17:* 43 (1977a).

Minah, G.E.; Loesche, W.J.: Sucrose metabolism by prominent members of the flora isolated from cariogenic and non-cariogenic dental plaque. Infect. Immunity *17:* 55 (1977b).

Nalbandian, J.; Freedman, M.L.; Tanzer, J.M.; Lovelace, S.M.: Ultrastructure of mutants of *Streptococcus mutans* with reference to agglutination, adhesion, and extracellular polysaccharide. Infect Immunity *10:* 1170 (1974).

Newman, H.N.: The host-organism interface in natural human dental plaque. J. Dent. *7:* 235 (1979).

Ritz, H.L.: Microbial population shifts in developing human dental plaque. Archs oral Biol. *12:* 1561 (1967).

Rosan, B.; Hammond, B.F.: Extracellular polysaccharides of *Actinomyces viscosus*. Infect. Immunity *10:* 304 (1974).

Saxton, C.A.: An electron microscope investigation of bacterial polysaccharide synthesis in human dental plaque. Archs oral Biol. *14:* 1275 (1969).

Saxton, C.A.: Scanning electron microscopic study of the formation of dental plaque. Caries Res. *7:* 102 (1973).

Schamschula, R.G.; Adkins, B.L.; Cooper, M.H.; Pearce, E.: Plaque minerals: concentration and stability. Biennial report, (Institute of Dental Research, Sydney 1980–1982).

Schroeder, H.E.; Boever, J. de: The structure of microbial dental plaque; in McHugh, Dental plaque, p. 49 (Livingstone, Edinburgh 1970).

Silverman, G.; Kleinberg, I.: Fractionation of dental plaque and the characterization of cellular and acellular components. Archs oral Biol. *12:* 1387 (1967).

Silverstone, L.M.; Johnson, N.W.; Hardie, J.M.; Williams, R.A.D.: Dental caries aetiology, pathology and prevention (Macmillan, London 1981).

Socransky, S.S.; Manganiello, A.D.; Propas, D.; Oram, V.; Houte, J. van: Bacteriological studies of developing supragingival dental plaque. J. periodont. Res. *12:*90 (1977).

Stephan, R.M.: Changes in hydrogen-ion concentration on tooth surfaces and in carious lesions. Am. dent. Ass. J. *27:* 718 (1940).

Stephan, R.M.: Intra-oral hydrogen-ion concentration associated with dental caries activity. J. dent Res. *23:* 257 (1944).

Tanzer, J.N.; Freedman, M.L.; Woodiel, F.N.; Eifert, R.L.; Rinehimec, L.A.: Association of *Streptococcus mutans* virulence with synthesis of intracellular polysaccharide; in Stiles, Loesche, O'Brien, Microbial aspects of dental caries, Sp. Suppl. Microbiology Abstracts, vol. 3, p. 597 (1976).

Theilade, J.; Fejerskov, O.; Horsted, M.: A transmission electron microscopic study of 7-day-old bacterial plaques in human tooth fissures. Archs oral Biol. *21:* 587 (1976).

Yamada, T.; Carlsson, J.: Regulation of lactic dehydrogenase and change of fermentation products in streptococci. J. Bact. *124:* 55 (1975).

6 Caries as a Specific Microbial Infection

Introduction

The development, structure and general characteristics of microbial dental plaques are considered in the previous chapter. Also, the heterogeneity and diverse metabolic reactions which characterize plaques are presented. In this chapter attention is focused on the bacterial species that contribute most to cariogenicity. The transmissibility of cariogenic bacteria and the evidence for bacterial specificity in caries etiology are discussed. Currently the *Streptococcus mutans* group occupies a dominant role in microbiological investigations of caries. Therefore, the metabolic characteristics which uniquely permit this group of organisms to play a cardinal role in the etiology of dental caries are emphasized.

Evidence of Bacterial Specificity in Caries Etiology

Transmissibility of Cariogenic Bacteria

One of the most important advances in the microbiology of dental caries was the demonstration by *Keyes* [1960] that dental caries in experimental animals is an infectious and transmissible disease. He observed that a strain of albino hamster which did not naturally develop caries when maintained on a caries-conducive high sucrose diet developed rampant decay when caged together with other caries-active strains of hamsters. Also, the offspring of caries-active dams became caries-inactive if the dams were given antibiotics such as penicillin or erythromycin during pregnancy and lactation. The mode of transmission of the bacterial components and the effects of antibiotics are illustrated in figure 6/1. This study indicated that carious lesions did not develop in the so-called 'caries-inactive' albino hamsters solely because these animals lacked cariogenic organisms, and such bacteria could be acquired from others. Conceptually, it demonstrated that an essential component accounting for familial patterns in caries activity was transmissible and not congenital and that this component was bacterial.

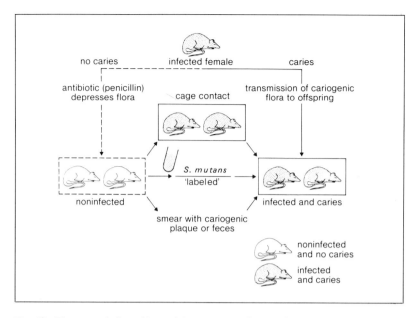

Fig. 6/1. The transmission of bacterial components from caries-active to caries-inactive animals. Caries was induced in caries-inactive animals by innoculation of a streptomycin-resistant strain of *S. mutans*, or by transfer of fecal or plaque flora from the caries-active aminals or by housing of caries-active and caries-inactive animals in the same cages [adapted from *Keyes*, 1960].

Since the albino animals harbored a complex bacterial flora that nevertheless lacked cariogenic potential, it was apparent that a high degree of microbial specificity was involved in the induction of carious lesions in such rodents. *Fitzgerald and Keyes* [1960] subsequently isolated specific streptococci from rodent carious lesions which would initiate rampant decay when inoculated intraorally into caries-inactive albino hamsters (fig. 6/2). Caries-inducing streptococci are now considered members of the *S. mutans* group. Concurrent with these experiments, *Fitzgerald* [1963] demonstrated that certain bacteria introduced in pure culture in gnotobiotic rats exhibited marked differences in their abilities to induce carious lesions.

Evidence of Bacterial Specificity in Animal Models
The subsequent testing of a number of bacteria isolated from human dental plaques have shown that various bacteria possess a spectrum of site-specific cariogenic potential in conventional and gnotobiotic animals (table 6/I). In hamsters, whose teeth do not contain occlusal fissures, only a lim-

Table 6/I. Cariogenic potential of bacteria tested in animal models [from *Gibbons and van Houte*, 1978]

Organisms	Pathogen-free albino hamster				Germ-free or conventional rat				
	bacterial accumulations — coronal	gingival	smooth enamel lesions	root surface lesions	bacterial accumulations — coronal	gingival	smooth enamel lesions	fissure lesions	root surface lesions
Streptococcus mutans	4+*	1+	4+	1+	1+	1+	3+	4+	1+
Streptococcus salivarius	?	?	–to 2+	–to 2+	±	–to 3+	–	–to 2+	–to 2+
Streptococcus sanguis	definitive data are not available				–to 2+	–to 2+	–	–to 1+	–
Streptococcus mitis	–	–	–	–	±	–	–	–to 1+	–
Enterococci	–	–	–	–	±	–	–	–to 1+	–
Filamentous organisms: *Actinomyces viscosus, A. naeslundii, Rothia* and *Nocardia* species	1+	4+	–	4+	1+	4+	–	–to 1+	4+
Various strains of *Lactobacilli*	–	–	–	–	±	–	–	–to 2+	–
Various diphtheroids	–	?	–	–	–	–	–	–	–
Strains of: *Neisseria*, fusiforms, gram-rods, others	?	?			?	?	?	–	–

* Arbitrary units. 4+ = most cariogenic.

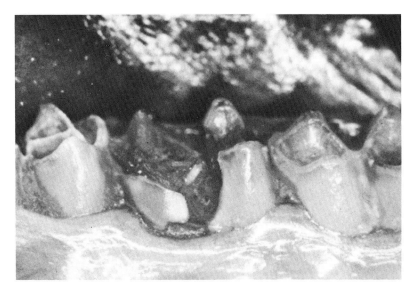

Fig. 6/2. Molar teeth of an albino hamster orally infected with a strain of *S. mutans* and fed a sucrose-containing diet. Note the streptococcal plaque and the decay developing in the second molar (courtesy of Dr. *P. Keyes*).

ited number of species have been found to initiate dental decay. Strains of *S. mutans* will consistently do this provided the animals are maintained on a diet rich in sucrose. Some *Actinomyces* species are able to attack the root surfaces of hamster teeth although they are generally unable to attack the enamel. In contrast, most other organisms are ineffective in initiating decay in the hamster.

Comparable observations have been made with gnotobiotic and with conventional rats. The molar teeth of rats contain occlusal fissures which are similar in size to those of human molars. Strains of *S. mutans* consistently produce decay in pits and fissures as well as on smooth enamel surfaces in such animals. Furthermore, *S. mutans* has also been shown to induce caries in monkeys, mice and gerbils. On the other hand, fewer of the tested strains of *S. sanguis*, *S. mitis*, *S. milleri*, enterococci, lactobacilli and *Actinomyces* initiate carious lesions in rats, and these are almost always restricted to fissures. The filamentous *Actinomyces*, however, heavily colonize the gingival crevice area and regularly induce root surface lesions (fig. 6/3).

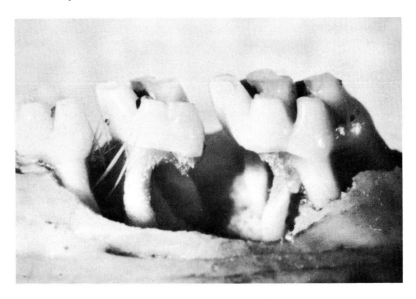

Fig. 6/3. Molar teeth of a gnotobiotic rat monoinfected with a strain of *A. viscosus*. Note the extensive root decay, but the enamel surfaces of the teeth are intact.

The enamel of erupting human and monkey teeth is about 20 times thicker and more fully mineralized at eruption time than the teeth of rodents. Therefore, posteruptive enamel maturation is an important factor but less critical in human and monkey experiments than in rodent models. For these reasons, conditions found in humans are better simulated in monkeys than in rodents. Long-term studies with monkeys (*Macaca fasicularis*) indicate that high caries activity develops if the animals are infected with *S. mutans* and fed a caries-conducive diet. In these animals, as in humans, *S. mutans* comprises a high proportion of the total streptococci at sites of caries activity. Uninoculated or *S. mutans*-free control monkeys fed the same caries-conducive diets develop little or no caries. Also of interest is the contrasting finding that both caries-active and caries-inactive monkeys fed caries-conducive diets harbor similar numbers of lactobacilli [*Bowen*, 1968].

It appears, therefore, that caries development in monkeys also involves a high degree of bacterial specificity. The oral flora of monkeys contains many organisms which are similar to those in the human mouth and therefore these observations are of special interest. The specific involvement of *S. mutans* in caries etiology is also supported by immuniza-

Table 6/II. Frequency distribution of S. *mutans* in carious and caries-free fissures [from *Loesche* et al., 1975]

Levels of S. *mutans* (% total flora)	Number of occlusal fissures	
	caries-free	carious
Not detected	70	30
Very low (<1%)	10	3
Moderate (1–10%)	17	32
High (>10%)	26	65
Total	123	130

tion experiments which have demonstrated that monkeys or rodents given S. *mutans* vaccines will develop significantly fewer carious lesions (vaccines are discussed in vol. 2, chapter 12).

Evidence of Bacterial Specificity in Humans

Studies in humans have mainly focused on the numerical relationship between various streptococci and lactobacilli and dental caries. The available data strongly suggest an active involvement of S. *mutans* in caries initiation. Strains of S. *mutans* isolated from humans have proved to be cariogenic in animal studies (table 6/I). While this illustrates the cariogenic potential of the organism, it provides only indirect evidence for the role of S. *mutans* in caries. The most substantial evidence for the hypothesis that S. *mutans* is responsible for caries development in humans is epidemiological. S. *mutans* can almost always be found in plaques over incipient lesions involving pits and fissures or smooth tooth surfaces (table 6/II). For example, in one study, 71% of carious fissures harbored S. *mutans* in concentrations of more than 10% of the viable bacterial count, whereas 70% of fissures with undetectable levels of S. *mutans* were free from caries [*Loesche* et al., 1975]. Also the proportions of S. *mutans* in plaque over carious areas are generally higher than in plaque over sound enamel. In studies of children (13–14 years old), and of older adults (17–22 years old), S. *mutans* was isolated from all carious lesions but only 23% of sound dental surfaces [*Littleton* et al., 1970]. In addition, the percentages of molar teeth infected with S. *mutans* correlates with dental caries experience of children in different communities (table 6/III). Longitudinal studies have further shown that the development of caries on initially sound tooth surfaces is most often preceded by colonization with elevated levels of S. *mutans* [*Ikeda* et al., 1973]. This finding has been substantiated by others [*Shklair* et al.,

Table 6/III. An example of the percentage of molar surfaces infected by *S. mutans* and the corresponding DMFS in children from two communities with vastly different caries experience [from *Gibbons* et al., 1974]

City	Number of children	DMFS	Percent molar surfaces infected		
			buccal	approximal	fissures
Charlotte	18	1.4	5.5	10.7	30.7
Danvers	20	7.6	26.0	46.7	80.2

DMFS = Decayed, missing and filled tooth surfaces.

1974; *Klock and Krasse*, 1978; *Loesche*, 1982] and indicates that *S. mutans* is associated with most, but not all, coronal carious lesions.

S. mutans has been found to be significantly increased in the saliva and dental plaques of patients with rampant caries due to xerostomia [*Brown* et al., 1978]. In addition, plaque samples from carious and sound tooth surfaces, as well as saliva from infants with nursing bottle caries contain unusually high levels of *S. mutans* [*Van Houte* et al., 1982].

It should be pointed out that *S. mutans* has also been isolated from plaques over sound enamel surfaces and from caries-free and caries-inactive individuals. However, such observations cannot be interpreted as indicating that the organism does not possess cariogenic potential or that it is not of major importance in caries etiology. Asymptomatic carrier states are common when considering many infectious diseases, and *S. mutans* or other pathogens must colonize the teeth sometime prior to the initiation of caries. Furthermore, the development of a carious lesion requires the interaction of the etiologic organisms and their metabolic end products with myriads of factors which include dietary components, frequency of eating, exposure to saliva, interactions with other plaque bacteria, the fluoride levels of dental enamel and the fluoride, calcium, and phosphate levels in plaque.

Not all studies support a unique or sole relationship between *S. mutans* and the initiation of caries in humans. In one major longitudinal investigation, *S. mutans* was isolated from some teeth after an incipient lesion had been detected, casting some doubt about a causal role for *S. mutans* [*Hardie* et al., 1977]. Nevertheless, the accumulated epidemiological data strongly implicate *S. mutans* as an important pathogen in caries etiology in humans while not excluding a cariogenic contribution by other species which is independent of *S. mutans*. The characteristics and properties that endow *S. mutans* with cariogenic potential are discussed next, followed by a consideration of other plaque species associated with caries.

Streptococcus mutans

Of all the oral bacteria, the streptococci have been studied most exhaustively. Mucous membranes in the mouth and in other parts of the body are characteristic habitats for streptococci. The most prominent species found in the oral cavity include: *S. mutans, S. sanguis, S. mitior, S. salivarius* and *S. milleri*. Although strains of *S. sanguis, S. milleri* and *S. salivarius* have occasionally been found to induce fissure caries in rats fed cariogenic diets, *S. mutans*-like bacteria comprise the most important group of streptococci implicated in caries etiology. An understanding of the ecology and the metabolism of this organism is important for understanding caries etiology.

Ecology

As discussed earlier, *S. mutans* does not colonize the mouths of infants prior to the eruption of teeth. Likewise it disappears from the mouth following the extraction of all teeth. Infants most likely become infected from their parents or from other individuals with whom they have frequent contact since the organism is not found free-living in nature and it has only been isolated from humans and certain animals. Studies which have utilized bacteriocin typing and serotyping to 'fingerprint' individual strains have shown that strains isolated from the newly erupted teeth of infants are often identical to those present in the saliva of the mother [*Berkowitz and Jordan*, 1975]. Furthermore, infants whose mothers harbor higher levels of *S. mutans* in saliva become colonized more readily than infants of mothers with low salivary *S. mutans* levels. One therapeutic approach to reduce *S. mutans* infection in infants could be to lower the salivary numbers in mothers by either dietary sucrose restriction, chemotherapy or a combination of both [*Köhler* et al., 1983].

S. mutans does not colonize teeth uniformly. The organism may be more frequently isolated from fissures and interproximal surfaces, those areas most frequently involved in caries, than from buccal or lingual smooth surfaces. In addition, some tooth surfaces may consistently harbor detectable concentrations of the organism whereas comparable surfaces on other teeth in the same mouth do not. This suggests that *S. mutans* does not spread readily from one tooth surface to another. This is also indicated by studies which have noted that streptomycin-resistant mutants of *S. mutans* artificially implanted on one side of the mouth cannot be isolated from teeth on the opposite side of the mouth. The reasons which account for the low rate of transmission of *S. mutans* include its relatively weak ability to adsorb to teeth and its low salivary concentrations available for attachment [*Gibbons and van Houte*, 1975].

The highly localized way in which *S. mutans* colonizes the teeth has important clinical implications. It has been demonstrated that dental explorers or dental floss often contain over 10^6 *S. mutans* cells following their oral use. Thus, these instruments may facilitate the spread of the organism. In fact, in a study to test this issue, strains of *S. mutans* artificially implanted in fissures on one side of the mouth did not spread to teeth on the opposite side of the mouth unless they were transferred by use of a dental explorer [*Loesche* et al., 1979].

The localized mode of colonization of *S. mutans* provides unique opportunities for chemotherapeutic control. For example, it has been shown that the application of potent disinfecting agents, such as iodine solution, to the teeth may eliminate *S. mutans* from previously colonized surfaces which may then remain uninfected for months thereafter due to the organism's low rate of transmission [*Caufield and Gibbons*, 1979]. Similarly, intensive application of chlorhexidine to the dentition decreases salivary *S. mutans* concentrations below that calculated to facilitate intraoral spread. Other approaches for the control of this organism will be considered in vol. 2, chapter 11.

Serological and Genetic Classification

Strains commonly called *S. mutans* derived from humans and various animals are generally similar on the basis of several phenotypic characteristics used in identifying streptococci. They ferment mannitol and sorbitol in addition to other common sugars. They also all synthesize water-insoluble glucans from sucrose and as far as is known, they all require teeth for oral colonization. Most induce carious lesions in experimental animals under appropriate conditions. However, strains from various sources exhibit considerable heterogeneity when analyzed genetically, serologically, and biochemically.

S. mutans has been divided into 5 genetic groups based on DNA base composition and hybridization [*Coykendall*, 1971; *Coykendall* et al., 1976]. Strains have also been divided into 8 serotypes designated 'a' through 'h' [*Bratthall*, 1970; *Perch* et al., 1974; *Beighton* et al., 1981]. The relationship between subspecies (which may be considered separate species in the future), genetic grouping and serological types is indicated in table 6/IV. The specific antigens for each serotype represent cell wall constituents which have been isolated and chemically characterized as polysaccharides [*Hamada and Slade*, 1980].

Table 6/IV. Relation between genetic groups and serotypes of organisms of the *Streptococcus mutans* group [from *Coykendall*, 1971; *Coykendall* et al., 1976; *Bratthall*, 1970; *Gibbons and van Houte*, 1975; *Beighton* et al., 1981]

Subspecies of *S. mutans* group	Genetic group	DNA base content (mol % G + C)	Serotypes	Approximate % of human isolates
S. mutans	I	36–38	c	80
			e	6
			f	4
S. rattus	II	42–44	b	<1
S. sobrinus	III	44–46	d/g/h	9
S. cricetus	IV	42–44	a	<0.1
S. ferus	V	43–45	c	?

The genetic differences between the *S. mutans* strains justifies subdivision of the group into different species or subspecies. Strains of *S. mutans* isolated from individuals in North America and in Europe most commonly belong to genetic group I, serotype c. Strains belonging to genetic group III have also been isolated from humans. Genetic group II and IV organisms are prominent in rats and hamsters, respectively, but are rare in humans. Organisms in genetic group V have thus far only been isolated from wild rat populations, and it is not known if similar organisms are present in humans.

In addition to taxonomy, there are other more pragmatic immunological implications which can be drawn from the studies of antisera to specific cell wall components of the different serotypes. For example, the antibody which is specific for serotype e *S. mutans* glucosyltransferase (GTase, considered in the next section of this chapter) almost completely inhibits the GTase activity of types c,e, and f *S. mutans*, but not GTase activity of a,d and g [*Hamada* et al., 1979]. Thus, theoretical possibilities exist for inhibiting glucosyltransferase of several serotypes by an antiserum against purified GTase of one single serotype. Much research remains to be done in order to apply this knowledge to caries prevention in humans (see vol. 2, chapter 12).

Sucrose Metabolism of Streptococcus mutans

The most important substrate for the involvement of *S. mutans* in the caries process is the disaccharide sucrose. Sucrose not only serves as a primary energy source but it also permits the initiation of additional biochemical events which are responsible for the cariogenic potential of this organism. The different pathways by which *S. mutans* may dissimilate sucrose are summarized in figure 6/4. The three pathways involved are:

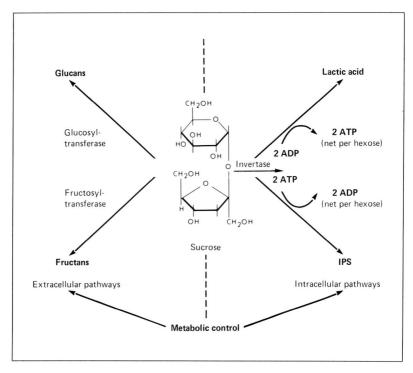

Fig. 6/4. Schematic representation of the metabolic fate of sucrose in a variety of *S. mutans* strains [modified after *Brown*, 1974]. IPS = intracellular polysaccharides.

(1) The conversion of sucrose to adhesive extracellular carbohydrate polymers by cell bound and extracellar enzymes.

(2) The transport of sucrose into the cell interior accompanied or followed by direct phosphorylation for energy utilization through the glycolytic pathway leading to lactic acid production.

(3) The degradation of sucrose to free glucose and fructose by invertase. The intermediary metabolites from sucrose enter the glycolytic cycle or may be utilized in intracellular polymer synthesis in order to provide a reservoir for energy.

Synthesis of Carbohydrate Polymers

Most of the sucrose metabolized by *S. mutans* is utilized for its energy requirement and results in the production of lactic acid. However, the su-

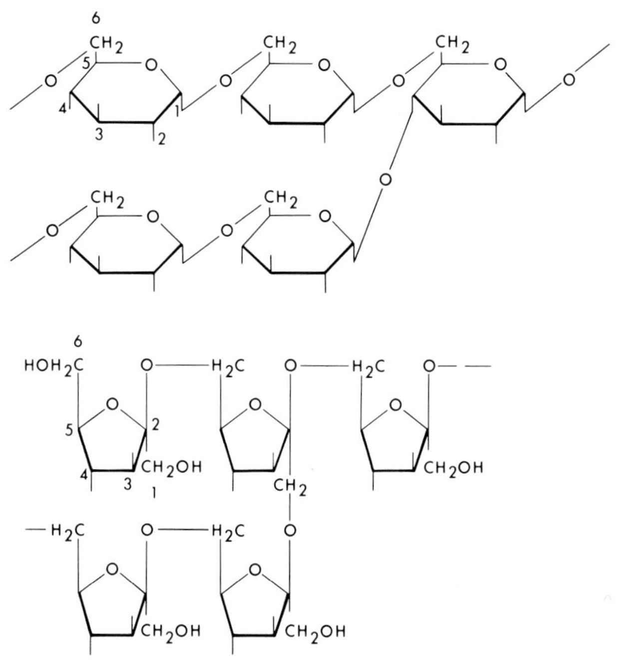

Fig. 6/5. Chemical structure of predominant polysaccharides produced in dental plaque, glucan (**a**) and fructan (**b**). The main linkages in the glucan polymers are $\alpha(1-6)$ core linkage and $\alpha(1-3)$ and $\alpha(1-4)$ branches. Common fructans are levans having a $\beta(2-6)$ core linkage. The length of the polymers and their cross-linkages are dependent upon the strain of *S. mutans* and the environment of the plaque.

crose which does not enter the cell may be used for the extracellular synthesis of carbohydrate polymers. Several investigators [reviewed by *Gibbons and van Houte*, 1975] observed that in the presence of sucrose, *S. mutans* formed adhesive colonies which adhered to the surfaces of culture flasks or to hard objects such as a tooth suspended in the culture medium (chapter 5; fig. 5/11). The ability of *S. mutans* to form adhesive plaques could explain its specific dependence on sucrose rather than other dietary carbohydrates.

It is known that *S. mutans* can polymerize the glucose and the fructose moieties of sucrose to synthesize two types of extracellular polymers, glu-

cans and fructans, respectively (fig. 6/5). Of the two classes of polysaccharides, the glucans are of more importance in promoting *S. mutans* accumulation on teeth. Two types of glucose homopolymers (glucans) are
formed by *S. mutans*: one type is called dextran and contains predominantly $\alpha(1-6)$ core linkages with lesser proportions of branches of $\alpha(1-2)$,
$\alpha(1-3)$, and $\alpha(1-4)$ linkages. A second type of glucan, called mutan, has a
core $\alpha(1-3)$ linkage with branches at $\alpha(1-4)$ and $\alpha(1-6)$ positions. Mutan
is an important constituent of the fibrillar plaque matrix and is less soluble and more resistent to enzymatic attack than is dextran. The $\alpha(1-6)$
polymers (dextrans) tend to be more water-soluble and degradable by enzymes produced by some other plaque bacteria than $\alpha(1-3)$ polymers
(mutan). These two classes of glucans, while tending to be rich in $\alpha(1-6)$
or $\alpha(1-3)$ linkages, also contain mixtures of the two linkage types and
thus present difficulties in precisely defining the compounds chemically.

The major component of the polysaccharide known as fructan or levan
is fructose. Fructans, unlike mutans, are generally highly soluble and can
be degraded by plaque bacteria. Fructan therefore does not persist in
plaque after its synthesis. It serves as a reservoir of fermentable sugars for
oral bacteria.

Lipoteichoic acid is another extracellular polymer that is found in cultures of *S. mutans*. This compound contains a glycolipid covalently linked
with a glycerol teichoic acid to which may be attached a carbohydrate moi-
ety. These highly negatively charged compounds may contribute to the
adhesiveness of bacteria but experimental evidence is incomplete.

Many *S. mutans* strains also produce an iodophilic intracellular polysaccharide which is a branched glycogen-amylopectin-like glucan with
$\alpha(1-4)$ and $\alpha(1-6)$ linkages and which is susceptible to amylase. Cells of
gram-positive cocci and other bacteria in the deep regions of the plaque
often contain numerous intracellular polysaccharide granules visible by
electron microscopy.

Intracellular glycogen and the extracellular polysaccharides (fructans
and glucans) serve as substrate reservoirs which the organism may utilize
for energy production as the exogenous supplies of readily metabolized
carbohydrate are depleted. In this manner both types of polysaccharides
may play a role in the survival of organisms and in their potential to prolong acid production via glycolysis well beyond meal time. Also, as has
been previously noted, extracellular polymer production by *S. mutans* is
limited at low sucrose concentrations in the growth medium, and under
these conditions most of the carbon catabolized is converted to lactic acid.
Sucrose-adapted *S. mutans* also possess significant levels of invertase activity which permits the organism to metabolize the dissacharide via its
hexose moieties.

Enzymes Involved in Synthesis of Glucans and Fructans

The enzymes responsible for the synthesis of extracellular glucans and fructans are called glucosyl and fructosyltransferases, respectively. The enzymes are formed constitutively (i.e. the presence of enzyme is independent of the presence of the principal substrate, sucrose) and they act by transferring glucosyl or fructosyl moieties from sucrose to primer molecules (fig. 6/5). The enzymes are highly specific for sucrose and have a wide pH optimum of 5.2–7.0 and a low Km indicating a high affinity between enzyme and substrate. No phosphorylated intermediates are involved. The energy required is derived from the energy-rich disaccharide bond of sucrose, and this explains why this sugar is the essential substrate. In the case of glucan synthesis, the glucose is incorporated into the polymer and the fructose is a reactant product. Accumulation of fructose inhibits this reaction. However, fructose is rapidly transported into the cell and utilized by the cell for energy or synthesis of intracellular polysaccharide. Separate glucosyltransferases are likely to be involved in the synthesis of the $\alpha(1–3)$ and $\alpha(1–6)$-linkages and it is probable that other transferases are involved in the synthesis of branch point linkages.

Lactic Acid Production

All *S. mutans* strains studied have been demonstrated to be homolactic fermenters converting over 90% of hexose to lactic acid [*Brown*, 1974]. The production of lactic acid from hexose by *S. mutans* proceeds strictly by the glycolytic pathway. At low concentrations of sucrose, both the fructosyl and glucosyl moieties are converted to lactic acid. Colonies, but not necessarily broth cultures of *S. mutans*, attain pH values lower than those produced by other common streptococci (table 6/V). The low pH produced in plaque, in the range of 4.2–5.7, creates conditions favoring demineralization of adjacent enamel (chapter 8). When different bacteria

Table 6/V. pH of broth cultures and of colonies of plaque streptococci grown on the surface of agar containing 5% sucrose [*Onose and Sandham*, 1976]

Organism	Number of strains	pH of		
		sucrose broth culture	colonies	underlying agar
Streptococcus mutans	10	4.2 ± 0.1	4.7 ± 0.1	4.8 ± 0.1
Streptococcus sanguis	9	4.4 ± 0.08	5.4 ± 0.2	5.9 ± 0.2
Streptococcus mitis	10	4.3 ± 0.05	5.7 ± 0.2	5.9 ± 0.1

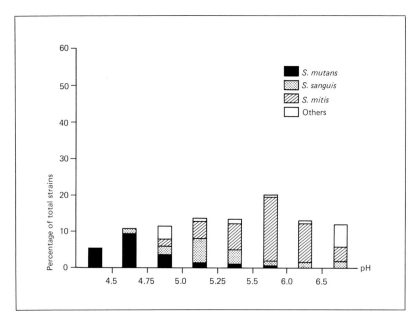

Fig. 6/6. The relative numbers (in percent) of different strains of bacteria associated with various terminal pH values. 394 strains of bacteria were obtained from caries-associated plaques and the strains grown on 5% sucrose-containing agar for 4 days and the pH under the colony measured. Note the predominance of *S. mutans* in colonies with low terminal pH values [from *Sandham and Phillips*, unpublished].

from caries-associated plaques are grown on 5% sucrose-containing agar the colonies with the lowest terminal pH are predominantly *S. mutans* (fig. 6/6).

Under slow growth conditions sugar transport by *S. mutans* is mediated by a phosphoenolpyruvate-dependent phosphotransferase system (PTS), specific for sucrose, as follows:

$$\text{Sucrose + phosphoenolpyruvate} \xrightarrow{\text{PTS}} \text{sucrose-6-phosphate + pyruvate.}$$

The phosphorylated sucrose is then cleaved by a sucrose-6-phosphate hydrolase (SPH) that yields glucose 6-phosphate and fructose as follows:

$$\text{Sucrose-6-phosphate} \xrightarrow{\text{SPH}} \text{glucose-6-phosphate + fructose.}$$

SPH has a high affinity for its substrate, sucrose-6-phosphate; therefore, low levels of sucrose-6-phosphate can be rapidly hydrolyzed.

The synthesis of SPH is constitutively regulated (independent of substrate) whereas PTS activity may be induced by growth of cells in a sucrose-containing medium. The activities of both PTS and SPH are greatly repressed when fructose, but not glucose, is used as a growth substrate [*St. Martin and Wittenberger*, 1979]. The sucrose PTS activity of sucrose-adapted cells may be completely inhibited by raffinose and lactose [*Slee and Tanzer*, 1979]. Low levels of fluoride have been shown to inhibit sugar translocation in cell membranes thus reducing the rate of carbohydrate metabolism [*Hamilton*, 1977].

Recent work indicates that *S. mutans* has at least one other sugar transport mechanism operative under higher growth rate, more abundant sucrose, and lower pH conditions than the PTS system. This system may operate somewhat like a pump, being linked to the expulsion of protons from the cell interior [*Hamilton and St. Martin*, 1982]. This ability to switch transport systems in response to substrate availability demonstrates *S. mutans'* efficient adaptation in a sucrose-dependent environment.

Invertase Activity in Streptococcus mutans

It is known that sucrose-adapted *S. mutans* strains possess significant levels of invertase activity [*Tanzer* et al., 1972a, b]. This enzyme hydrolyzes sucrose intracellularly to free glucose and fructose. Invertase in these organisms is subject to control by the cell and is activated by inorganic phosphate. Since phosphate accumulation is coupled to acid production it is probable that one of several mechanisms by which sucrose degradation is regulated in *S. mutans* is the activation of invertase by inorganic phosphate.

A detailed knowledge of the cellular control mechanisms that play a role in the utilization of sucrose and other fermentable sugars by *S. mutans* is lacking. Furthermore, a complete picture of the metabolic characteristics which account for the high cariogenic potential of *S. mutans* is not available. However, some important metabolic traits can be summarized as follows:

- *S. mutans* has the metabolic potential to produce a low pH (acidogenic) and to survive in a low pH environment (aciduric). The terminal pH of *S. mutans* grown in glucose or sucrose-enriched media is well below pH 4.5. Surface colonies of *S. mutans* also attain a lower pH than colonies of other common plaque streptococci. Transport systems operative at low pH may contribute to its relative aciduricity.
- *S. mutans* is known to utilize sucrose at faster rates than other organisms such as *S. mitior, S. sanguis* and *A. viscosus*.

Table 6/VI. Comparison of source metabolism of different plaque species with *Streptococcus mutans* [adapted from *Loesche*, 1980]

Species	Acid production	Growth initiation below pH 5.5	Extracellular polymers				ICP	PTS	MOH	LTA
			fructan	dextran	mutan	other				
S. sanguis	+	−		+			+	+	−	+
S. mitis	+	−		±			+	+	−	−
S. salivarius	+	−	+	±			+	+	−	+
A. viscosus	+	−	±			+	+		−	−
A. naeslundii	+	−				+	+		−	−
A. israelii	+	−					+		+	
L. casei	+	+					+		+	+
Neisseria sp.	+	?		±		+	+			
S. mutans	+	+	+	+	+		+	+	+	+

ICP = Intracellular polysaccharide; PTS = phosphotransferase system; MOH = mannitol fermentation; LTA = lipoteichoic acid.

– *S. mutans* can synthesize complex mixtures of extracellular glucans and fructans from sucrose, and the glucans permit cells of the organism to accumulate on teeth.

– *S. mutans* has the ability to store intracellular glycogen-amylopectin type polysaccharides which provide it with a reservoir of substrate and enable prolonged periods of increased metabolic activity.

– The major fermentation product of *S. mutans* is lactic acid. At low glucose concentrations formic and acetic acids and ethanol may also be produced.

A comparison of the sucrose metabolism of different plaque bacteria is shown in table 6/VI. The metabolic versatility of *S. mutans* sets it apart from many other plaque bacteria.

Other Plaque Bacteria Associated with Caries

Lactobacilli

As early as 1915, *Kligler* reported the presence of higher numbers of lactobacilli in carious lesions than in noncarious sites. Lactobacilli are strong acid producers and are among the most aciduric and acidogenic bacteria. Their aciduric characteristics have been utilized for the development of selective growth media for caries activity based on *Lactobacillus* counts. These are considered further in vol. 2, chapter 10.

Lactobacilli are found in carious lesions and their numbers in plaque and in saliva often correlate with caries experience. Furthermore, restrictions of dietary carbohydrate intake [*Jay*, 1947] or the restoration of carious lesions often lead to the diminution of oral *Lactobacillus* populations. It is thought that the acidic conditions existing within a carious lesion and its retentiveness lead to the selection of these acid-tolerant organisms, especially in deep dentinal lesions where they often predominate. It appears that a preexisting lesion favors, or is even required for, their colonization. This argues that lactobacilli may not be involved in caries initiation but rather may become secondary invaders which contribute to the progression of already existing lesions. This possibility is supported by the observations that lactobacilli are not detectable in plaques covering white spot lesions on smooth tooth surfaces and by longitudinal studies which have indicated that lesions may develop on teeth which do not harbor lactobacilli [*van Houte*, 1980].

On the other hand some *Lactobacillus* strains (*L. acidophilus* and *L. casei*) have been shown to produce caries in gnotobiotic rats. Further studies of the cariogenicity of human plaque lactobacilli showed that 17 of 32 strains tested were moderately to highly cariogenic in such animals [*Fitzgerald* et al., 1981]. The predominant sites of caries attack were fissures. Thus, while lactobacilli may contribute to the progression of deep dentinal lesions in humans, it also seems probable that these organisms may initiate caries in those sites which favor their retention, such as in deep fissures or in enamel defects. Additional studies are required to substantiate this possibility.

Filamentous Bacteria

Several types of filamentous organisms will initiate root surface carious lesions in experimental animals. *Actinomyces* and *Rothia* species have been found in human dental plaque and dental calculus in significant numbers and they have been isolated in high proportions from decayed root surfaces of human teeth [*Sumney and Jordan*, 1974]. *Actinomyces viscosus*, an acidogenic bacterium which also stores intracellular polysaccharides, is almost always among the predominant flora of plaque overlying root lesions, but its role in initiating these lesions is difficult to assess because *A. viscosus* is also often predominant on sound root surfaces in both persons experiencing and resisting root caries. It is obvious that more definitive studies of the association of specific bacteria with human root caries initiation must be conducted, but such studies have been hampered by the lack of rapid techniques which permit the confident enumeration of species other than streptococci and lactobacilli. These two genera compose only a moderate proportion of the flora on roots where incipient lesions are developing.

Gram-Negative Cocci

Veillonella. Of the gram-negative cocci, *Veillonella* is the genus most commonly found in plaque. Interest in this group relates to its possible anticariogenicity. These organisms lack key enzymes involved in glycolysis and the hexose monophosphate shunt and therefore do not utilize sugars as an energy source. *Veillonella* utilizes lactic acid by converting it to propionic and other weak acids as follows:

$$2CH_3CHOHCOOH \longrightarrow CH_3CH_2COOH + CH_3COOH + CO_2 + H_2$$

lactic acid	propionic acid	acetic acid
(pKa = 3.08)	(pKa = 4.75)	(pKa = 4.78)

This reaction does not result in a total reduction of acid molecules; rather, the stronger lactic acid with a pKa of 3.08 (pH at which an acid is half-dissociated) is converted to a less dissociated acid. Thus, the net effect of *Veillonella* metabolism of lactic acid could be to diminish the overall hydrogen ion concentration of dental plaque.

It has been observed that *Veillonella* strains increase in numbers in dental plaque after lactic acid producing organisms have first colonized [*Ritz*, 1967]. A positive correlation between *Veillonella* and caries activity has been reported in some studies but contradicted in others. Elevated levels of *Veillonella*, slightly lower levels of lactic acid and higher levels of propionic and acetic acid can be found in plaques from noncarious surfaces relative to plaques from carious sites. The weaker acidic end products resulting from *Veillonella* metabolism could reduce the potential for tooth demineralization. Some experimental confirmation of this hypothesis exists. Gnotobiotic rats co-infected with *S. mutans* and *Veillonella alcalescens* were found to have fewer carious lesions than animals monoinfected with *S. mutans* [*Mikx* et al., 1972].

Streptococci Other than S. mutans

Streptococcus sanguis. This α -hemolytic *Streptococcus* species was originally isolated from the blood of patients with bacterial endocarditis. In humans, this organism's main habitat is the oral cavity, especially dental plaque. The species does not colonize the oral cavity until the first teeth erupt at about 6 months of age.

Serological studies of *S. sanguis* indicate the presence of at least three or four types. While the serology is complex, the organism is easy to identify on sucrose-containing media, because it produces small, firm colonies which become embedded in and deform the surrounding agar. Many strains of *S. sanguis* are typable as group H by the method of Lancefield.

Being so ubiquitous, *S. sanguis* is consistently present in plaque obtained from both carious and noncarious sites. However, its proportions of the plaque microflora relative to *S. mutans* usually show a high association with sound rather than carious sites. Moreover, *S. sanguis* has a very low cariogenicity in experimental animals, with lesions limited to occlusal fissures.

Streptococcus mitior. Often called *S. mitis*, this organism does not hydrolyze arginine and esculin as does *S. sanguis.* It produces soft, round and black-brown colonies on mitis salivarius medium which contains sucrose. Many oral strains of *S. mitior*, like *S. sanguis* and *S. mutans*, produce an extracellular glucan from sucrose. A characteristic of the organism is the absence of significant amounts of rhamnose in the cell wall. Some strains share common antigens with *S. sanguis* but many are serologically distinct.

S. mitior is one of the most commonly isolated bacteria in the oral cavity. It is the most predominant species on the buccal mucosa. It and *S. sanguis* are among the most predominant organisms in dental plaque. Its significance in human caries is unknown and assumed to be very minor.

Streptococcus salivarius. This species is found predominantly on the tongue, soft tissue and in saliva but is not found in high numbers in plaque. *S. salivarius* adheres well to epithelial cells but not to hard tissues, especially pellicle-coated enamel. *S. salivarius* forms unique large, dome-shaped colonies on sucrose-containing agar. The species produces copious amounts of a very viscous extracellular polymer which is a levan (fructan). Some strains of this organism have been shown to produce some caries in experimental animals. However, its low numbers in human plaque suggest that it is not of great significance in human caries.

Streptococcus milleri. This species was originally isolated from localized dental, brain and liver abscesses. The organism has also been isolated from the gingival crevice and cervical plaque but does not predominate in other intraoral sites. *S. milleri* strains are frequently resistant to sulfonamides and bacitracin and are often found on the selective medium used for isolation of *S. mutans*.

S. milleri is a fairly homogeneous group based on its morphological characteristics but serologically it is very heterogeneous. Although some strains induce fissure caries in experimental animals, its importance in dental caries in humans is not known at present.

Microflora of Dentinal Caries

In this and in the preceding chapter, emphasis thus far has been placed on the microflora involved in plaque formation and in enamel caries. Studies relating to these areas are numerous and much information is available. On the other hand, only a few studies have considered the microflora of an advanced dentinal lesion. Such information is important in providing clues about the mechanism of destruction of dentin and the pathogenesis of caries leading to pulp exposure.

Early studies concerned with the microflora of dentinal lesions showed that the common bacteria found were 'gram-positive pleomorphic rods' or 'gram-positive filaments'. More definitive studies to identify the flora of an advanced lesion in dentin have now been undertaken. The mean percent of the bacterial groups in deep dentinal lesions is shown in table 6/VII. The dominant organisms are gram-positive rods and filaments, especially the lactobacilli. It is interesting to note that proportions of lactobacilli are not known to be elevated in deep root lesions. This demonstrates further site specificity in dental caries. The frequent isolation and high levels of acidogenic bacteria like *Lactobacillus* suggest that these organisms may be involved in the initial decalcification of dentin prior to the necrosis of the organic matrix.

Table 6/VII. Mean percent of bacterial types in deep dentinal caries [from *Edwardsson*, 1974]

Gram-positive anaerobic rods	44%
facultatively anaerobic rods	38
anaerobic cocci	7
facultatively anaerobic cocci	6
Gram-negative anaerobic cocci	<1
anaerobic rods	<1
Genera: *Lactobacillus* spp.	33%
Arachnia	12
Eubacterium	11
Propionibacterium	11
Bifidobacterium	9
Peptostreptococcus	7
Streptococcus	6
Actinomyces	5
all others	<1 each

Note the dominance of gram-positive over gram-negative forms and especially the high prevalence of *Lactobacillus*. Only 6% of the genera are comprised of streptococci of which *S. mutans* forms only a small part.

Specific and Nonspecific Plaque Hypothesis

There is no question that dental caries is an infection. In the past, and as an extension of *Miller's* chemicoparasitic theory, the total plaque was viewed as a pathogenic structure which had to be eliminated or reduced if caries was to be prevented. If all plaques were similar in their potential to induce caries, the main difference between health and disease states might be expected to be in the quantitative aspects of plaque accumulation. This possibility carries with it the implication that mechanical debridement should be the dominant method of disease control [*Loesche*, 1982]. Further, specific antimicrobial agents would be limited in their efficacy since the accumulation or activity of the whole plaque would require suppression. On the other hand, evidence is impressive that the qualitative nature of the flora in plaque determines the metabolism and the potential for caries production. This view is termed the specific plaque hypothesis. Inherent in this concept is that certain plaques are more cariogenic than others because they contain higher numbers of specific bacterial species that cause caries. The species implicated most often in enamel caries are *S. mutans* and lactobacilli and in root caries *A. viscosus* [*Loesche*, 1982]. According to this hypothesis, most but not necessarily all carious lesions are due to specific bacterial species. Further, the hypothesis implies that plaque in some sites is not disease-producing. The concept of the specific plaque hypothesis suggests the development and implementation of preventive procedures that treat dental caries as a specific bacterial infection. These concepts will be discussed further in vol. 2, chapter 11.

References

Beighton, D.; Russell, R.R.; Hayday, H.: The isolation and characterization of *Streptococcus mutans* serotype h from dental plaque of monkeys (*Macaca fascicularis*). J. gen. Microbial. *124:* 271 (1981).

Berkowitz, R.J.; Jordan, H.V.: Similarity of bacteriocins of *Streptococcus mutans* from mother and infant. Archs oral Biol. *20:* 725 (1975).

Bowen, W.H.: Dental caries in monkeys. Adv. oral Biol. *3:* 185 (1968).

Bratthall, D.: Demonstration of five serological groups of streptococcal strains resembling *Streptococcus mutans*. Odont. Revy *21:* 143 (1970).

Brown, A.T.: Carbohydrate metabolism in caries-conducive, oral streptococci; in Sipple, McNutt, Sugars and nutrition, chap. 38, p. 689 (Academic Press, New York 1974).

Brown, L.R.; Dreizen, S.; Daly, T.E.; Drane, J.B.; Handler, S.; Riggan, L.J.; Johnston, D.A.: Interrelations of oral microorganisms, immunoglobulins and dental caries following radiotherapy. J. dent. Res. *57:* 882 (1978).

Caufield, P.W.; Gibbons, R.J.: Suppression of *Steptococcus mutans* in the mouths of humans by a dental prophylaxis and topically applied iodine. J. dent. Res *58:* 1317 (1979).

Coykendall, A.L.: Genetic heterogeneity of *Streptococcus mutans*. S. Bact. *106:* 192 (1971).

Coykendall, A.L.; Bratthall, D.; O'Connor, K.; Dvarskas, R.A.: Serological and genetic examination of some nontypical *Streptococcus mutans* strains. Infect Immunity *14:* 667 (1976).

Edwardsson, S.: Bacteriological studies on deep areas of carious dentine. Odont Revy *25:* suppl. 32 (1974).

Fitzgerald, R.J.: Gnotobiotic contribution to oral microbiology. J. dent. Res. *42:* 549 (1963).

Fitzgerald, R.J.; Adams, B.O.; Fitzgerald, D.B.; Knox, K.W.: Cariogenicity of human plaque lactobacilli in gnotobiotic rats. J. dent. Res. *60:* 919 (1981).

Fitzgerald, R.J.; Keyes, P.H.: Demonstration of the etiologic role of streptococci in experimental caries in the hamster. J. Am. dent. Ass. *61:* 9 (1960).

Gibbons, R.J.; Houte, J. van: Bacterial adherence in oral microbial ecology. A. Rev. Microbiol. *29:* 19 (1975).

Gibbons, R.J.; Houte, J. van: Bacteriology of dental caries; in Shaw, Sweeney, Cappuccino, Meller, Textbook of oral biology, p. 975 (Saunders, Toronto 1978).

Gibbons, R.J.; Paola, P.F. de; Spinell, D.M.; Skobe, Z.: Interdental localization of *Streptococcus mutans* as related to dental caries experience. Infect. Immunity *9:* 481 (1974).

Hamada, S.; Slade, H.D.: Mechanisms of adherence of *Streptococcus mutans* to smooth surfaces in vitro; in Beachey, Receptors and recognition bacterial adherence, ser. B, vol. 6, p. 105 (Chapman & Hall, London 1980).

Hamada, S.; Tai, S.; Slade, H.D.: Serotype-dependent inhibition of glucan synthesis and cell adherence of *Streptococcus mutans* by antibody against glucosyltransferase of serotype e *S. mutans*. Microbiol. Immunol. *23:* 61 (1979).

Hamilton, I.R.: Effects of fluoride on enzymatic regulation of bacterial carbohydrate metabolism. Caries Res. *11:* suppl. 1, p. 262 (1977).

Hamilton, I.R.; St. Martin, E.J.: Evidence for the involvement of proton motive force in the transport of glucose by a mutant of *Streptococcus mutans* strain DR0001 defective in glucose-phosphoenolpyruvate phosphotransferase activity. Infect. Immunity *36:* 567 (1982).

Hardie, J.M.; Thomson, P.L.; South, R.J.; March, P.D.; Bowden, G.H.; McKee, A.S.; Fillery, D.; Slack, G.L.: A longitudinal epidemiological study on dental plaque and the development of caries – interim results after two years. J. dent. Res. *56:* 90 (1977).

Houte, J. van: Bacterial specificity in the etiology of dental caries. Int. dent. J. *30:* 305 (1980).

Houte, J. van; Gibbs, G.; Butera, C.: Oral flora of children with 'nursing bottle caries'. J. dent. Res. *61:* 382 (1982).

Ikeda, T.; Sandham, H.J.; Bradley, E.L., Jr.: Changes in *Streptococcus mutans* and lactobacilli in relation to the initiation of dental caries in Negro children. Archs oral Biol. *18:* 555 (1973).

Jay, P.: The reduction of oral Lactobacillus counts by the periodic restriction of carbohydrate. Am. J. Orthod. *33:* 162 (1947).

Keyes, P.H.: The infectious and transmissible nature of experimental dental caries. Findings and implications. Archs oral Biol. *1:* 304 (1960).

Kligler, I.J.: Chemical studies of the relations of oral microorganisms to dental caries. J. allied Dent. Soc. *10:* 141 (1915).

Klock, B.; Krasse, B.: Effect of caries-preventive measures in children with high numbers of *S. mutans* and lactobacilli. Scand. J. dent. Res. *86:* 221 (1978).

Köhler, B.; Bratthall, D.; Krasse, B.: Preventive measures in mothers influence the establishment of the bacterium *Streptococcus mutans* in their infants. Archs oral Biol. *28:* 225 (1983).

Littleton, N.W.; Kakehashi, S.; Fitzgerald, R.J.: Recovery of specific caries-inducing streptococci from carious lesions in the teeth of children. Archs oral Biol. *15:* 461 (1970).

Loesche, W.J.: Oral microbiology (University of Michigan Press. Ann Arbor 1980).

Loesche, W.J.: Dental caries. A treatable infection (Thomas, Chicago, 1982).

Loesche, W.J.: Rowan, J; Straffon, L.H.; Loos, P.J.: Association of *Streptococcus mutans* with human dental decay. Infect Immunity *11:* 1252 (1975).

Loesche, W.J.: Svanberg, M.L.: Pope, H.R.: Intraoral transmission of *Streptococcus mutans* by a dental explorer. J. dent. Res. *58:* 1765 (1979).

Mikx, R.H.M.; Hoeven, J.S. van der; König, K.G.; Plasschaert, M.; Guggenheim, B.: Establishment of defined microbial ecosystems in germfree rats. I. Effect of interaction of *Streptococcus mutans* or *Streptococcus sanguis* with *Veillonella alcalescens* on plaque formation and caries activity. Caries Res. *6:* 211 (1972).

Onose, H.; Sandham, H.J.: pH changes during culture of human dental plaque streptococci on Mitis-Salivarius Agar. Archs oral Biol. *21:* 291 (1976).

Perch, B.; Kjems, E.; Ravin T.: Biochemical and serological properties of *Streptococcus mutans* from various human and animal sources. Acta pathol. microbiol. scand., B, Microbiol. Immunol. *82:* 357 (1974).

Ritz, H.L.: Microbial population shifts in developing human plaque Archs oral Biol. *12:* 1561 (1967).

Shklair, I.L.; Keene, H.J.; Cullen, P.: The distribution of *Streptococcus mutans* on the teeth of two groups of naval recruits. Archs oral Biol. *19:* 199 (1974).

Slee, A.M.; Tanzer, J.M.: Phosphoenolpyruvate-dependent sucrose phosphotransferase activity in *Streptococcus mutans* NCTC 10449. Infect. Immunity *24:* 821 (1979).

St. Martin, E.J.; Wittenberger, C.L.: Characterization of a phosphoenolpyruvate-dependent sucrose phosphotransferase system in *Streptococcus mutans*. Infect. Immunity *24:* 865 (1979).

Sumney, D.L.; Jordan, H.V.: Characterization of bacteria isolated from human root surface carious lesions. J. dent. Res. *53:* 343 (1974).

Tanzer, J.M.; Brown, A.T.; Meyers, K.I.: Sucrose dissimilation by *Streptococcus mutans* indeptendently of glucosyl and fructosyl transferase. Int. Ass. dent. Res. Abstr. No. 232 (1972a).

Tanzer, J.M.; Chassy, B.M.; Krichevsky, M.I.: Sucrose metabolism by *Streptococcus mutans* SL-1. Biochem. biophys. Acta *261:* 379 (1972b).

7 Nutrition, Diet (Local Substrate) and Dental Caries

Nutritional Status and Dental Caries

Since man broke from the natural food chain, developed new energy resources and applied technology to food processing our dietary habits have undergone major changes. Both the qualitative nature of our diet and pattern of eating have changed and are changing.

Ingestion of food may affect oral-dental health by both systemic and local mechanisms. Nutritional effects are mediated systematically; dietary effects are mediated locally in the oral cavity. The systemic effects result from the absorption and circulation of nutrients to all cells and tissues and may be mediated through influences on development of teeth, the quality and quantity of salivary secretion, improved host resistance and improved function. Dietary constituents exert their local effects by influencing the metabolism of the oral flora and by modifying salivary flow rates and, indirectly, the qualitative aspect of salivary secretions. Also important is the manner in which food items affect taste perception and condition dietary preferences and patterns of eating. A schematic representation of the mechanism of metabolic preeruptive, and local, posteruptive effect of food on oral health is shown in figure 7/1.

Numerous epidemiological studies have failed to show any clear-cut relationship between nutritional status and dental caries. Indeed, in a study of the caries prevalence of populations in Ethiopia, Thailand, Vietnam and Alaska nutritional deficiences in thiamine, vitamin A and riboflavin have been documented, but the caries levels in these countries was found to be relatively low [*Russell*, 1963]. Neither the great variation in the levels of caries nor its widespread nature (chapter 2) correlates with nutritional status. Paradoxically, the populations of highly industrialized, well nourished nations have a higher prevalence of dental caries than the less affluent peoples of the world and caries can be regarded as a disease arising from the local effects of overconsumption of certain foods. There is no support for the premise that overt malnutrition and high caries experience coexist [*Navia*, 1979]. However, this statement should not be construed as implying that teeth never differ in structure and composition and, therefore, in caries resistance as a result of nutritional influences.

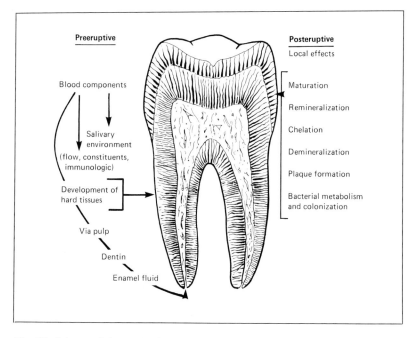

Preeruptive

Blood components

Salivary environment
(flow, constituents, immunologic)

Development of hard tissues

Via pulp

Dentin

Enamel fluid

Posteruptive
Local effects

Maturation

Remineralization

Chelation

Demineralization

Plaque formation

Bacterial metabolism and colonization

Fig. 7/1. Schema of the mechanism of preeruptive (metabolic) and posteruptive (local) effects of food factors on teeth.

What is the reason for this seeming paradox? The reader must be perplexed that studies to date have not yielded concrete evidence demonstrating an increased resistance to caries as a function of proper nutrition. Let us explore this riddle.

A significant point is that dental caries is an interaction between diet, cariogenic flora and the tooth of the host. Significant, also, is the fact that the tooth is relatively passive in the caries process. The environmental challenge to teeth from products of bacterial-substrate reactions is often the most important variable in the caries process. Thus, even teeth that are well-formed and mineralized cannot withstand a strong environmental challenge from the chemical by-products of a highly cariogenic flora and a high concentration of substrate in the oral cavity. Conversely, poorly mineralized teeth may not decay if the local substrate and therefore the concentrations of acidic metabolic by-products of oral bacteria are relatively low.

One should also recognize that nutritional and dietary influences present during the development of teeth are chronologically years apart from the environmental influences that operate on erupted teeth. Diets and eat-

ing patterns change with age, making it difficult to assess nutritional influences on dental tissues.

Chemical analysis of the inorganic constituents of dental tissue has not
disclosed significant differences between carious and noncarious teeth, except for differences in fluoride concentratioins in teeth with a low caries
susceptibility from residents living in a fluoride community as compared to
those in a nonfluoride community. This is a more difficult problem than
might appear at first sight. If enamel from a caries-free tooth is taken for
analysis there is no proof that it would remain caries-free if it had remained
in the mouth. When the apparently sound enamel of a carious tooth is
sampled it is always possible that changes have already occurred as a result
of mild acid attack or from caries of a neighbouring tooth. If there are
subtle differences between teeth that develop under ideal nutritional and
metabolic conditions resulting in a high caries resistance, compared to tissue that develops when nutritional or metabolic deficiencies exist, these
have not yet been uncovered by chemical analysis. More and profitable
may be studies at a molecular level of the crystallinity, degree of dislocation of enamel crystals and degree to which apatite crystals may be calcium
deficient. The suggestion, based on a sophisticated but indirect method
(study of electron spin resonance), that microcrystalline spatial alignment
of hydroxyapatite in enamel may determine the caries resistant properties
of the tissue is intriguing [*Cevc* et al., 1980] but needs corroboration with
more carefully selected enamel samples. There is evidence from animal
experiments that if the diet is so deficient in the nutrients concerned with
mineralization (Ca, P and vitamin D) that highly defective bone is produced, the teeth may be almost normal. The teeth develop as if they had a
priority for taking up deficient nutrients at the expense of bone [*Gaunt and
Irving*, 1940; *Ferguson and Hartles*, 1963]. This is at least partly explained
by the fact that bone may be resorbed to release calcium and phosphorus to
meet general body needs but this does not occur in the teeth.

There are, at least, three dramatic exceptions to the statement that
nutritional status and caries prevalence and unrelated. The first, already
referred to, is that ingestion of trace quantities of fluoride during dental
development enhances the resistance of teeth against caries attack; more
about fluoride in prevention of caries in volume 2. Secondly, vitamin D
affects the development of teeth and, as some unconfirmed evidence suggests, the susceptibility of teeth to caries. Pieces of the fascinating vitamin
D puzzle are only now falling into place although its influence on teeth and
caries has been neglected. Thirdly, it is known from animal experiments,
and suggested by clinical trials in man, that the nutritional and dietary
environment of the tooth immediately after eruption influences its caries
resistance (see Posteruptive Maturation, chapter 4).

Nutritional Influences on Dental Tissues and Caries

Vitamin D

Metabolism of Vitamin D. Vitamin D along with parathyroid hormone and calcitonin play primary roles in regulating the concentration of calcium and inorganic phosphate in the plasma and extracellular fluids, in regulating the movement of these ions into and out of cells and in controlling the mineralization of bones and teeth. Until recently it was believed that vitamin D was the active hormonal compound that cured rickets. It is now clearly established that vitamin D has to be converted by a controlled mechanism to a hormone that regulates calcium and phosphorus metabolism.

The chemistry of vitamin D and its derivatives has been slowly elucidated. Vitamin D_2 is derived by radiation of the naturally occurring substance ergosterol and has for many years been the major synthetic form of vitamin D used for the prevention and cure of rickets in man. Subsequently, the form of vitamin D occurring in the human body, namely D_3 or cholecalciferol (CC), was produced by radiation of 7-dehydrocholesterol which is present in the skin.

It is known that both vitamin D_2 and vitamin D_3 are themselves inactive in vivo. They must first be converted to an hormonal end product by means of two enzymatic hydroxylations before they can exert physiological actions at a target cell. The first metabolic step which takes place in the liver is the conversion of vitamin D to 25-hydroxy vitamin D (25-OH-D_3) by a specific enzyme, vitamin D-25-hydroxylase. The 25-OH-D_3 subsequently undergoes conversion to 1,25 dihydroxy D_3 ($1,25(OH)_2D_3$) in the kidney by the enzyme 25-hydroxyvitamin D-1-hydroxylase. Of the metabolites identified to date, $1:25 (OH)_2D_3$ has the greatest and most rapid effect on the transport of calcium. This compound has all the characteristics of a hormone in that it is produced in the kidney, is transported by the blood to its target tissues (small intestine, bone and kidney) where it has specific effects (calcium and phosphate regulation) and its production is under precise feedback regulation. The metabolic scheme whereby vitamin D is converted to its hormonal end products is illustrated in figure 7/2.

Along with the elucidation of the chemistry considerable progress has been made in the understanding of the physiological functions of the vitamin. It is now well established that small amounts of vitamin D are essential for normal calcium homeostasis. One action that has been conclusively demonstrated is that vitamin D specifically improves intestinal absorption of calcium probably by increasing the synthesis of a calcium-binding protein in the mucosa which is concerned with calcium absorption.

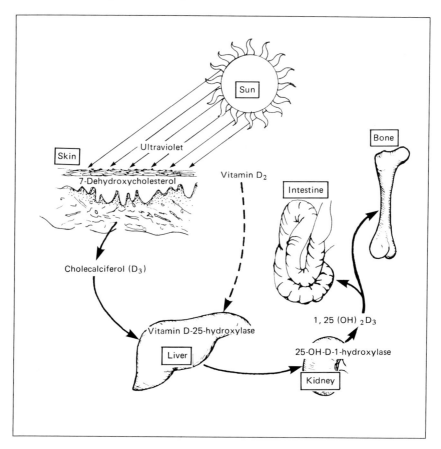

Fig. 7/2. The known metabolic pathways of vitamin D metabolism to its active hormone 1, 25-(OH)$_2$D$_3$.

For a long time now it has been known that in rachitic conditions enamel hypoplasia was frequently observed though it is frequently associated with other systemic conditions (see below). A brief discussion of enamel hypoplasia, its prevalence, etiology and relationship to caries follows.

Enamel Hypoplasia. Enamel hypoplasia is the most common abnormality of development and mineralization of human teeth. The lesion is characterized by a quantitative defect in enamel tissue resulting from an

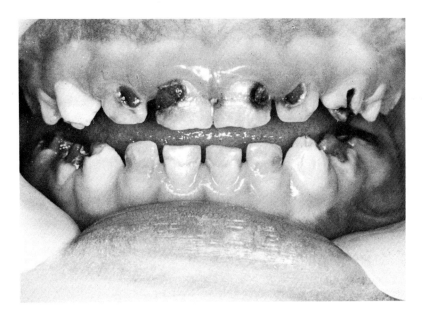

Fig. 7/3. Enamel hypoplasia of primary dentition resulting from hypocalcemia associated with vitamin D dependency rickets [from *Nikiforuk and Fraser*, 1979].

undetermined metabolic injury to the formative cells – the ameloblasts (a rare hereditary type exists but is not discussed here). Clinically, enamel hypoplasia is seen as a roughened surface with discreet pitting or circumferential band-like irregularities which posteruptively acquire a yellow-brown stain. A dentition with typical lesions is depicted in figure 7/3. Enamel hypoplasia is endemic in many countries of the world and is commonly reported in association with diseases of childhood. Although the specific biochemical determinant of this lesion has not been definitely elucidated, recent evidence suggests that it is linked specifically to defects in the homeostasis of calcium [*Nikiforuk and Fraser*, 1981].

Some years ago population surveys in several countries showed that 3–15% of children exhibited some degree of enamel hypoplasia in permanent teeth [*Pindborg*, 1970]. However, the incidence of this lesion is significantly higher in vitamin D deficiency, hereditary vitamin D dependency rickets, hypoparathyroidism, and a wide spectrum of perinatal disorders. Earlier reports which implicated German measles (Rubella) during pregnancy as a major factor in enamel hypoplasia have been definitely disproven [*Grahnén*, 1958; *Lundstrom* et al., 1962].

A specific type of enamel hypoplasia of primary teeth called linear enamel hypoplasia (LEH) is common in some economically underdeveloped countries (chapter 1, fig. 1/3). For example, its prevalence has been reported to be about 30–40% in Guatemala and in parts of the Caribbean coast. In children, who have signs of severe malnutrition, linear hypoplasia was present in up to 73% of the population [*Sweeney* et al., 1971]. Enamel hypoplasia resembling the linear type has been reported in association with acute diarrheal disease in preschool Apache Indian children [*Infante* et al., 1975; *Woodward* et al., 1974]. Although the pathophysiology of LEH is undetermined, many authors have suggested the synergistic action of malnutrition and infection as the most probable causative factors. A more probable factor is hypocalcemia induced by gastrointestinal diarrhea as discussed below.

Hypocalcemia, a Specific Cause of Enamel Hypoplasia. Recently evidence has suggested that the etiology of enamel hypoplasia is highly specific and linked with disorders of calcium homeostasis. In a study of children with chronic disorders of calcium and phosphate homeostasis, enamel hypoplasia was found in conditions characterized by hypocalcemia (hereditary vitamin D dependency rickets and hypoparathyroidism), but not in those characterized by hypophosphatemia (X-linked hypophosphatemic rickets) [*Nikiforuk and Fraser*, 1981]. The occurrence of enamel hypoplasia, therefore, bore no relation to the serum phosphate concentration. Enamel hypoplasia has also been reported in many other pediatric disorders in which hypocalcemia is a major sign, for example severe vitamin D deficiency, prematurity, gastroenteritis, and neonatal tetany. These observations lead to the general hypothesis that low serum calcium concentration during enamel formation is a specific determinant of enamel hypoplasia; this mechanism is illustrated in figure 7/4.

Enamel Hypoplasia and Caries. Enamel hypoplasia is clinically significant not only because it is disfiguring and the restorative treatment costly, but because it may affect caries susceptibility. *Mellanby* [1936] reported that there was a strong correlation between hypoplasia in the teeth of British schoolchildren (which she thought was caused by vitamin D deficiency) and caries susceptibility. For example, out of a collection of 1,500 extracted teeth, 74% of very hypoplastic teeth were carious, whereas 80% of the nonhypoplastic teeth were caries-free. Several other surveys have supported this conclusion [*Allen*, 1941; *Bibby*, 1943; *Carr* 1953]. Caries has also been associated with hypoplasia in many parts of the Third World [*Schamschula* et al., 1978]. There is no information about the chemical composition of hypoplastic enamel so the exact reason for its greater

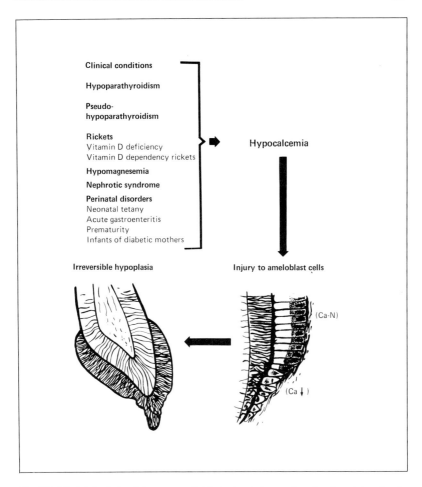

Fig. 7/4. Model depicting injury to ameloblasts due to hypocalcemia. A variety of systemic diseases such as rickets, hypoparathyroidism and perinatal disorders are associated with hypocalcemia and enamel hypoplasia (Ca-N, normal calcium) [*Nikiforuk and Fraser*, 1981].

proneness to caries is uncertain, but it is possible that its irregularity and pits may favor the development of more plaque compared with smooth well-formed enamel.

In an important study of children with LEH, *Infante and Gillespie* [1977] found a significantly higher incidence of caries even in the posterior hypoplasia-free teeth of children whose incisors had LEH than in those who did not have this condition. Also, the prevalence of enamel hypoplasia and dental caries is higher in prematurely born children than in controls [*Rosenzweig and Sahar*, 1962]. Thus, evidence is strong that the factor responsible for hypoplasia of the linear type also predisposes to dental caries. Prevention of enamel hypoplasia in the Third World would portend a major reduction in caries prevalence in the affected populations.

Vitamin A

In vitamin A-deficient animals, atrophic changes in the ameloblasts, subsequent abnormalities in tooth morphology and a reduced number of salivary acini in the major and minor salivary glands has been observed. Addition of vitamin A to the diet of animals, posteruptively, does not affect the number or extent of the carious lesions. In a study of persons with vitamin A deficiency sufficiently severe to cause xerophathalmia, slight hypoplasia was found in only one quarter of the sample and many had perfectly formed teeth in spite of their deficiency. Evidently in man, severe vitamin A deficiency during tooth formation does not necessarily lead to defective enamel.

Other Vitamins and Caries

The only member of the vitamin B complex which has been associated with caries is pyridoxine (vitamin B_6). This vitamin has been stated to reduce caries in rats but the effect was not confirmed on monkeys [*Cole* et al., 1980]. Very high doses (some 10 times the normal dose) have been reported in two small scale experiments in human subjects (pregnant women and schoolchildren) to reduce caries. It is not suggested that a deficiency of pyridoxine is responsible for caries but that large unphysiological doses, in which pyridoxine is being used as a drug rather than as a vitamin, reduced caries by modifying the oral flora.

Lipids

Deficiency of essential fatty acids in man is rare and evaluation of the role of these nutrients on caries rates is not available. As more food is processed it is possible that nutritional deficiencies may increase in the population that subsist primarily on such foods.

Fat, consumed posteruptively in diets of animals, has been correlated with caries reduction. The mechanism of action of fats in reducing caries may be due to a combination of several factors. The enamel surface may be protected from demineralization by the formation of fatty films but this is unlikely in approximal areas. Another factor may be that contact between carbohydrate foods and bacteria is reduced in the presence of fat. Certain fatty acids in the diet have an antimicrobial action, but whether this occurs in the mouth has not been adequately studied [*Williams* et al., 1982].

Protein Deficiency

Gross protein deficiencies are rare in modern industrialized countries but occur in many economically deprived regions where kwashiorkor is prevalent. The caries rate of this population is considerably less than in populations on an adequate diet. This is probably related to the low intake of cariogenic food, and reduced frequency of eating of refined carbohydrate. The effect of protein and calorie deficiencies in animal caries models is discussed below.

It is almost certain that the last word has not been written about optimal nutrition in man and its role in host (tooth and salivary secretions) resistance to caries. This statement is supported by evidence that severe nutritional deficiencies in experimental animals are known to affect development of teeth and salivary glands and increase their susceptibility to dental caries [*Navia*, 1979].

Experimental Animal Studies

Protein and Calorie Deficiency and Dental Caries

Several studies, reviewed by *Shaw* [1970] and *Navia* [1979], show that in rats, protein deficiency during dental development induced by underfeeding the mothers during pregnancy and lactation led to smaller teeth, a delay in eruption, and a greater susceptibility to caries. Restriction of caloric intake by the mothers to 80% of normal led to lower body weight of the offspring but none of the dental effects of protein deficiency occurred. In a series of experiments *Navia* [1979] produced a protein calorie deficiency in rat pups by reducing the milk output of rat dams through a low protein (8%) diet. The results of the these studies indicated that protein deficiency in suckling pups produced severe retardation in development and eruption of teeth. The dental defects could be reversed by the administration of a protein supplement to the malnourished pups; however, a caloric supplementation, per se, did not correct the dental abnormalities. Total salivary volume and salivary protein levels were also significantly reduced. A logical extension of these findings was to determine if a protein malnutrition during tooth development affects caries susceptibility. When experimental and control rat pups were placed on a cariogenic diet it was found that the animal previously malnourished due to a protein deficiency had a significantly higher caries susceptibility than the controls.

The precise mechanism by which protein deprivation in animals induces a higher caries susceptibility is not clear. The following factors probably contribute: reduced salivary flow and therefore reduced total buffering capacity, a reduced remineralizing and antibacterial activity; altered morphology of dentition; decrease in the immune response as mediated by both the humoral T-cell immune mechanisms. A decrease in immune response due to protein deficiency has been reported in man as well as experimental animals.

Calcium and Phosphate in Diet and Tooth Composition
There is no evidence that deficiencies in calcium and phosphate in westernized countries are severe enough to affect composition of the teeth. The mechanisms controlling the calcium concentration of plasma are such that only very severe deficiencies are likely to affect the supply of minerals to the developing tooth. Early work suggesting that hard water reduced caries has not been reinvestigated by modern epidemiological methods but if true is likely to be explained by trace elements (e.g. fluoride or strontium) or by effects of the calcium of the hard water on the environment of the tooth than on enamel structure. While severe deficiencies in calcium and phosphorus are rare in industrialized countries, hypocalcemia may occur in conjunction with some diseases of childhood, such as severe diarrhea during infancy and celiac disease, as noted earlier in this chapter.

Dietary Studies on Controlled Human Populations

In chapter 4 it is noted that caries-immune teeth do not exist. Even teeth formed under ideal nutritional conditions are prone to dental caries if the local conditions are highly cariogenic. Therefore, the single most important determinant of cariogenicity in the oral cavity is the availability of a suitable local substrate for the oral flora. The conclusion that foodstuffs and plaque bacteria interact locally on tooth surfaces to cause caries logically leads to several questions. Is diet the major factor contributing to the dramatic rise in the prevalence of dental caries during the last 150 years? What constituents or properties of foods determine their cariogenicity? What is the mechanism by which wartime diets reduced dental caries? Is sucrose the unique dietary constituent that potentiates caries? These questions are explored next.

As described in detail in chapter 2, carious lesions were sparse in ancient man but increased dramatically in the industrialized world. The increase in carious lesions observed in isolated populations such as the Canadian Eskimo correlated with their adoption of dietary habits of the mainland. Epidemiological studies in many parts of the world support the hypothesis that the increase in caries was associated with dietary changes. Three major studies on controlled human populations have greatly extended and refined our knowledge about the role of diet and dental caries. These studies are summarized and the practical aspects emphasized.

Hopewood Study in Australia

Studies on children living under controlled conditions are difficult enough, but to find a group whose diet is devoid of refined carbohydrates is indeed a rare opportunity. In 1942 an eccentric, wealthy Australian businessman transformed what was formerly a spacious country mansion, Hopewood House, into a 'motherhouse' for young children at Bowral, N.S.W., Australia. Since the businessman had attributed his own dramatic recovery in health to a drastic change in dietary habits, he stipulated that the children of Hopewood House should be raised on a natural diet that excluded refined carbohydrates. A population of 80 children equally divided as to sex, were admitted to the home in early infancy. They ranged in age from 7 to 14 years at the end of a 10-year period [*Sullivan and Harris*, 1958; *Harris*, 1963].

The basically vegetarian diet of these children was adequate but spartan with regard to sugars. It consisted of the carbohydrates contained in wholemeal bread, wholemeal porridge, biscuits, wheatgerm, fresh and dried fruit, vegetables (cooked and raw), along with butter, cheese, eggs, milk and fruit juices. A small amount of meat was included in the diet up to 1948–1949, after which meat was practically excluded from the diet. The meals were supplemented by vitamin concentrates and an occasional serving of nuts and a sweetening agent such as honey or molasses. The food was uncooked as far as possible in order to retain its natural state. The most striking feature of this diet was the notable absence of white or brown sugar and sugar-flour confections. The fluoride content of the water and food was insignificant and no tea was consumed. All meals and between-meal eating were controlled with great regularity. Now there's a toothsome diet!

At the end of a 10-year period, the 13-year-old children of Hopewood House had a mean DMF per child of 1.6; the corresponding figure for the general child population of the State of N.S.W. was 10.7. Only 0.4% of the 13-year-old state school children were free from dental caries, whereas 53% of the Hopewood children experienced no caries (fig. 7/5). The general health of the children was considered good but not superior to the general population; more of the Hopewood children were in the lower percentiles of height and weight than was expected.

The childrens' oral hygiene was poor, dental calculus was uncommon, but gingivitis was prevalent in about 75% of the children. This work shows that in institutionalized children, at least, dental caries can be reduced to

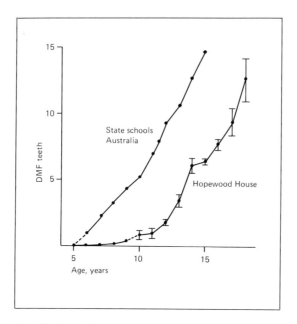

Fig. 7/5. Plot of the mean number of DMF teeth per child versus chronological age in state schools of Australia and in children of Hopewood House [adapted from *Marthaler*, 1967].

insignificant levels by a spartan diet, and without the beneficial influence of fluoride and in the presence of unfavorable oral hygiene. It is usual for children living in communal homes even on a normal diet to have a lower caries rate than comparable children living with their parents, probably because sugar-containing foods are not available between meals. Only part of the difference found in Hopewood House can, therefore, be attributed to the nature of the diet.

Vipeholm Study in Sweden
   In 1939, the Swedish Government requested the Royal Medical Board to investigate 'what measures should be taken to reduce the frequency of the most common dental disease in Sweden'. This request led to a study at the Vipeholm Hospital, Lund, an institution for mentally defective individuals, of the relationship between diet and dental caries. This hospital, with its large numbers of practically permanent patients, provided an opportunity for a longitudinal study under well-controlled conditions. The

purpose of the study was to find answers to the following questions: (1) 'Does an increase in carbohydrate (mostly sugar) intake cause an increase in dental caries? If so, is caries acitivity influenced by: (a) the ingestion at meals of refined sugar in a nonsticky form; (b) the ingestion at meals of sugar in a sticky form: and (c) the ingestion between meals of sugar in a sticky form. (2) Does a decrease in carbohydrate (sugar) intake produce a decrease in dental caries?'

A comparable study on human subjects will almost certainly never be repeated as it now would be regarded as unethical to alter diets experimentally in directions likely to increase caries (or any other disease). Because of the significance of the Vipeholm study, it is described in detail.

The 436 patients involved in this study were divided into 1 control and 6 experimental groups. In order to maintain strict control over the diets they were allocated to patients in different wards of the hospital. Four meals were eaten daily. All patients received for 1 year a diet relatively low in sugar, with no sugar in-between meals, during which the average number of new carious lesions was extremely low (0.34 new carious surfaces per patient). Subsequently, the effects on caries of dietary changes, involving the addition of large sucrose supplements in sticky and nonsticky form, either with or between meals, were assessed. The plan and results of the Vipeholm study are described by *Gustafsson* et al. [1954], and summarized by *Davies* [1955]. A description of the groups follows.

The control group consisted of 60 males, average age 34.9 years who, for 2 years, received a low carbohydrate (mostly starch), high fat diet practically free from refined sugar. Caries activity was almost completely suppressed. After 2 years this diet was replaced by an ordinary diet to which was added 110 g of sugar a day at mealtimes which was accompanied by a small but statistically significant rise in caries activity (fig. 7/6).

The procedures in the other groups were as follows: The sucrose group received 300 g (later raised to 370 g) of sucrose in solution at mealtimes which did not result in a significant rise in caries.

The bread group was subdivided into male and female groups and received once daily with their afternoon coffee during the first 2 experimental years, 345 g of sweet bread containing 50 g of sugar which did not produce a demonstrable increase in caries. During the second 2 years, 4 portions of sweet bread were given daily with all meals resulting in a significant increase in caries, more in the males than in the females.

The chocolate group received the same sugar with meals (300 g) as the sucrose group during the first 2 years which was reduced to 110 g supplemented by 65 g of milk chocolate between meals during the second 2 years, resulting in a 4-fold increase in caries.

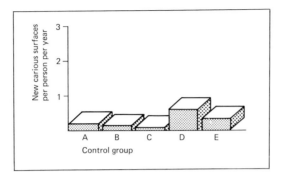

Fig. 7/6. The effect of frequency and form of carbohydrate intake on dental caries activity. Control group in the Vipeholm study (see text) [*Davies*, 1955].

After 2 control years, the caramel group received 22 caramels daily in 2 portions between meals during the third year, changed in the fourth year to 22 caramels in 4 portions between meals. Caries increased during the third year and more so during the fourth year, and than dropped to the control level in the fifth year when the caramels were withdrawn and replaced by an isocaloric quantity of fat with meals.

The 8-toffee group showed a similar rise in caries during the third, fourth and fifth years when they received 8 toffees in two portions (third year) and in four portions (fourth and fifth years).

The 24-toffee group showed the greatest increase in caries of all the groups, a rise of DMF of 6, during the 2 years in which they received 24 toffees between meals followed by a sharp drop in the fifth year when the toffees were withdrawn (fig. 7/7). The effects of carbohydrate type and frequency of eating on caries in all groups are summarized in figures 7/8 and 7/9a, b.

The main conclusions of the Vipeholm study summarized by the authors are as follows:

'The risk of sugar increasing caries activity is great if the sugar is consumed in a form with a strong tendency to be retained on the surfaces of the teeth.

The risk of sugar increasing caries activity is greatest if the sugar is consumed between meals and in a form in which the tendency to be retained on the surfaces of the teeth is pronounced with a transiently high concentration of sugar on these surfaces (fig. 7/9a, b).

Increase in caries activity due to the intake of sugar-rich foodstuffs consumed in a manner favoring caries disappears on withdrawal of such foodstuffs from the diet.

Carious lesions may continue to appear despite the avoidance of refined sugar, maximum restriction of natural sugars and total dietary carbohnydrates.

The risk of an increase in caries activity is intensified with an increase in the duration of sugar clearance from the saliva.'

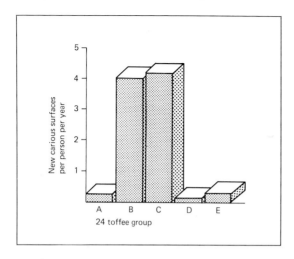

Fig. 7/7. Caries experience in 48 males in the Vipeholm study who used a basic diet in years A and D and ingested 24 toffees between meals during years B and C [*Davies*, 1955].

These important conclusions will be applied and expanded within the context of dietary management of caries in vol. 2, chapter 8. In spite of being probably the most ambitious experiment ever carried out on human caries the Vipeholm experiment did suffer from some inherent defects in design. This is not surprising considering that it was planned in the 1940s – a time at which very few large-scale clinical experiments had been attempted. The various groups were made up from the patients in individual wards, consequently with no possibility of matching the age or initial caries of the subjects, although this objection was partly met by the plan that each group acted as its own control. The patients were mentally handicapped and did not always understand or follow the instructions correctly. Also, the dietary regimes of the various groups were not changed in a consistent pattern, some groups having longer periods of sugar with meals than others.

Turku Study
Another large-scale and important experiment on caries in human subjects was carried out in Turku, Finland, and reported in detail by *Scheinin and Makinen* [1975] – the aim being to compare the cariogenicity of sucrose, fructose and xylitol. The basis of the experiment is that xylitol is a sweet substance not metabolized by plaque organisms (for a general account of xylitol, see vol. 2, chapter 9). 125 subjects of average age 27.6 years (with an undesirably wide range from younger than 15 to over 45 and with more

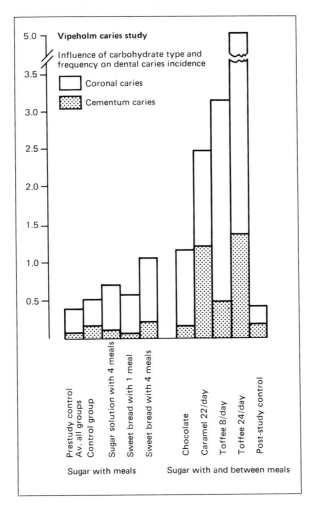

Fig. 7/8. Summary of the Vipeholm caries study of the influence of carbohydrate type and frequency on dental caries [from *Burgess*, unpublished].

than half over the age of 25, i.e. an age usually with a low caries increment) were divided into three groups partly on a basis of their own preference. One group received their ordinary sucrose-containing diet, in the second group sucrose was almost entirely replaced by xylitol and in the third group by fructose. About 100 food items including pastries, candies, chewing gum, pickles, mustard and even cough mixture were made with the two alternative sugars.

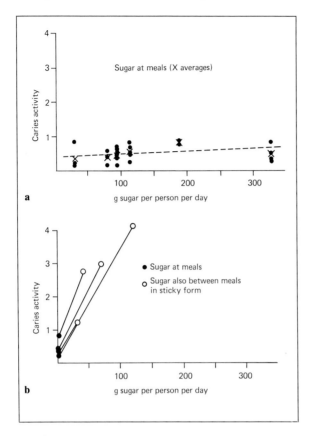

Fig. 7/9a, b. The relationship between sugar consumption at meals and between meals, and caries activity observed in the Vipeholm study [*Gustafsson* et al., 1954].

One set of the published results included scores for very early white spot ('incipient') lesions which were much more numerous than the frank 'lesions with defect', i.e. cavitation. This accounts for the very high scores– an annual DMFS of 3.6 in the sucrose group, higher than other figures for caries in Finland even for children. The results after 1 year (fig. 7/10) suggested that sucrose and fructose had equal cariogenicity whereas xylitol produced almost no caries. By the second year, caries had continued to increase in the sucrose group but remained unchanged in the fructose group implying that sucrose was more cariogenic than fructose. The DMFS in the xylitol group fell to zero at 2 years; evidently some early white spot lesions had been remineralized to a point where they could not be scored.

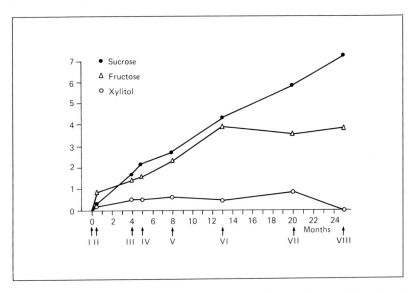

Fig. 7/10. Increase in DMFS surfaces in the three groups in the Turku experiment based on clinical and radiographic findings and including white spots [from *Scheinin and Makinen*, 1975, with permission].

These results of the comparison of sucrose and fructose were ambiguous but xylitol was shown to be either noncariogenic (i.e. does not promote caries) or because of the number of reversals even anticariogenic (actively preventing caries).

Later, the 2-year results based on advanced cavities, disregarding white spots, were published [*Scheinin*, 1979], and although they showed a lower DMFS increment for xylitol (1.47) than for sucrose (3.33), the difference (56%) was much smaller than in the previous result. The average score for fructose (3.57) implied that it had virtually the same cariogenicity as sucrose.

In a second 1-year trial to test the effects of a xylitol-containing chewing gum, 102 subjects, average age 22.2 years, were assigned randomly to two groups – one chewing a gum containing sucrose (an average of 4.2 sticks a day) and the other using a xylitol-containing gum (4.9 sticks a day). The caries score rose from the initial value with the sucrose gum and fell in the xylitol group (fig. 7/11). Evidently, the saliva stimulated by the gum remineralized early existing lesions at a greater rate than new lesions formed or, less likely, xylitol exerted an anticariogenic effect.

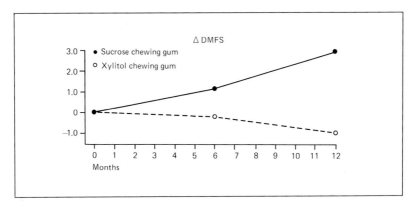

Fig. 7/11. Changes in DMFS during 1 year in which chewing gum containing either sucrose or xylitol was used [from *Scheinin and Makinen*, 1975, with permission].

Experimental Production of Caries in Man

A method for inducing 'white spots', presumed to be incipient dental caries, on a short-term basis, in volunteer dental students, has been tried in Denmark [*von der Fehr* et al., 1970] and Britain [*Edgar* et al., 1978]. The procedures followed in these studies were 9 daily rinses with 10 ml of 50% sucrose and discontinuance of active oral hygiene procedures. The original experiments lasted for 3 weeks and white-spot lesions on smooth surfaces were produced in the experimental group. The British workers obtained a similar result within 2 weeks (or even two separate 9-day periods with tooth-brushing after the end of the first 9 days). The rapidity with which initial carious lesions were observed, in contrast to the slow rate of caries progression under normal clinical conditions, is related to the high cariogenic challenge. The dense bacterial plaque accumulation when oral hygiene procedures are suspended and the protracted high concentration of substrate produce a highly cariogenic environment. At the end of the experiment meticulous oral hygiene measures were reinstituted along with a daily mouthrinse of 0.2% NaF. These procedures resulted in remineralization of the white spots and a reversal of the caries index scores to the same values as in the control group.

The method employed in this clinical study on humans may have merit in short-term investigations of cariogenic properties of food or the potential of caries-inhibiting agents. A difficulty is that different subjects in the same group do not always respond in the same way and it is difficult to recruit and organize sufficiently large groups to provide statistically significant results.

Effect of Wartime Dietary Restrictions on Caries

A unique situation arose in several European countries involved in the Second World War, and in Japan, as a result of rationing. Wartime dietary restrictions in these countries, but analyzed particularly in Norway and Switzerland, resulted generally in an increase in consumption of potatoes, fish, cod liver oil, vegetables and unrefined flour and a decrease in the consumption of fat, meat, sugar, sugar products, syrup, and flour of low extraction. An analysis of the dental caries rates in the Scandinavian countries by *Toverud* [1957] (fig. 7/12) indicates that in 7- and 8-year-old children the caries rates in permanent molars decreased dramatically about 1-3 years after reduction in sugar intake. The caries rates increased sharply 1-2 years after the rise of sucrose in the postwar diets of children. Similar findings were reported in Japan and Switzerland [*Takeuchi*, 1961; *Marthaler*, 1967].

Some authors have interpreted the lag period between the reduction of sugar consumption and the maximum caries reduction as related to the nutritional influences of wartime diets upon the development of teeth and not simply due to the local dietary effects of substrate reduction. However, careful analysis of the data does not support this view. The lag period is more easily explained on the basis of local factors: the time period required for the reduction of plaque cariogenic flora and especially the time required for cavitation to develop. It is possible that those teeth that erupted during the period of maximum sucrose reduction had prolonged periods of surface maturation that was not interrupted by carious attacks and that this may have resulted in increased resistance to subsequent caries attack. However, the interpretation that teeth developing and mineralizing during the period coinciding with the greatest restriction in sugar intake benefited from the improved nutritional influences of wartime diets is questionable. The withdrawal of local substrate in the form of sucrose is more probably the dominant factor that reduced cariogenicity of wartime diets.

Carbohydrate Intolerance and Dental Caries

Several hereditary conditions in man have been described which result in an inability to metabolize a specific sugar. Intolerance to disaccharide or monosaccharide occurs because of a deficiency of a specific enzyme involved in the metabolism of the sugar. A condition known as hereditary fructose intolerance provides evidence of a direct link between sugar ingestion and dental caries.

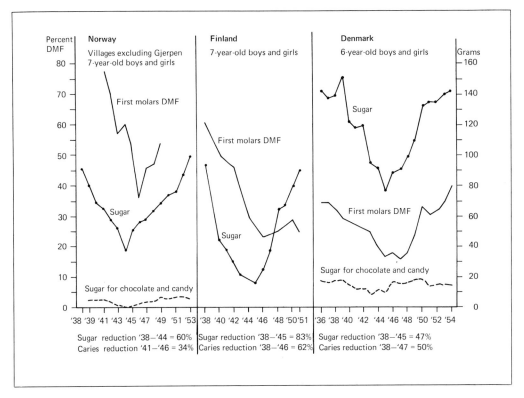

Fig. 7/12. The percentages of decayed, missing and filled first permanent molars among 7-year-old boys and girls in Norway, Finland, and Denmark are shown for the years during and immediately after World War II. In addition, the average percentage reductions in the amount of total sugar and the sugar available for chocolate and candy manufacture are shown for the same interval [*Toverud*, 1957].

Hereditary Fructose Intolerance

In 1959, *Froesch* described an inborn error of fructose metabolism transmitted by an autosomal recessive gene. This condition results in episodes of pallor, nausea, vomiting, coma and convulsion following ingestion of fruit containing fructose or cane sugar. In persons with this condition fructose tolerance tests show marked hypoglycemia (as low as 8 mg/ 100 ml); the hypoglycemia is characterized by its unresponsiveness to glucagon, a hormone known to raise blood glucose by a stimulation of the glycogen breakdown in the liver. There is, also, a sharp rise in blood fructose concentration and a drop in serum phosphorus levels. The metabolic

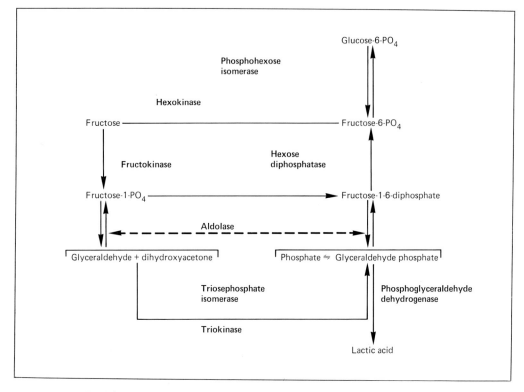

Fig. 7/13. Metabolism of fructose showing that the main deficiency in hereditary fructose intolerance is a deficiency of fructose-1-phosphate aldolase (heavy dotted line).

error in this condition is due to deficiency of hepatic fructose-1-phosphate aldolase as depicted in figure 7/13. This causes a cellular accumulation of fructose-1-phosphate which in turn inhibits fructose phosphorylation.

Persons afflicted with hereditary fructose intolerance (HFI) develop, early in life, symptoms of the condition when given a formula or diet containing sucrose. Treatment consists of complete dietary exclusion of sucrose; although other carbohydrates, such as glucose, lactose, and galactose, may be included. It is important that early diagnosis and treatment be initiated in order to prevent cerebral damage that may follow the hypoglycemia.

Persons with HFI show a strikingly reduced dental caries experience when compared to a control population of the same age [*Marthaler*, 1967]. Reports on persons with HFI are not detailed enough to express the caries experience in terms of DMFT scores, but reveal that about 50% of the population are caries-free. If carious lesions are present they are limited to the most susceptible pit and fissure surfaces.

In addition to HFI several other intolerances to disaccharides or monosaccharides have been reported although their significance in relation to dental caries experience is unknown. Of particular interest are individuals who are deficient in carbohydrate-splitting enzymes such as intestinal sucrose-isomaltase, and maltase. Improvement is rapid following removal of sucrose and starch from the diet of these patients. These conditions are relatively uncommon and the dental caries information of afflicted individuals is lacking. It would be interesting to know whether caries data on such persons confirm the role of sucrose in caries production.

Dietary Constituents and Cariogenicity

Beyond the classical Hopewood and Vipeholm studies, data on cariogenicity of foods in humans are sparse. It is not practical to subject the myriads of foods developed by new technological processes to clinical trials. We have to rely upon epidemiological studies, laboratory data, dental plaque studies, nutritional and dietary surveys and other relevant data in order to define cariogenic determinants of food. We shall now synthesize a large volume of information, often inadequate, in order to determine the main dietary constituent(s), dietary properties and patterns of food consumption that are associated with dental caries.

Constituents: Polysaccharides and Sugars

The four carbohydrates starch, sucrose, fructose and glucose comprise the greatest proportion of foods consumed by man. The main polysaccharide (starch) is not highly cariogenic in animals or man at least in some circumstances. Populations in countries such as Japan and Italy are known to consume large amounts of starch in the form of rice, macaroni and spaghetti, but their caries rates are relatively low. On the other hand, controlled studies in experimental animals and in humans have confirmed that excessive and frequent use of highly fermentable mono- and disaccharides is correlated with high caries rates. While glucose, fructose, lactose and mannose have been shown to be cariogenic in animal experiments they are usually minor constituents of human foods as they are present only in dried fruits, honey and milk. Sucrose is by far the commonest dietary sugar. In North America this single dietary item contributes to more than one half of the total carbohydrate consumed and because sucrose dominates dietary sugar it is the carbohydrate most related to caries. Because of the significance of carbohydrates in caries chapter 8 is devoted to a discussion of the patterns of consumption of carbohydrates in American diets and to the role of sucrose.

Physical Properties of Foods and Cariogenicity

We know little about the significance of physical properties of foods and their effect on cariogenicity, since few studies involving human subjects have been conducted to explore this relationship. Some important physical properties that determine food texture are: (1) mechanical properties: hardness, cohesiveness, viscosity, adhesiveness; (2) geometric properties: particle size and shape; (3) others: moisture and fat content.

Texture of food and subjective descriptions of food items by the use of terms as soft-hard, crumbly-brittle, tender-tough, sticky-gooey, gritty-coarse, dry-moist arise from their physical properties [*Caldwell*, 1970].

From a dental standpoint the physical properties of food may have significance by affecting food retention, food clearance, solubility and oral hygiene (plaque reduction). The incorporation of dyes into toffee [*MacGregor*, 1958] demonstrated the tenacious retention of candy on enamel surfaces. Adhesive properties of food have been measured and correlated with their retention in the mouth after ingestion.

The high fibrous, cellulose content of plant food exerts a mechanical cleansing action on teeth and eating of raw fruits and vegetables has long been recommended as an aid to oral hygiene and also as a caries preventive measure. Clinical studies have not confirmed that physical parameters are as important as the frequency of eating, in determining cariogenicity of foods. A study on the effect of apples and dental health gave indications of caries reduction, but initial differences in caries score of the 'control' and 'apple' group made comparisons more difficult [*Slack and Martin*, 1958]. Other fibrous vegetables as raw carrots and celery also exert mechanical cleansing effects, and are not as strongly acidic as apples. A clinical study [*Reece and Swallow*, 1970] in which carrots were eaten after the midday meal did not result in a significant reduction in caries in schoolchildren. On the other hand, addition of water to an experimental animal diet, or modification of particle size of a diet, is known to induce significant effects on caries in animals.

The physical texture and chemical composition of food is known to effect salivary flow rates. Saliva that is rapidly flowing is more alkaline than resting saliva and more supersaturated with calcium and phosphate, and thus may be more caries-inhibitory.

Physical properties of food, particularly those that improve the cleansing action and reduce the retention of food within the oral cavity and increase saliva flow, are to be encouraged in everyday diets. However, clinical evidence that consumption of these food items will significantly reduce caries, per se, is lacking.

Natural versus Processed Foods. The concept that natural, unrefined foods contain protective factors against dental caries has long been expounded. The idea originated with experiments which indicated that saliva incubated with refined foods caused a greater dissolution of tooth enamel than when incubated with unrefined foods. Mixtures that included bran, wheat germ and unrefined treacle and cane juice contained protective factors. The protective substance in the studies with cereals was identified as phytate – a polyphosphate. Phytate when applied to tooth enamel reduces its solubility and has caries-inhibiting effects when added to animal diets but its effect on caries in man has not been tested [reviewed by *Jenkins*, 1966].

Acidity of Foods

Some dietary items are highly acidic and therefore affect, usually in a transient manner, the pH in plaque and saliva. Natural foods, such as lemons, apples, fruit juices and carbonated beverages, are sufficiently acidic as to cause demineralization of enamel that is in prolonged contact with them. These items, under normal dietary use, are of no consequence in the dental caries process. However, excessive (habitual) use of these foods and beverages may cause etching of enamel with cavitation. Reports of excessive frequency of consumption of carbonated beverages, having a low pH, and continuous chewing or habitual sucking of lemons as a cause of dental erosion is well documented. Thus, habitual use of highly acidic foods should be discouraged.

Distinction should be made between destruction of teeth by a carious process and dissolution of enamel by chemical erosion. In the former process, the production of acids by bacteria acting on a substrate is essential; in the latter, enamel is dissolved by excessive and frequent contact with ingested fluids of low pH (usually below 4).

References

Allen, I.: A survey of nutrition and dental caries in 120 London elementary schoolchildren. Br. med. J. *i:* 44 (1941).

Bibby, B.G.: The relationship between microscopic hypoplasia (Mellanby) and dental caries (abstract). J. dent. Res. *22:* 218 (1943).

Caldwell, R.C.: Physical properties of foods and their caries-producing potential. J. dent. Res. *49:* 1293 (1970).

Carr, L.M.: Correlation between Mellanby hypoplasia and dental caries. Dent. J. Aust. *25:* 158 (1953).

Cevc, G.; Cevc, P.; Schara, M.: The caries resistance of human teeth is determined by the spatial arrangement of hydroxyapatite microcrystals in the enamel. Nature, Lond. *286:* 425 (1980).

Cole, M.F.; Eastoe, J.E.; Curtis, M.A.; Korts, D.C.; Bowen, W.H.: Effects of pyridoxine, phytate and invert sugar on plaque composition and caries activity in the monkey (*Macaca fascicularis*). Caries Res. *14:* 1 (1980).

Davies, G.N.: An appreciation of the Vipeholm study of dental caries. N.Z. dent. J. *51:* 153 (1955).

Edgar, W.M.; Geddes, D.A.M.; Jenkins, G.N.; Rugg-Gunn, A.J.; Howell, R.: Effects of calcium glycerophosphate and sodium fluoride on the induction in vivo of caries-like changes in human dental enamel. Archs oral Biol. *23:* 655 (1978).

Fehr, F.R. von der; Löe, H.; Theilade, E.; Experimental caries in man. Caries Res. *4:* 131 (1970).

Ferguson, H.W.; Hartles, R.L.: The effect of vitamin D on the bones of young rats receiving diets low in calcium or phosphorus. Archs oral Biol. *8:* 407 (1963).

Gaunt, W.E.; Irving, J.T.: The influence of dietary calcium and phosphorus upon tooth formation. J. Physiol., Lond. *99:* 18 (1940).

Grahnén, H.: Maternal rubella and dental defects. Odont. Revy *9:* 181 (1958).

Gustafsson, B.E.; Quensel, C.E.; Lanke, L.S.; Lundqvist, C.; Grahnén, H.; Bonow, B.E.; Krasse, B.: The Vipeholm dental caries study. The effect of different levels of carbohydrate intake on caries activity in 436 individuals observed for five years. Acta odont. scand. *11:* 232 (1954).

Harris, R.S.: Biology of the children of Hopewood House, Bowral, Australia. IV. Observation of dental caries experience extending over five years 1956–61. J. dent. Res. *42:* 1387 (1963).

Infante, P.F.; Gillespie, G.M.: Enamel hypoplasia in relation to caries in Guatemalan children. J. dent. Res. *56:* 493 (1977).

Infante, P.F.; Owen, G.M.; Russell, A.L.: Dental caries in preschool Apache Indian children. J. dent. Res. *54:* 915 (1975).

Jenkins, G.N.: The refinement of food and caries. Adv. oral Biol. *2:* 67 (1966).

Lundström, R; Lysell, L.; Berghagen, N.: Dental development in children following maternal rubella. Acta paediat., scand *51:* 155 (1962).

MacGregor, A.B.: A new method of demonstrating the foodstuffs in the mouth, with special reference to different forms of sweets. Proc. R. Soc. Med. *51:* 41 (1958).

Marthaler, T.: Epidemiological and clinical dental findings in relation to intake of carbohydrates. Caries Res. *1:* 222 (1967).

Mcllanby, M.: The influence of diet on caries in children's teeth. Spec. rep. ser. No. 211 (Medical Research Council, London 1936).

Navia, J.M.: Nutrition in dental development and disease; in Winick, Human nutrition – a comprehensive treatise, vol. I, p. 333 (Plenum Publishing, New York 1979).

Nikiforuk, G.; Fraser, D.: Etiology of enamel hypoplasia and interglobular dentin: the roles of hypocalcemia and hypophosphatemia. Metab. Bone Dis. Rel. Res. *2:* 17 (1979).

Nikiforuk, G.: Fraser, D.: The etology of enamel hypoplasia: a unifying concept. J. Pediat. *98:* 888 (1981).

Pindborg, J.J.: Pathology of hard tissues, p. 88 (Saunders, Philadelphia 1970).

Reece, J.A.; Swallow, J.N.: Carrots and dental health. Br. dent. J. *128:* 535 (1970).

Rosenzweig, K.A.: Sahar, M.: Enamel hypoplasia and dental caries in the primary dentition of prematuri. Br. dent. J. *113:* 279 (1962).

Russell, A.L.: International nutrition surveys: a summary of preliminary dental findings. J. dent. Res. *42:* 233 (1963).

Schamschula, R.G.; Adkins, B.L.; Barmes, D.E.; Charlton, G.; Davey, B.G.: WHO Study of Dental Caries Etiology in Papus New Guinea, publ. No. 40 (WHO, Genève, 1978).

Scheinin, A.: Influence of the diagnostic level on caries incidence in two controlled clinical trials. Caries Res. *13:* 91 (1979).

Scheinin, A.; Mäkinen, K.K.: Turku sugar studies I-XXI. Acta odont, scand. *33:* suppl. 70, p. 1 (1975).

Shaw, J.H.: Preeruptive effects of nutrition on teeth. J. dent. Res. *49:* suppl., p. 1238 (1970).

Slack, G.L.; Martin, W.J.: Apples and dental health. Br. dent. J. *105:* 366 (1958).

Sullivan, H.R.; Harris, R.: The biology of the children of Hopewood House, Bowral, N.S.W. II. Observations extending over five years (1952–1956). 2. Observations on oral conditions. Aust. dent. J. *3:* 311 (1958).

Sweeney, E.A.; Saffir, A.J.; DeLeon, R.: Linear hypoplasia of deciduous incisor teeth in malnourished children. Am. J. clin. Nutr. *24:* 29 (1971).

Takeuchi, M.: Epidemiological study on dental caries in Japanese children – before, during and after World War II. Int. dent. J. *11:* 443 (1961).

Toverud, G.: Influence of war and post-war conditions on the teeth of Norwegian schoolchildren. I. Eruption of permanent teeth and status of deciduous dentition. Milbank Mem. Fund Q. *34:* 354 (1956).

Toverud, G.: Influence of war and post-war conditions on the teeth of Norwegian schoolchildren. II. Caries in the permanent teeth of children aged 7–8 and 12–13 years. Milbank Mem. Fund Q. *35:* 127 (1957).

Toverud, G.: Influence of war and post-war conditions on the teeth of Norwegian schoolchildren. III. Discussion of food supply and dental conditions in Norway and other European countries. Milbank Mem. Fund Q. *35:* 373 (1957).

Williams, K.A.; Schemehorn, B.R.; McDonald, J.L.; Stookey, G.N.; Katz, S.: Influence of selected fatty acids upon plaque formation and caries in the rat. Archs oral Biol. *27:* 1027 (1982).

Woodward, W.E.; Hirschhorn, H.; Sack, R.B.; Cash, R.A.; Brownlee, I.; Chickadonz, G.H.; Evans, L.K.; Shepard, R.H.; Woodward, R.C.: Acute diarrhoea on an Apache Indian reservation. Am. J. Epidem. *99:* 281 (1974).

8 The Role of Sucrose in Dental Caries

In the previous chapter, we noted that the widespread nature of dental caries in the industrialized world is related to dietary changes. Of the many dietary changes that have occurred over the past century, the qualitative and quantitative changes in the consumption of carbohydrates, and specifically sucrose are the most significant. The changing patterns of sucrose consumption in industrialized societies and the properties of sucrose that contributed to the unique cariogenic role of sucrose are discussed in this chapter. Since foods containing sucrose are apt to contribute most to the cariogenic potential of diets eaten by modern man the methods for assessing cariogenicity is also discussed in this chapter.

The Beginnings of the 'Sweet-Tooth' Habit

During the early and later millennia associated with the development of agriculture, cereals and roots, such as wheat, barley, rice and potatoes, were the main source of calories and nutrients in human diets. Sweet food was a delicacy and was originally provided by honey; sugar from cane or beet was unknown. The statutes governing bee hives and the sale of honey in the early civilizations of Western Asia attest to the fact that bee-keeping or apiculture is an ancient art. The honey from the mountain of Hymettus was famous during Ancient Greek times [*Ackroyd*, 1974].

Sugar extracted from the cane of a grass, and during the last two centuries from sugar beet, is a late-comer to the list of human dietary constituents. The agricultural records of the Ancient Greek and Roman Empires do not mention sugar cane. The Biblical authors who described the Promised Land of 'milk and honey' may have never heard of sugar. Sugar cane was probably first cultivated in the Ganges Valley in India where the alluvial soil was particularly suitable for growing cane, and then spread to China around the first century, AD.

The cultivation of sugar spread slowly from India and China along the Persian Gulf and later to the west of the Caspian Sea reaching the Mediterranean about the sixth century AD. The fertile Nile Valley in

Egypt was renowned for its fine quality sugar. Sugar, also called 'honey and reeds', was probably first introduced into central and western European countries by the Crusaders. During the 11th and until the 15th century sugar became a well-known dietary item, albeit scarce and expensive, and consumed primarily by nobility and kings.

One of the earliest uses of sugar was to disguise the acrid taste of the medicines of this period. Slowly the desirable taste attribute of sugar was recognized, and the demand and production grew in a spectacular fashion.

The rapidity with which the growth and production of sugar increased over a span of about 500 years is illustrative of the importance of sweetness as an attribute of diets of industrialized nations. The insatiable demand for sugar played a significant role in the unfortunate chapter in human history associated with the slave trade that provided cheap labor for the sugar plantations in South America, the Caribbean and later in North America [*Ackroyd*, 1967].

Not until the cultivation of sugar spread to tropical lands, and not until the discovery of a new source – the sugar beet – did sugar become an abundant, cheap, and universal food item. Since beet sugar may be grown in temperate zones, it is produced in large amounts in North America and Europe. In the 1980s about 60% of all sugar produced is obtained from cane and 40% from beet.

Levels of Consumption of Carbohydrates and Sugars in American Diets

Carbohydrates as a class of foods are abundant, cheaply produced relative to fats and protein and are consumed in larger amounts than other foods by most populations in the world. Carbohydrates constitute an average of 50% of calories with free choice of foods. The two carbohydrates, starch and sucrose, comprise the greatest proportion of all foods consumed by man; the other sugars, lactose, glucose and fructose, are minor constituents. In societies that depend upon cereals for their major food source, carbohydrates in the form of starch contribute most of the caloric intake. In North America, during the earlier period for which statistics are available (1909–1913), the daily carbohydrate consumption fell from an average of 500 g/person (representing over 56% of the total calories) to about 380 g today [*Page and Friend*, 1974]. A reduction in the use of flour and cereal products is largely the reason for this decline. The proportion of carbohydrates in the form of starch has declined and of refined sugar (cane and beet) increased, during the past seven decades (fig. 8/1). In the early 1900s about one third of the total carbohydrates consumed was sugar; now it is about one half (fig. 8/2).

Fig. 8/1. Per capital civilian consumption of total sugars, refined sugar, starch and carbohydrate, 1909 – 1913 to 1972 [*Page and Friend*, 1974].

Changes in Levels and Sources of Sugar Consumption

World production of factory-processed sugar has increased from 8 million tons in 1900 to 70 million tons in 1970, and projected to have increased to 93 million tons in 1980 (fig. 8/3). The magnitude of the increase in a single food item has no parallel and has far outstripped the population growth during the same period.

Current consumption of sugar is equal to about 200 g (7 oz)/person/day. About 66% of this is consumed as pure sucrose and as various sugars in syrups; about 13% each from dairy products and fruits and the remainder from other food items (fig. 8/4). Apart from a rise of about 25% in total sugar intake between 1900 and 1930, the proportion of sugar provided by these broad categories did not fluctuate widely for the past 50 years. In 1909–1913 the amount of sucrose comprised 64.8% of total sugars; in 1972 the figure was 61.8% [*Page and Friend*, 1974].

Over the past three quarters of a century the pattern of sucrose consumption has shifted from that of direct consumer use to an increased use of 'hidden sugar' in foods and beverages (fig. 8/5). The per capita increase in

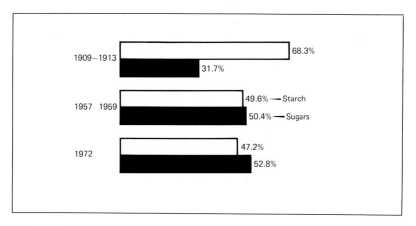

Fig. 8/2. Proportion of carbohydrate in the national food supply provided by starch and sugars for selected periods. Note that sugar comprises about one half of the total carbohydrate consumed in recent times [*Page and Friend*, 1974].

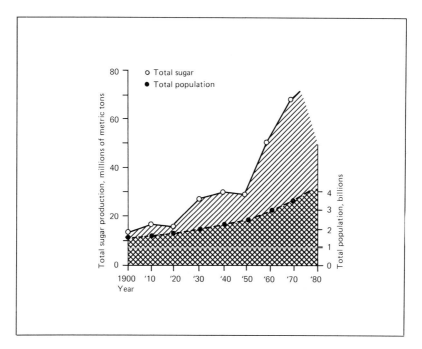

Fig. 8/3. World sugar production 1899 – 1900 to 1969 – 1979 and world population during the 20th century [after *Wretlind*, 1974, and *Ackroyd*, 1974].

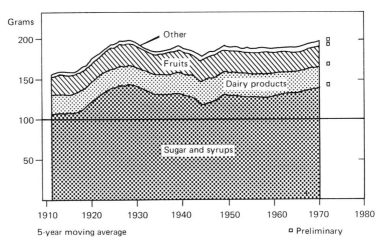

Fig. 8/4. Per capita daily consumption of sugar and the sources of the sugar in the major food supply, 1909 – 1913 to 1972 [*Page and Friend*, 1974].

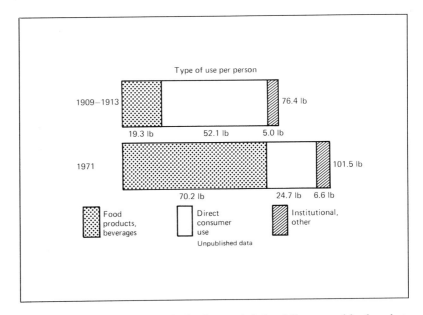

Fig. 8/5. Per capita per year use of refined sugars in industrially prepared food products and beverages, direct consumer use, and use by institutional and other users. Note the significant increase in the use of sugar in processed foods and beverages [*Page and Friend*, 1974].

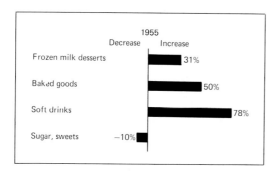

Fig. 8/6. Change in household use of selected types of foods, 1955 – 1965 [*Page and Friend*, 1974]. The 1965 consumption is expressed as a percentage of 1955.

the use of refined sugar in foods and beverages is about 350% over the past six decades (about 80% of sugar consumed by Americans comes in processed food) while direct consumer use of sugar has declined by about 50%. Food products and beverages account for about two thirds of refined sugar consumed. The 'soft drinks' industry is now the largest single industrial user of refined sucrose (nearly 23 lb/capita/year or about one fifth of the refined sugar in US. diet). This represents almost a 7-fold increase in the use of sugar in beverages since the turn of the century. Cereals and bakery foods account for the largest use of sugar by the food processing industry. The change in the household use of refined sugar in summarized in figure 8/6.

Factors Affecting Cariogenicity of Sucrose in Diets

Frequency of Eating

There is no simple, direct, proportionality between sucrose content of food and its caries-producing potential. A partial explanation for this related to the finding first clearly shown by the Vipeholm experience that the frequency of consumption of sugars and the oral clearance time for sugars (i.e. retentivity) are important factors affecting cariogenicity. In addition, the salivary stimulation brought about by food and its mastication, the role of saliva in demineralization and remineralization of enamel all affect the rate of caries production.

The importance of frequency of eating as a factor in cariogenicity of foods has been explored in experimental animals by *König* et al. [1968],

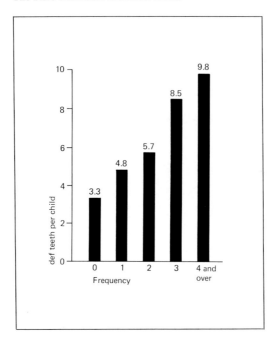

Fig. 8/7. The relationship between caries activity (def) and between-meal eating in 5- to 6-year-old children [*Weiss and Trithart*, 1960].

who developed a caging system which permits control over the amount and frequency of eating (for more detail, see p. 229). These animal studies clearly confirmed the conclusion of the Vipeholm experiment that the frequency with which experimental diets containing sugars is consumed is significant in caries development. In a study of more than 1,000 children in Tennessee, USA, *Weiss and Trithart* [1960] indicated that the frequency of between-meal snacks of candies, cookies, chewing gum or carbonated beverages correlated with the DMF rates (fig. 8/7) although not all similar surveys have given such clear results. The availability of sweets at school canteens has also been related to the prevalence rate of caries in children [*Fanning* et al., 1969]. These findings assume an added significance in that 'coffee' breaks, often supplemented with a sweet snack, are virtually a contractual right of many employees. A break from monotonous work is desirable, the frequent ingestion of sweets is not.

The mechanism by which frequency of eating translates into increased caries acitivity is best explained by terms of intraplaque events. When sucrose is ingested frequently (over 5 times per day), even a relatively low concentration of 1.25%, will cause a drop in pH to between 4 and 5 depending on the site and method of measurement. The pH periodicity of plaques with respect to eating sweets is discussed in vol. 2, chapter 8.

Oral Sugar Clearance

The concept that a prolonged clearance of a local substrate potentiates caries has long been suspected and was clearly shown in the Vipeholm study. A significant correlation was found between a high sugar concentration in saliva with a prolonged clearance time and caries activity (fig. 7/9) [*Lundqvist*, 1952]. This finding implies that retentive, sticky, sweet foods with little detergency or self-cleaning properties may be potentially more cariogenic than foods that are detergent and rapidly clear the oral cavity. A partial list of foods arranged according to their caries potentiality associated from oral sugar clearance is given in table 8/I. This is a guide in dietary counselling but ignores acid production from stored polysaccharides (discussed in vol. 2, chapter 8).

Effective Concentration of Sucrose

There is no question about the significance of frequency of consumption of sucrose-containing foods on caries, but what specific concentration of sucrose is most detrimental from a caries standpoint is not simply decided. The reasons for this relate to the availability of sucrose for support of bacterial metabolism in plaque which is influenced by the texture, consistency of the food, the stimulation of saliva illicited by chewing and the rapidity of clearance of the substrate.

Prior to the introduction of industrialized methods of food processing humans ingested sugar in natural forms primarily in fruits. The concentration of sugars in natural fruits is of the order of 5–10%, dried fruits may contain as much as 50–60% sugar. Ancient man ingesting these levels of sugar had low levels of caries (usually less than 10% of the teeth were affected) and the lesions were predominantly in the highly susceptible occlusal surfaces. Thus, it can be concluded that ingestion of levels of sugar found in fruits (5 to 10%, but greatly diluted in vivo by saliva) predispose humans to caries in highly susceptible surfaces only.

With the advent of highly concentrated processed cane sugar the level of sucrose consumption as well as the concentration of sucrose in food items increased dramatically. *Kleinberg* [1961] showed that in vivo 5% (300 mM of glucose) gave optimal acid production in the absence of saliva and that a 3M solution had a detectable inhibitory effect on acid production.

Many processed foods and sweet snacks contain sucrose in the range of the concentrations tested (5–50%) (vol. 2, chapter 8). Therefore,

Table 8/I. Foods are listed according to a caries potentiality index based on oral sugar clearance times [adapted from *Lundqvist*, 1952]

Food product	Sugar content %	Clearance time (min) for total sugar above concentration levels of:				Caries potentiality index
		0.02%	0.2%	2%	20%	
Fluids						
Fruit juice	11.5	2	1			3
Tea +2 sugar lumps	11.2	3	1			4
Chocolate (milk) + sugar	14.2	4	1	0.25		5
Solids						
Fruit jelly	11.0	2	1.5			4
White bread + butter	1.5	4.5	2			7
Biscuits (sugar-containing)	9.0	11.25	5	1.5		18
Milk products						
Cheese	0.2	–	–	–		0 (lowest)
Ice cream	2.4	5	2.5	1		9
Fruits						
Apples	7.5	3.5	1			5
Pears	9.0	4.0	2			6
Marmalade + bread and butter	16.3	6.25	2.5	0.5		9
Marmalade	65.3	5.75	3.5	1.0		10
Vegetables						
Potatoes (boiled)	0.8	4.5	2	0.5		7
Honey						
Honey	72.8	11.25	5	1.5		18
Honey + bread and butter	19.0	15	7.5	1.5		24
Candy						
Chocolate (dark)	33.7	7.5	3.5	1.5		13
Sweets	80	11.25	6.25	3	1.5	22
Caramel	64	18.75	5	2.5	0.5	27
Toffee	78	11.25	11.25	5.0	2.0	30 (highest)

Other methods of ranking may give different results.

ingestion of these sweet foods would result in maximum acid production in plaque indicating that the multi-enzyme system of plaque flora would be saturated. At saturation level any further increase in substrate concentration may briefly extend the time during which low pH levels persist but does not cause a greater drop in pH. This may be the reason why in some studies the addition of sucrose to a basal diet that initially contains high levels of sucrose does not result in a further increase in caries [*King* et al., 1955]. The current level of sucrose consumption in industrialized countries, in all probability, results in plaque saturation during the time that the sweet foods are ingested until the sugar is cleared from the oral cavity. This explains why total sugar content of a food only grossly relates to caries. On the other hand, intermittent, frequent utilization of sucrose replenishes substrate concentration as it is being used up and drives the reaction rate at a maximum velocity. It should be noted that most of the sucrose consumed in food is cleared from the oral cavity and is unavailable to plaque flora. Only the soluble, diffusible portion is utilized by plaque bacteria.

Is Sucrose a Unique Substrate for Cariogenic Flora?

Certain monosaccharides, including the digestion products of sucrose, are universally utilized by living cells as a source of energy to fuel the glycolytic cycle for the synthesis of ATP. Many oral bacteria utilize sucrose, glucose, fructose and other simple sugars to produce organic acids (lactic, acetic and propionic) in sufficient concentration to lower the pH of plaque to levels that may result in some demineralization of enamel. It is only from sucrose, however, that most bacteria are able to synthesize both soluble and insoluble extracellular polymers (dextrans and mutans) which increase the bulk of plaque and facilitate the attachment of bacteria, especially *Streptococcus mutans*, to it. Unlike other disaccharides, such as maltose or lactose, sucrose can serve directly as a glycosyl donor in the synthesis of extracellular polymers. The high free energy of hydrolysis of sucrose permits this reaction to proceed without other sources of energy (chapter 6). This property along with the high specificity of the enzymes involved in the synthesis of the extracellular polymers has led some workers to regard sucrose as having a unique role in caries.

Animal experiments on the relative cariogenicity of sucrose and other sugars have led to contradictory results depending on many factors such as the type of basal diet, whether fissure or smooth surface caries were compared and whether the animals had been infected with *S. mutans*. In general, sucrose has been shown to be more cariogenic than monosaccharides or other disaccharides but the differences have only been large and consistent when the rats were infected with *S. mutans*, which forms smooth surface plaques heavily loaded with glucans when sucrose is eaten. In experiments with conventional rats, sucrose showed a trend towards being more cariogenic (fig. 8/8) but all the sugars tested were cariogenic and, under some conditions, as cariogenic as sucrose.

Only two experiments on human caries in which sucrose has been compared with other sugars have been reported. In the Turku experiment in which the cariogenicity of xylitol and sucrose were compared, a third group used fructose in place of sucrose for 2 years. Apart from the lower caries

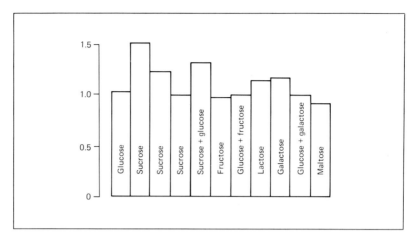

Fig. 8/8. Relative cariogenicity of various sugars (sucrose = 1.0) in conventional rats [*Green and Hartles*, 1969].

effects from xylitol the results were indecisive (fig. 7/10). In the second experiment [*Frostell* et al., 1981], caries increment was compared in the deciduous teeth of 150 children who were either on a normal sucrose diet or on a similar diet in which sucrose had been completely replaced by invert sugar (glucose and fructose in equal proportions) for 2 years. As in the Turku experiment, there was little difference after the first year, but a significantly lower dmfs score with invert sugar at the end of the second year (fig. 8/9).

Although these animal and human experiments do suggest that sucrose is more cariogenic than other sugars, the results are not all in agreement and are probably valid only in experimental conditions in which only one sugar was in each diet. A more cautious conclusion is that all the common sugars are cariogenic but that sucrose can, in some conditions, be more so than other sugars. Only because sucrose is the sugar eaten most often and in greatest quantity can it be regarded as uniquely associated with caries.

pH Changes in Plaques from Foods

The localization of large numbers of bacteria on the tooth surface in dental plaque also results in a concentration of their metabolic by-products at these sites where interaction with tooth enamel readily occurs. Such a

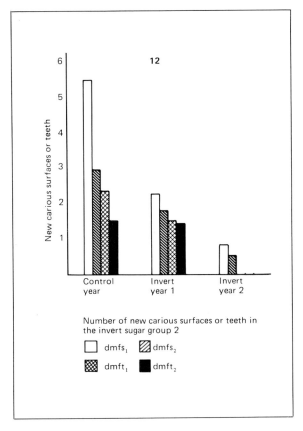

Fig. 8/9. The number of new carious surfaces or teeth in children on invert sugar and sucrose after 1 and 2 years [*Frostell* et al., 1981].

concentrated and complex mixture of bacteria give rise to a wide variety of glycolytic products which cause the plaque pH to drop. In chapter 5 the concept of a critical pH in plaque was introduced and a typical Stephan curve (relationship between time of ingestion of a glucose or sucrose and pH drop) was discussed. During the 1970s improvements in techniques for measuring plaque pH in vivo has resulted in considerable investigation of food substances and factors affecting changes in plaque pH.

Methods of Measuring Plaque pH
The usual procedure consists of measuring the pH of plaque, which has accumulated during several days with no tooth brushing, at intervals of,

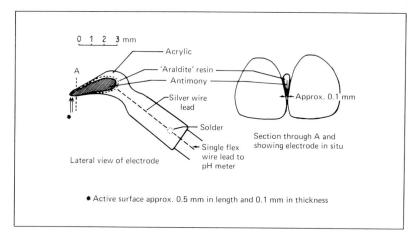

Fig. 8/10. Edge type of antimony pH electrode for use in interproximal plaques [*Klein-berg*, 1958].

say, 5 min after eating the food and graphing the results (a Stephan curve; chapter 5). Several methods are in use for measuring the plaque pH. Electrodes (fig. 8/10) may be placed on the plaque ('touch method') or approximately 1-mg amounts of plaque, representative of the smooth surface plaque as a whole, may be collected at each time interval with a scaler and their pH measured outside the mouth ('harvesting' or 'sampling method'). For the study of interproximal plaque, electrodes are built into extracted or artificial teeth mounted on a denture ('indwelling electrode', fig. 8/11) and attached either by wire to a pH meter (wire telemetry) or to a microtransmitter inside the mouth, the signal being received outside the mouth (radio telemetry). The touch and sampling methods give similar results – the classical Stephan curve of a pH drop reaching a minimum of about 5.0 within about 5–10 min and with most foods returning to baseline within 30 min (fig. 5/18). The indwelling electrodes give slower responses and reach lower pH values (about 4.0) sometimes requiring 1–2 h for return to baseline (fig. 8/12). It is still uncertain whether this result indicates real differences between the pH changes of smooth surfaces and interproximal plaque or whether it is an artifact arising from 'poisoning' of the electrode by prolonged contact with the proteins of plaque. When two similar electrodes were placed in the same mouth, one buccally and the other in the interproximal area (fig. 8/11) the Stephan curves of the interproximal electrode

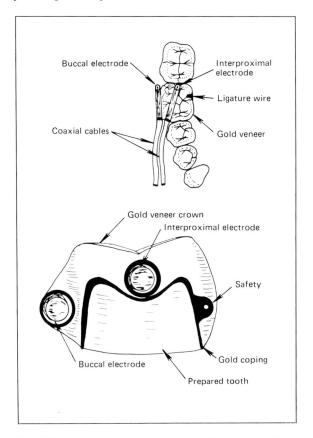

Fig. 8/11. An appliance used for wire telemetry with 2 electrodes to compare the Stephan curves in interproximal and buccal areas [*Schachtele and Jensen*, 1982].

showed the same differences found with other methods, i.e. the minimum pH was lower and the return to baseline slower than with the buccal electrode. This suggests that the differences are real.

Artificial Mouths

Various attempts have been made to reproduce in vitro an environment surrounding teeth as near as possible to that present in vivo. Extracted teeth are mounted, sometimes close together to form a contact point, in a closed chamber and saliva is allowed to drip onto the teeth at controlled rates. The environment of the teeth can be altered by placing different foods or cultures

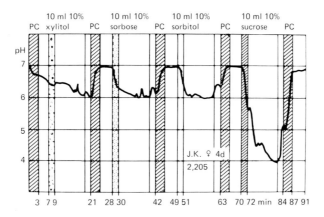

Fig. 8/12. The effect of sucrose and of 3 nonfermentable substances on Stephan curves measured with an indwelling electrode. PC = Effect of paraffin chewing which stimulates saliva and neutralizes the acids forming in the plaque so that the rise in pH is more rapid than in most results with indwelling electrode [*Firestone*, 1982].

of different organisms in the system. The results are studied by examining the teeth either intact or in section or by measuring the calcium and phosphate going into solution.

Acid Production from Foods

Since carbohydrates and more specifically sugars have been definitely implicated in caries etiology, acid production from these food substances has been extensively studied in human plaque in situ. Generally monosaccharides and disaccharides result in the greatest fall in plaque pH. On the other hand, the application of solutions of raw starch or cooked starch suggests that acid formation is slower than occurs with sugars, and the amount of acid formed does not exhaust the buffering capacity of the plaque. One explanation for this result is that the diffusion of the larger starch molecules is considerably slower than for mono- and disaccharides, and acid production can only occur from the comparatively low concentration of maltose released from starch by amylase which diffuses into plaque. The marked differences in plaque pH response to sucrose as compared to sorbitol and xylitol are depicted in figure 8/12. Telemetrically recorded pH of plaque supports the concept that xylitol and sorbitol (except after prolonged incubation of plaque, see vol. 2, chapter 8) lack the cariogenic potential of sucrose.

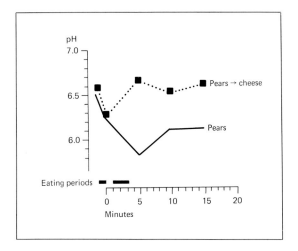

Fig. 8/13. The effect of cheese immediately after eating pears (an acid sugar-containing food) in preventing a typical Stephan curve [from *Edgar*, 1981, with permission].

In addition to testing the cariogenicity of foods, plaque pH data may be used for testing the ability of some foods to reduce the pH drop in plaque. As an example, it has been observed that cheese and butter reduce the cariogenicity of bread in rats. *Rugg-Gunn* et al. [1975] showed that ingestion of cheddar cheese caused the pH of buccal plaque, measured by the harvesting method, to be raised from the low level caused by consumption of an acidogenic food (fig. 8/13). Other workers have stated that if certain types of cheese are eaten 30 min before rinsing with a sucrose solution, a significantly reduced fall in plaque pH occurred compared to a sucrose rinse prior to cheese consumption [*Jensen* et al., 1982]. The mechanism of the effect of cheese in raising the plaque pH is still uncertain but one possibility is that the bicarbonate in the alkaline saliva secreted in response to cheese ingestion diffuses into plaque and neutralizes the acids. An additional anticaries action of cheese (not related to plaque pH) is that calcium and phosphate ions are extracted from it during mastication and enter plaque, thus reducing demineralization and favoring remineralization. The finding by one group of workers that cheese taken 30 min before sucrose reduces the pH drop has not been investigated by others and remains unexplained.

The importance of stimulus sequence in plaque pH has been demonstrated by several workers [*Edgar*, 1982]. If a sugar-containing food is followed by nonacidogenic food, the pH drop, measured by the harvesting method, is much smaller than if a meal ends with the acidogenic sugary food. The saliva stimulated by the nonacidogenic food neutralizes the acid being formed in plaque, thus reducing the pH drop. It is unfortunate that the usual custom is to eat sweets at the end of a meal often followed by a sweetened tea or coffee which have been shown to prolong the Stephan curve. If meals began with sweets and ended with a savory food, there is reason to believe that the pH drop in plaque and therefore caries would be greatly reduced. The effect on caries of such a drastic change has, of course, never been tested clinically.

From these results it is apparent that the nature of the substrate is one of the main determinants of plaque pH. The availability of fermentable carbohydrate is important but given the complexity of the composition and form of the foods consumed by humans it is very difficult to predict the pH response of a particular food item. The important substrate factors which affect the acidogenic potential of a food are summarized in table 8/II.

In addition to the importance of substrate concentration it should be noted that microbial factors also significantly influence the acidic potential of food. This is particularly significant with respect to the cariogenic potential of cooked starch foods. It has been repeatedly shown that cooked starch solutions or cooked flour products cause a drop in plaque pH in humans. However, the acidogenicity of starch products, as determined by pH studies, and their apparent noncariogenicity in rats when fed without sugar, is a longstanding contradiction. On the other hand, when rats were inoculated with *S. mutans* prior to the experiment, the fissure and smooth surface caries produced by the cooked wheat starch diet was greater than

Table 8/II. Substrate factors capable of influencing the acidogenic potential of a food at the time of ingestion [*Schachtele and Jensen*, 1982]

Total fermentable carbohydrate content
Concentrations and types of mono-, di-, oligo-, and polysaccharides
Concentrations and types of proteins
Concentrations and types of lipids
Physical form including factors that affect oral retention
Presence of fluoride, calcium, phosphate, and other elements
Presence of organic phosphates
Total buffering capacity
Presence of sialogogues, metabolic inhibitors, and flavors
Acidity of the food
Sequence of ingestion relative to other foods
Frequency of ingestion of sweet foods

---

that produced by sucrose. In man, the sugar in the diet favors the growth of organisms such as *S. mutans* and, in their presence, the plaque bacteria may form acid from the digestion products of starch. This consideration may explain the low caries rate of the high starch diets in the control group in the Vipeholm experiment or the xylitol group in the Turku experiment; in the complete absence of sugar, a cariogenic flora will not develop.

In interpreting these findings it is important to recognize that the pH levels in plaque are a function of complex interrelationships between carbohydrate concentration, plaque bacteria, salivary flow, food clearance, pH of the ingested food or beverages, plaque buffering capacity, solubility of foods, rate of diffusion into and from plaque and other factors.

Tests for Cariogenicity of Foods

As a rational basis for giving dietary advice in order to maintain optimum dental health, it is obviously important to know which foods favor or inhibit plaque formation and caries. Many different approaches have been made in attempts to compare the cariogenicity of different foods but the results are often contradictory (e.g. starchy foods), and in most of the tests it is uncertain to what extent the results apply to the natural environment of the human mouth. During the 1970s many techniques for assessing cariogenicity of foods have been developed and these are now briefly reviewed.

Chemical Tests
Sugar Concentration. The simplest test is chemical analysis of a food. If a food does not contain more than traces of carbohydrate and is not itself acid then it can be assumed to be noncariogenic. If it contains starch, and especially sucrose, a food may be cariogenic but its effect is not necessarily proportional to the concentration of sugar it contains as the solubility and stickiness and other constituents may be important factors. Also, the mode of ingestion of the food (frequency of eating) is important in determining cariogenicity on a clinical level (see vol. 2, chapter 8).

Rate of Acid Production from Food-Saliva Mixtures. When foods containing carbohydrates are incubated with saliva, the pH falls as acids are formed by bacterial glycolysis. The rates of acid production, especially if associated also with measures of retention of the food on the tooth surface (table 8/I), are thought to give some indication of the relative cariogenicity of foods but, as with most of these tests, there is no means of deciding on their reliability in man.

When the incubated mixtures of cariogenic food and saliva are shaken with powdered enamel, some enamel will dissolve ('enamel solubility test') and the amount dissolved may be a more accurate indicator of cariogenicity than acid production alone. The solvent action is not necessarily proportional to the pH fall because some foods contain substances which protect the enamel in vitro (white and brown bread produce very similar pH drops but less enamel dissolved with the incubated brown bread-saliva mixture). The effectiveness of these substances in preventing caries in vivo is unknown.

Plaque pH Measurements
A more physiological method of comparing the acidogenicity of foods is to measure the pH change in plaque by one of the methods described on p. 221 after a food has been eaten. This takes into account the ability of plaque bacteria to form acid from the food and the effect of the saliva flow resulting from its ingestion but gives no information on the effect of individual foods on the dissolution of enamel.

Table 8/III. Snack foods (USA) grouped by category and acidogenic potential [*Edgar*, 1981]

Group	Beverages	Fruit, etc.	Baked goods	Sweets
Least acidogenic	1 milk	peanuts		sugarless gum
	2 chocolate milk	crisps apple	bread + butter Graham crackers	caramels sugared gum chocolate liquorice
	3 carbonated beverages	banana	cream-filled cakes sandwich cookies crackers bagel	orange jellies
	4 apple juice orange juice	dates raisins sweetened cereal	doughnut bread + jam whole wheat bread cakes plain sweet biscuits	
	5		apple pie chocolate grahams angel food cake	rock candy clear mints
Most acidogenic	6			sourballs fruit gums fruit lollipops

Tables have been compiled in which foods are ranked according to their effect on either the minimum pH or on the total area enclosed by the Stephan curve which it is assumed are related to their cariogenicity [*Edgar* et al, 1975; *Rugg-Gunn* et al., 1978] (table 8/III).

In Switzerland, candies are tested by this method and if, after eating it, the plaque pH does not fall below 5.7 (a typical figure for the 'critical pH' above which enamel does not dissolve in plaque or saliva), it is labelled as 'safe for the teeth'. This assumes that acidogenicity (acid formation) can be equated with cariogenicity (caries formation) which may not be true with all foods. In vitro experiments suggest that some foods may produce acid but not caries, but there is no evidence that foods can cause caries if they are incapable of producing acid.

Animal Tests

Tests on animals in which dental caries can be induced (hamsters and some strains of the laboratory rat) have been used to compare the cariogenicity of foods or the protective effects of additives. In the early experiments, the food or additive being tested was mixed with the basic cariogenic diet and the results were therefore influenced by the taste and intake of the food. A food might appear to be more cariogenic simply because the animals liked it and ate it more frequently. *König* et al. [1968] developed a sophisticated way of studying the influence of eating frequency on dental caries. They designed an apparatus for the controlled feeding of laboratory rats. Each animal was housed in a separate cage and given access to its own food supply (fig. 8/14). The food was presented to each rat in a circular tray which had 18 separate depressions or dishes stamped into it. A programming system caused the trays to rotate to the next dish after any desired time interval. This made it possible to offer the animal its daily food allowance in any number of meals, up to 36 per day, or study the effects of alternating different foods, such as a cariogenic sugar diet with cheese. Another technique is to provide the basic diet by stomach tube and allow only the food under test to be taken by mouth and hence have contact with the teeth. The caries is scored usually by assessing the extent of demineralization in sections of the teeth stained with murexide. The experiments usually last only 3–4 weeks and only the first stages of caries are reached, i.e. the initiation rather than the progression of caries is measured. It is not known whether these two stages are controlled by the same factors.

The applicability of the results of animal tests to human caries has been called in question by the finding in over a hundred experiments by various workers that the addition of 1–2% of inorganic phosphates to a cariogenic diet reduced caries in rats but similar additives had little or no effect in experiments on human subjects.

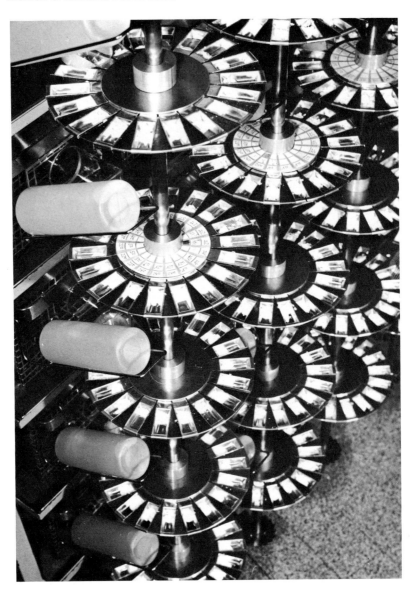

Fig. 8/14. The machine for controlling the frequency of feeding cariogenic diets to rats [with permission from *König* et. al., 1968].

The ideal method of comparing the cariogenicity of foods is by clinical trials, but these are extremely expensive and raise ethical problems if a positive control group receives a diet or food likely to increase caries. Also, it is not always possible to alter the intake of a basic nutrient, like starch, which is bound to be a major constituent of all balanced diets. The Vipeholm study and the Turku experiment (discussed in chapter 7) on xylitol are the two most ambitious clinical trials in the caries field.

Intraoral Caries Test

In view of the difficulties of such experiments, other more limited tests in human subjects have been developed. The intraoral caries test (ICT) [*Ostram and Koulourides*, 1976] consists of measuring the hardness changes resulting from demineralization of small sterilized slabs of human or bovine enamel mounted on dentures or detachable appliances placed on the teeth for periods of 1 week (fig. 8/15a, b). The usual method is to cover the enamel with Dacron gauze which increases plaque formation. The enamel slabs from one side of the mouth are placed into extraoral solutions of test substrate. The slab from the other side is placed into control solutions, usually 3% sucrose or water. They are then replaced in the mouth and thus the foods react with a reasonably normal plaque formed in the mouth but there is no contact between the experimental foods and the natural teeth, so obviating the risk of caries. The effects of the experimental diet on the enamel slabs are evaluated by microscopically examining the enamel surface and by microhardness test of the enamel. The degree of indentation into enamel is a measure of the porosity and demineralization of the enamel. The method has been used to compare the cariogenicity of various sugars, usually taking sucrose as a standard [*Koulourides* et al., 1976], and to demonstrate the effectiveness of fluoride-containing rinses saturated with calcium phosphate in remineralizing enamel presoftened by exposure to acids [*Pearce*, 1982].

Short-Term Clinical Tests on Humans

In another type of experiment pioneered by *von der Fehr* et al. [1970] (chapter 7) but which has been used only to a limited extent, the subjects abstain from toothbrushing for 21 days (later it was found that 2 separate periods of 9 days abstention is adequate) during which half the subjects take up to 9 daily rinses of the cariogenic substance under test. At the end of the experimental period, the accumulated plaque is removed and small areas of 'white spot' demineralization which have been produced are counted and their areas estimated and compared in the two groups. The scoring can be facilitated by photographing the teeth. Fluoride rinses are then used daily for 1–2 months during which many of the white spots

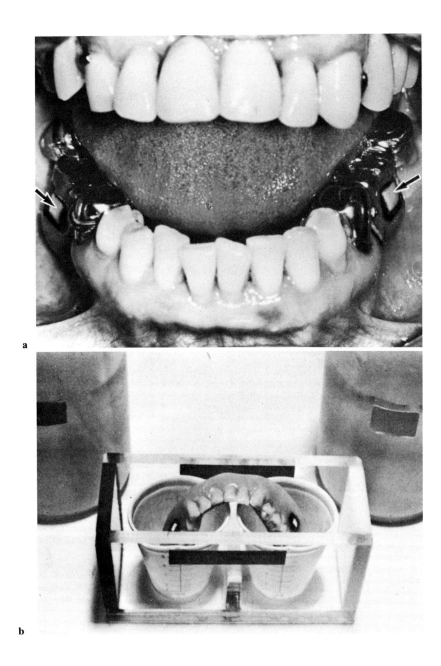

Fig. 8/15. a The device for carrying out the intraoral caries text (ICT). The enamel slabs are placed on the buccal side of the partial denture and are covered with Dacron (arrows) to facilitate plaque formation. **b** Similar device using a full denture which may be immersed in two separate extraoral substrate supplements [from *Koulourides*, 1980, with permission].

become smaller or disappear as a result of their remineralization. Repeated trials in the same individual by this type of experiment is not feasible because the most susceptible areas of enamel become etched, and presumably changed in susceptibility during the remineralization phase. In both this and the ICT methods, individual variation in caries susceptibility greatly affects the result. This is less important in the ICT as the subjects can act as their own controls by testing in successive periods sucrose and the other test sugars.

It is only possible from the sum total of evidence from these tests to classify foods into broad categories, such as noncariogenic (if they contain little carbohydrate), 'probably slightly' or 'highly cariogenic'. Some foods are in one category with one test but another category by a different test and there are also intersubject differences (foods which are highly acidogenic in 1 subject may be less so to another subject). In all probability a combination of the plaque pH response and the ICT test combined with animal dietary studies will provide a reasonably accurate evaluation of the cariogenicity of foods. Chapter 8 in vol. 2 is devoted to a discussion of reducing cariogenicity of substrate on a clinical basis.

Carbonated Beverages (Soft Drinks) and Dental Caries

The high level of consumption of 'soft drinks' in the industrialized countries, especially among the teenage groups, is sufficient reason to consider the cariogenic potential of these beverages. In a 1965 survey (fig. 8/6), about 60% of persons reported using soft drinks every day. The consumption in 18- to 19-year-old males reaches the highest level, about 300 g of drink per day, which is equivalent to about 1.6 6-oz bottles per day. Again, averages for a given age group are meaningless since it is known that consumption may vary widely from individual to individual.

In addition to the high level of consumption, two other properties of 'soft drinks' are significant as potentially cariogenic. Soft drinks contain about 10% sucrose (except for the diet variety). This is equivalent to about 16 g of sugar per 6-oz bottle, a not insignificant amount if individuals are ingesting high levels of soft drink. Also, the pH of most soft drinks such as Cola is low, about 2.4–2.5. The acidity is due to the presence of carbonic and phosphoric acids. This pH is sufficient to cause deminerlization of enamel, and has been repeatedly demonstrated in laboratory animals whose fluid intake was limited to carbonated beverages. It is not possible to extrapolate these experiments to humans. Since oral sugar clearance from soft drinks is rapid, the pH changes in the plaque resulting from ingestion of soft drinks is transitory. However, both the sucrose content and the low pH of carbonated beverages may play a role in the caries process in habitual users of acid beverages.

The juices of some fruits (e.g. apple and orange) not only contain sugar and have a low pH but are also heavily buffered. Their effect on plaque pH is more prolonged than is that of some other soft drinks.

Additional Reading

Hefferren, J.J.; Koehler, H.M. (eds): Foods, nutrition and dental health, vol. 1 (Pathotox Publishers, Park Forest South 1981).
Imfeld, T.N.: Identification of low caries risk dietary components. Monogr. oral Sci., vol. II (Karger, Basel 1983).

References

Ackroyd, W.R.: Sweet malefactor: sugar, slavery and human society (Heinemann, London 1967).
Ackroyd, W.R.: Sugar in history; in Sipple, McNutt, Sugars in nutrition, p. 3 (Academic Press, New York 1974).
Edgar, W.M.: Plaque pH assessments related to food cariogenicity; in Hefferren, Koehler, Foods, nutrition and dental health, vol. 1 (Pathotox Publishers, Park Forest South 1981).
Edgar, W.M.: Duration of response and stimulus sequence in the interpretation of plaque pH data. J. dent. Res. *61:* 1,126 (1982).
Edgar, W.M.; Bibby, B.G.; Mundorff, S.; Rowley, J.: Acid production in plaques after eating snacks: modifying factors in foods. J. Am. dent. Ass. *90:* 418 (1975).
Fanning, E.A.; Gotjamanos, T.; Vowles, N.J.: Dental caries in children related to availability of sweets at school canteens. Med. J. Aust. *i:* 1,131 (1969).
Fehr, F.R.; von der Löe, H.; Theilade, E.: Experimental caries in man. Caries Res. *4:* 131 (1970).
Firestone, A.R.: Human interdental plaque-pH data and rat caries tests: results with the same substances. J. dent. Res. *61:* 1,130 (1982).
Frostell, G.; Blomqvist, T.; Bruner, P.; Dahl, G.M.; Fjellström, A.; Henrikson, C.-O.; Larje, O.; Nord, C.-E.; Nordenvall, K.-J.; Wik, O.: Reduction of caries in pre-school children by sucrose restriction and substitution with invert sugar. The Gustavsberg study. Acta odont. scand. *39:* 333 (1981).
Green, R.M.; Hartles, R.L.: The effect of diet containing different mono- and dissaccharides on the incidence caries in the Albino rat. Archs oral Biol. *14:* 235 (1969).
Jensen, M.E.; Harlander, S.K.; Schachtele, C.F.; Halambeck, S.M.; Morris, H.A.: Evaluation of the acidogenic and antacid properties of cheeses by telemetric monitoring of human dental plaque pH; in Hefferren, Koehler, Food, nutrition and dental health, vol. 4 (Pathotox Publishers, Park Forest South 1982).
King, J.D.; Mellanby, M.; Stones, H.H.; Green, H.N.: The effect of sugar supplements on dental caries in children. Privy Council, spec. rep. ser. No. 288 (Medical Research Council, London 1955).
Kleinberg, I.: The construction and evaluation of modified types of antimony microelectrodes for intra-oral use. Br. dent. J. *104:* 197 (1958).

Kleinberg, I.: Studies on dental plaque. I. The effect of different concentrations of glucose on the pH of dental plaque in vivo. J. dent. Res. *40:* 1,087 (1961).

König, K.G.; Schmid, P.; Schmid, R.: An apparatus for frequency-controlled feeding of small rodents and its use in dental caries experiments. Archs oral Biol. *13:* 13 (1968).

Koulourides, T.: Dynamics of biologic mineralization applied to dental caries; in Menaker, The biologic basis of dental caries, p. 419 (Harper & Row, Hagerstown 1980).

Koulourides, T.; Bodden, R.; Keller, S.; Manson-Hing, L.; Lastra, J.; Housch, T.: Cariogenicity of nine sugars tested with an intraoral device in man. Caries Res. *10:* 427 (1976).

Lundqvist, C.: Oral sugar clearance and its influence on dental caries activity. Odont. Revy *3:* suppl. I, p.1 (1952).

Ostram, C.A.; Koulourides, T.: The intraoral cariogenicity test in young subjects. Caries Res. *10:* 442 (1976).

Page, L.; Friend, B.: Level of use of sugars in the United States; in Sipple, McNutt, Sugars in nutrition, p. 93 (Academic Press, New York 1974).

Pearce, E.I.F.: Effect of plaque mineralization on experimental dental caries. Caries Res. *16:* 460 (1982).

Rugg-Gunn, A.J.; Edgar, W.M.; Geddes, D.A.M.; Jenkins, G.N.: The effect of different meal patterns upon plaque pH in human subjects. Br. dent. J. *139:* 351 (1975).

Rugg-Gunn, A.J.; Edgar, W.M.; Jenkins, G.N.: The effect of some British snacks upon the pH of human dental plaque. Br. dent. J. *145:* 95 (1978).

Schachtele, C.F.; Jensen, M.E.: Human plaque pH: evaluating the acidogenic potential of foods. IADR Progr. Abstr. *60:* No. 217 (1981).

Schachtele, C.F.; Jensen, M.E.: Comparison of methods for monitoring changes in the pH of human dental plaque. J. dent. Res. *61:* 1,117 (1982).

Weiss, R.L.; Trithart, A.H.: Between meal eating habits and dental caries experience in pre-school children. Am. J. publ. Hlth *50:* 1,097 (1960).

Wretlind, A.: World sugar production and usage in Europe; in Sipple, McNutt, Sugars in nutrition, p. 81 (Academic Press, New York 1974).

9 Saliva and Dental Caries

Saliva from the major and minor salivary glands constitutes one of the largest secretions of the human body as about 700–800 ml is secreted daily. The involvement of the oral tissues in such diverse functions as mastication and deglutition of food, taste sensations, speech, and initial digestion of carbohydrates would not be possible without salivary secretions. The interface between saliva and oral tissues is the site of many dynamic reactions which affect the integrity of both the soft and hard tissues of the mouth and saliva constitutes one of the main natural defense systems of the oral cavity. Also, since the caries process involves local, exogenous causal factors it is not surprising that salivary secretions can dramatically affect the rate of caries development.

Effect of Desalivation and Hyposalivation on Dental Caries

Total or partial aplasia of salivary glands is rare but, where present, is accompanied by a high caries prevalence. In experimental animals extirpation of salivary glands markedly accelerates the caries process and this procedure has been a common practice in experimental caries research. An analogous situation in man results when the salivary glands are removed as in cases of tumor growth. Radiation therapy in the region of the salivary glands may also severely impair their function. A clinical condition known as xerostomia arises from severely restricted salivary flow in which the oral soft tissues are dry and inflamed and patients complain of soreness of the mucosa. As much as a 10-fold increase in enamel and root caries has been reported in patients whose salivary glands have been irradiated to reduce tumor growth [*Dreizen* et al., 1977].

Reduced salivary secretion (hyposalivation), despite normal salivary glands, is a more common consequence of pathological conditions or the use of medications with antisialagogue effects. In man, salivary flow is almost entirely under parasympathetic neural rather than hormonal control. Therefore, drugs such as atropine, which affect the cholinergic parasympathetic nerves, exert a depressing effect on saliva flow. Hyposalivation also occurs in patients who are dehydrated due to such conditions as fever or prolonged diarrhea. Hyposalivation is commonly associated with diabetes, anemia, hypovitaminosis A or B, uremia and dehydrating disease of old age. Patients with hyposalivation experience difficulty in mastication, swallowing, the wearing of dentures and sometimes in speaking. Sjögren's syndrome is an autoimmune disease in which the acinar cells of the salivary glands are destroyed and replaced by lymphocytes. Such patients not only have xerostomia but also may have dry eyes due to lacrimal gland destruction as well as symptoms of rheumatoid arthritis.

A restriction in salivary flow leads to exacerbation of dental caries, periodontal disease and other soft tissue afflictions. In order to understand the mechanisms by which the above conditions are potentiated when salivary flow is restricted, it is necessary to consider the constituents of saliva and their function.

Salivary Clearance from the Oral Cavity

One of the most important functions of saliva with respect to caries is its role in the removal of bacteria and food debris from the mouth.

Bacteria

When saliva is swallowed, any bacteria contained therein are removed from the oral cavity and pass into the stomach. The average unstimulated salivary flow rate is about 0.3 ml/min and the amount of saliva present in the mouth prior to swallowing is of the order of 3 or 4 times that volume. Thus, the half-life in the oral cavity for any inert material suspended in saliva is only a few minutes and is certainly very much less than the mean generation time of oral microorganisms. Thus, if any species of microorganism did not have the ability to adhere to either the teeth or the mucosa, it would rapidly be lost from the mouth. Surprisingly, it is only during the last decade that the importance of bacterial adherence in both the mouth and the small intestine has been appreciated.

Despite the continuous flow of saliva, dental plaque can accumulate at a rapid rate (10–20 mg/day) in the absence of oral hygiene procedures but the rate of plaque accumulation appears to be even more rapid in patients with xerostomia [Llory et al., 1972].

Food Debris

When food debris is retained in the mouth it remains available as a substrate for the metabolic activity of the oral microorganisms. Thus, if clearance of food debris is retarded for any reason, this will tend to promote the development of caries. Although most solid foods show some

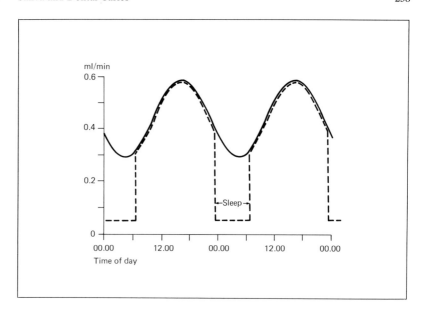

Fig. 9/1. Diagrammatic representation of the circadian rhythm in the flow rate of unstimulated whole saliva [from *Dawes*, 1972].

adherence to the teeth or oral mucosa, some types such as caramels or toffees are notorious for their prolonged retention.

Dawes [1983] has recently developed a mathematical model of salivary clearance from the oral cavity of sugar in solution. The model incorporates the process of swallowing and as the volume of saliva remaining in the mouth after swallowing is never zero the assumption is made that the volume will oscillate between a maximum (immediately prior to swallowing) and a minimum (immediately after swallowing). The other assumption is that the salivary flow rate will be dependent on the salivary sugar concentration and will vary between some maximum value and some minimum value which will be the unstimulated flow rate.

Analysis of the model leads to the conclusion that when a sufficient amount of nonretentive sugar is consumed so that it can be tasted, the time required for the sugar concentration to fall to some low value below which plaque bacteria cannot form acid is independent of the initial amount of sugar consumed. The explanation for this rather surprising result is that increased amounts of sugar stimulate a higher flow rate of saliva which increases the rate of clearance. In effect, a negative feedback system is operating to clear the mouth of sugar. Thus, for amounts of sugar in a nonretentive form as in soft drinks, the cariogenicity may be unrelated to the sugar concentration. However, the frequency of sugar intake will still play a critical role in caries development.

When the effects of varying all the different parameters in the model are studied, the results show, as might be expected, that the unstimulated salivary flow rate is the most important variable. Small decreases from the average unstimulated salivary flow rate can greatly prolong sugar clearance time. This partly explains the great increase in caries which occurs in patients with xerostomia. The results also point to the danger of consuming carbohydrate-containing foods just prior to bedtime since the salivary flow is greatly decreased during sleep (fig. 9/1) and sugar clearance time will be increased.

Before discussing the constituents of saliva it is appropriate to discuss briefly the difficulties of collecting and analyzing saliva.

Collection of Human Saliva

Saliva is the very antithesis of a pure chemical compound and it would indeed be difficult to prepare a more heterogeneous mixture. Whole saliva is a composite of the secretions of the paired parotid, submandibular and sublingual salivary glands. The numerous minor mucous glands also contribute to the salivary pool as does gingival crevice fluid and the fluid transudate from the oral mucosa. Whole saliva also contains desquamated epithelial cells, leukocytes, bacteria and food debris. The salivary glands not only secrete fluids which differ from each other in composition but which are affected by a variety of factors, such as the flow rate, the duration of stimulation, the diet and the time of day when the saliva is collected. Further, the unstimulated salivary flow rate exhibits a circadian rhythm as shown in figure 9/1 and virtually stops during sleep. It is precisely because of the numerous factors involved in the regulation of salivary composition that many of the early studies on whole saliva are conflicting and difficult to interpret. More meaningful results have been obtained by studying secretions collected from the individual salivary glands under carefully standardized conditions.

Unstimulated saliva is the term used to describe the saliva which can be collected by subjects who are awake but are undergoing no apparent exogenous stimulation. The average flow rate is about 0.3 ml/min. Stimulated whole saliva is usually collected by allowing the subject to chew inert materials such as paraffin wax. As saliva accumulates in the mouth it is expectorated into a test tube prior to analysis.

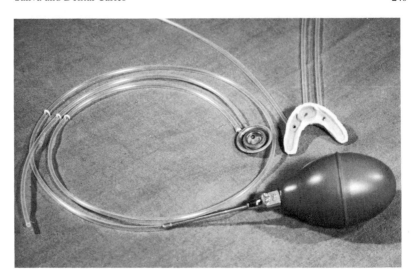

Fig. 9/2. Carlson-Crittenden device (Lashley cannula) for collecting saliva from the parotid gland (left side). Collection device for submandibular and sublingual saliva (upper right side).

Saliva from the parotid duct is usually obtained by the use of the Carlson-Crittenden device (also referred to as a Lashley cannula) illustrated on the left of figure 9/2. This device has outer and inner concentric depressions. The inner hollow of this device is placed over Stenson's duct and the saliva is able to flow down a polyethylene tube into a collecting receptacle. The outer hollow is connected to a vacuum suction bulb; negative pressure ensures a tissue seal for the collecting device.

Submandibular saliva is more difficult to obtain but is usually collected by direct cannulation of the ducts or by a custom-made device of silicone rubber which fits over the openings of both submandibular ducts (upper right of fig. 9/2) and simultaneously allows collection of sublingual saliva.

The major contribution to unstimulated whole saliva is derived from the submandibular glands. However, as exogenous stimulation is applied the contribution from the parotid glands approaches that from the submandibular. Minor salivary gland secretions and sublingual gland secretions each contribute about 7–8% of the total volume of saliva.

Inorganic Constituents of Saliva

Water is the main constituent of saliva. In man saliva is always hypotonic with respect to plasma. Unstimulated saliva may have as low as one tenth of the plasma osmolarity, but at very high flow rates the osmolarity may be about three quarters that of plasma. The specific gravity of saliva is about 1.007, with about 0.6% solid matter, 0.3% organic and 0.3% inorganic. The main inorganic constituents in whole mixed saliva, and for comparison those in blood serum and in plaque fluid from humans are listed in table 9/I.

The main electrolytes of saliva are potassium, sodium, calcium, chloride, bicarbonate and inorganic phosphate. Other electrolytes that are present in low concentrations, less than 1 mM, include fluoride, sulfate, thiocyanate, iodide and magnesium. The saliva secreted in the acinar regions of the glands has an electrolyte composition similar to that of an ultrafiltrate of plasma (table 9/I). However, the composition is markedly altered as the saliva passes along the duct system, mainly due to reabsorption of sodium and chloride and secretion of potassium and inorganic phosphate. The concentrations of both cations and anions are affected by factors such as flow rate (fig. 9/3), the duration of stimulation [Dawes, 1969] and the time of day of saliva collection [Dawes, 1972]. The concentration of sodium increases with increased flow rate from the major salivary glands. In unstimulated parotid saliva the sodium concentration may be as low as 1 mM but increases to about 100 mM at high flow rates. The effect of flow rate on the concentration of chloride in the saliva is similar except at low flow rates (fig. 9/3). At slow flow rates the increased time available for reabsorption of both sodium and chloride in the salivary ducts causes a decrease in their concentrations; the opposite occurs at higher flow rates. The concentration of potassium in unstimulated parotid saliva may be as high as 7 times that of plasma. At higher flow rates the concentration of potassium decreases but is still 3–4 times higher than in plasma. Although figure 9/3 illustrates the general effects of flow rate on salivary composition, it should be stressed that at any given flow rate there is a high degree of interindividual variation in the concentration of virtually all components of saliva.

Salivary pH and Buffering Capacity

The bicarbonate is the most important buffer system in the saliva and the pH of saliva is governed by the ratio between the combined and free carbonic acid as expressed by the Henderson-Hasselbalch equation:

$$pH = pK_a + \log \frac{[HCO_3^-]}{[H_2CO_3]},$$

where $[H_2CO_3] = 0.03 \cdot pCO_2$, and the pK_a is approximately 6.1.

Table 9/I. A comparison of the concentrations of selected constituents of blood, saliva and plaque fluid serum in humans[1]

	Blood serum, plasma or whole blood (B)	Saliva[2] parotid U	S	submandibular U	S	whole (mixed) U	S	Plaque fluid
pH	7.35–7.45 (B)	5.8	7.7	6.5	7.4	6.7	6.8–7.5	6.5
Bicarbonate, mM	23–32 (B)	1.0	22–30	2–4	14–16	5	15–50	
Sodium, mM	135–145	1.5–2.5	30–55	3–4	25	4–6	26	35 (mM)
Potassium, mM	3.5–5.5	24–28	13–22	14–15	13	22	20	61.5 (mM)
Calcium, mM	2–2.5	1.0	1.0	1–1.6	1.6–2	1.5–4	1.5–3	6.5 (mM)
Magnesium, mM	1–1.5	0.1–0.2	0.02	0.05–0.1	0.035	0.2	0.15–0.2	3.7 (mM)
Chloride, mM	95–105	17–22	17–33	11–12	16–26	15	30–100	
Phosphorus (inorg.), mM	1–1.5	10	3	4–6	2	6	4	14.2 (mM)
Glucose, mg/100 ml	70–100 (B)	0.8	0.2	0.5		0.5–1.0	1.0	
Ammonia, mg/100 ml	0.08–0.11 (B)	0.9	0.06	0.7	0.04	12	4–8	
Urea, mg/100 ml	14–40 (B)	30	22–27	10	5	20	13–22	18 (mM)
Thiocyanate, mg/100 ml	0.1–1.5		3			15	7–16	
Total protein, mg/100 ml	6.5–8.2 (g/100 ml)	250	270–320	110	150	225–350	280–300	1.49 (g/100 ml)
Iodide, µg/100 ml	3–8 (bound)	4–10	2–15	12	6	4–24	15–180	
Fluoride, µg/100 ml	10–20	3	2			8–25	2–20	2 (µM)

[1] Means or ranges for means are given. No entry indicates lack of data.
[2] Values are for unstimulated (U), or stimulated (S) flow rates approximating 1.0 ml/min for pure secretions, usually exceeding 1.0ml/min for whole saliva.
The blood and saliva values are reprinted from *Suddick* et al. [1980]. The plaque fluid values are from *Tatevossian and Gould* [1976].

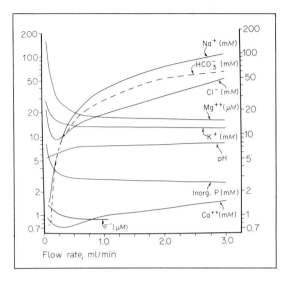

Fig. 9/3. The effect of flow rate on the composition of parotid saliva [*Dawes*, 1975].

Since the partial pressure of CO_2 in saliva is relatively constant and in equilibrium with that in venous blood from the glands, variations in bicarbonate concentration are the chief determinant of salivary pH. As seen in figure 9/3, the bicarbonate concentration is very low in unstimulated saliva and such saliva is poorly buffered with a pH as low as 5.3. However, at high flow rates the salivary bicarbonate concentration may reach as high as 60 mM (fig. 9/3) and this type of saliva is well buffered with a pH as high as 7.8.

By virtue of the volatile nature of CO_2 gas, the breakdown by acids of bicarbonate leads to the eventual escape of CO_2 from solution. This confers additional buffering power to the bicarbonate system in excess of that due only to the concentration of bicarbonate present. The loss of the CO_2, in effect, removes the acid element of the bicarbonate-carbonic acid system and reduces the change in the ratio of bicarbonate to carbonic acid. About 85% of the total buffer capacity of the saliva comes from the bicarbonate system [*Wah Leung*, 1951]. Phosphate and proteins in saliva constitute the other buffer systems, but the concentrations of these substances are too low to be of significance.

Saliva contains O_2, N_2 and CO_2, in solution. Most of the CO_2 is in the form of bicarbonate, carbonate and dissolved CO_2. Ductal saliva has a pCO_2 of about 46 mm Hg. When the saliva is exposed to atmospheric air ($pCO_2 = 0.3$ mm Hg) in the mouth or in a beaker, there is a loss of dissolved CO_2 and an increase in pH which may reach higher than 9.0 in saliva present as a thin film in a beaker. Further, loss of carbon dioxide occurs due to the presence of carbonic anhydrase in saliva which catalyzes the reaction:

$$H_2CO_3 \rightleftharpoons CO_2 + H_2O.$$

The rapid loss of CO_2 from freshly secreted saliva, and the rise of pH may be sufficient to cause the solubility product for hydroxyapatite to be exceeded leading to precipitation of this compound, as well as other calcium phosphate salts (dicalcium phosphate). These properties of saliva may be significant in explaining why calculus formation is greatest in the area approximating the orifices of the parotid and the submandibular ducts.

Buffering capacity of saliva is a very significant property that affects the dental caries process. The bicarbonate in saliva is able to diffuse into the dental plaque to neutralize the acid formed from carbohydrate by the microorganisms. Exposure of plaque to stimulated saliva reduces the extent to which the pH falls after carbohydrate consumption [*Abelson and Mandel*, 1981]. The higher the salivary flow rate, the greater will be its buffering capacity.

Calcium and Phosphate Concentrations in Saliva

The inorganic phase of enamel consists essentially of crystalline hydroxyapatite. The solubility product, or Ksp, is determined for hydroxyapatite by the relation:

$$Ksp = [a_{Ca^{2+}}]^5 \, [a_{PO_4^{3-}}]^3 \, [a_{OH^-}]$$

in a saturated solution, where a indicates the activity of the appropriate ion (measured in mol/l) and the Ksp has a value of about 3.72×10^{-58}. The ion product in any given sample of saliva is defined by:

$$Ip = [a_{Ca^{2+}}]^5 \, [a_{PO_4^{3-}}]^3 \, [a_{OH^-}]$$

and may be less than, equal to or greater than the solubility product. If the Ip = Ksp, then the saliva is saturated with respect to hydroxyapatite. If Ip < Ksp, the saliva is unsaturated whilst if Ip > Ksp it is supersaturated. If the Ip were less than the Ksp the teeth would slowly solubilize. Thus, calcium and phosphate in saliva form an important natural defense mechanism against dissolution of teeth.

The Ip for a given sample of saliva is actually very difficult to calculate since calcium and phosphate in saliva exist in ionized and un-ionized forms. Some of the ions are bound to macromolecules and some exist as inorganic pairs or complexes such as $CaHPO_4$ and $CaHCO_3$. In resting saliva over 80% of the calcium is in the ionized form.

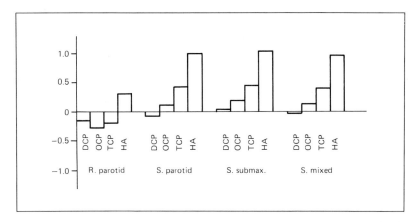

Fig. 9/4. Relative degree of saturation of resting parotid saliva and stimulated parotid, submaxillary, and mixed saliva with respect to dicalcium phosphate (formula $CaHPO_4 \cdot 2H_2O$, indicated as DCP), octacalcium phosphate (formula $Ca_8[PO_4]_6H_2 \cdot 5H_2O$ indicated as OCP), tricalcium phosphate (formula $Ca_3[PO_4]_2$, indicated as TCP), and hydroxyapatite (formula $Ca_{10}[PO_4]_6[OH]_2$, indicated as HA). The ordinate is calculated as the logarithm of the ratio between the salivary activity product and the solubility product divided by the number of ions in the solid. The zero line indicates saturation, positive values indicate supersaturation, and negative values undersaturation [from *Grøn and Hay, 1978*, with permission].

The activity of the ions is dependent on the ionic strength of the saliva, calculation of which demands a knowledge of the concentrations of all the other ions in saliva besides those of calcium, phosphate and hydroxyl.

As seen in figure 9/3, the phosphate concentation tends to fall as flow rate increases whilst the calcium concentration falls initially but then rises at higher flow rates. Despite the fall in total phosphate concentration as flow rate increases, paradoxically the Ip increases. This is due to the associated increase in pH at higher flow rates. The pH affects the Ip in two ways. Firstly, the fraction of total phosphate present as PO_4^{3-} ions (as opposed to HPO_4^{2-} or $H_2PO_4^-$ ions or H_3PO_4) increases markedly with pH. Secondly, the hydroxyl ion concentration also increases with pH.

Enamel contains predominantly hydroxyapatite but four different types of calcium phosphate salts have been detected in dental calculus. These are dicalcium phosphate dihydrate, octacalcium phosphate, tricalcium phosphate and hydroxyapatite. The relative degree of saturation of mixed saliva and resting saliva obtained from separate glands with respect to these four calcium phosphate compounds is depicted in figure 9/4. It will be noted that stimulated salivary secretions are all supersaturated with respect to octacalcium phosphate, tricalcium phosphate and hydroxyapatite.

Since saliva is supersaturated with respect to hydroxyapatite [*Grøn*, 1973], one might expect random precipitation of this salt to occur. However, this does not usually happen because saliva contains several types of proteins which inhibit the precipitation of calcium phosphates by binding to the surface of early crystal nuclei thereby preventing their further growth. The functions of these proteins are discussed in more detail later in the chapter.

The presence of calcium, phosphate and other inorganic ions, particularly fluoride, permits saliva to play an important protective role in maintaining the integrity of dental tissues. Saliva plays a key role in the posteruptive maturation of enamel. A calcium- and phosphate-rich environment also facilitates remineralization of incipient carious lesions or demineralized zones of enamel. Accessibility of saliva is an important factor in permitting remineralization of incipient carious lesions. Remineralization is discussed in detail in vol. 2, chapter 3.

Fluoride Concentration in Saliva

The level of fluoride ions in ductal saliva in man on a moderate fluoride intake is very low, in the range of 0.01–0.03 ppm which is slightly lower than that in plasma [*Shannon*, 1977]. Fluoride ion levels of whole saliva appear to be about double those in parotid and submandibular ductal saliva, probably due to the increased fluoride concentration in cellular debris, or (less likely) due to high fluoride levels in secretions of minor salivary glands. Fluoride levels in saliva are largely independent of salivary flow rate and are determined by the amount ingested. Administration of 3.0–10.0 mg of fluoride daily results in a significant increase in fluoride concentrations in secretions from the major salivary glands, even 24 h after the dose administration [*Shannon*, 1977]. Although the salivary fluoride concentration appears low, it is in fact between about 3 times and several hundred times the hydroxyl ion concentration (depending on flow rate). The ion product for fluorapatite is defined by:

$$Ip = [a_{Ca^{++}}]^5 \, [a_{PO_4^{3-}}]^3 \, [a_{F^-}],$$

and in both unstimulated and stimulated saliva it always exceeds the Ksp for fluorapatite. Thus, fluorapatite is essentially insoluble in all types of saliva, which is why it is so beneficial to have as high a proportion of fluorapatite in surface enamel as possible.

The small concentration of fluoride in saliva as well as in potable water promotes the formation of fluorapatite in surface enamel. Higher stable concentrations of fluoride in the enamel surface accrue very slowly from the salivary environment and perhaps dental plaque [*Jenkins and Edgar*, 1977], but may be reached more rapidly by topical fluoride applications.

The importance of maintenance and augmentation of fluoride in the enamel surface is obvious when we consider what happens to persons who are transferred from a fluoridated to a nonfluoridated community. In such persons the fluoride concentration in the enamel surface is reduced as is the protection against caries. More on this subject in volume 2, chapter 2, dealing with fluorides and dental health.

Organic Constituents of Saliva

Saliva secreted by the salivary glands mixes in the oral cavity with small volumes of crevicular fluid and transudate from the oral mucosa. Enmeshed in saliva are bacteria, desquamated epithelial cells and leukocytes. The proteins in whole saliva may be modified by hydrolytic enzymes from bacteria and cells. In order to understand the nature of saliva proteins it is therefore best to study salivary proteins as they are secreted by the glands prior to mixing with other components.

Over 20 different proteins and glycoproteins have been found in both parotid and submandibular saliva using electrophoretic and column chromatographic techniques. The total protein in saliva may range from 0.025 to 1 g/100 ml as compared to the narrower limits of about 7 g/100 ml in serum. Of the different components identified in parotid saliva by gel electrophoresis a number have been purified. Many of the proteins appear to be closely related to each other but the task of identifying and purifying them is difficult and much remains to be learned about their characteristics and significance.

Salivary Proteins with Digestive Functions

Amylase and Other Hydrolytic Enzymes

α-Amylase constitutes about 30% of the total protein in parotid saliva but its concentration is considerably lower in submandibular saliva. α-Amylase is a hydrolytic enzyme which cleaves the $\alpha(1-4)$ glycosidic linkages in starch and glycogen. It contains about 1 g atom of calcium per mole of enzyme and requires chloride ion for its activity. There is always sufficient chloride in saliva for full enzymic activity and the optimum pH is about neutrality.

Amylase in saliva is present as about 6 isozymes [*Merritt and Kahn*, 1978]. Two major families of enzymes have been identified; a glycosylated group which has a molecular weight of 62,000 and a nonglycosylated group with a molecular weight of 56,000 [*Keller* et al., 1971]. The difference in the molecular weight is accounted for by the carbohydrate content. Within each of the families, different isozymes can be identified on the basis of electrophoretic mobility and they appear to differ only in the degree of amidation. It is possible that the isoenzymes originate from the same protein by postribosomal modifications. The different isozymes have identical amino acid compositions and presumably primary structures. They possess the same catalytic activity and the biological significance of the multiple forms of the enzyme has not been determined.

The main functions of amylase in the oral cavity may be to increase the rate of dissolution and removal of starch-containing food debris retained around the teeth and on the oral mucosa. It does not contribute significantly to digestion as it is inactivated by the acid in gastric juice.

In addition to amylase, small amounts of other enzymes with digestive functions have been detected. These include acid phosphatase, ribonuclease, esterase, β-glucuronidase and amino peptidase. These hydrolases may have little physiological significance in digestion. Lipase activity of saliva is very low and is probably of no significance.

Salivary Antibacterial Substances

A number of antibacterial factors, such as lysozyme, lactoperoxidase, lactoferrin and immunoglobulin A, are present in saliva. Given the fact that the mouth is always populated by a great variety of bacterial species it is self-evident that in spite of these antibacterial factors, organisms commonly encountered in the mouth manage to survive. The role of the salivary antibacterial factors in the oral microbial ecology is largely unknown but possibly they function to prevent the establishment of more pathogenic transient invaders.

Lysozyme
Lysozyme is an enzyme which has the property of cleaving the cell walls of certain microorganisms, thereby causing their lysis. The enzyme cleaves the β 1–4 bond between *N*-acetylmuramic acid and *N*-acetylglucosamine which constitute the repeating disaccharide unit of the cell wall peptidoglycan. The antibacterial action of lysozyme apparently does not depend completely on cell lysis. *Streptococcus mutans* BHT lose their viability in the presence of lysozyme and either detergent or sodium chloride without lysis of the cell wall peptidoglycan. On the other hand, some organisms appear to be resistant to salivary lysozyme action. While the action of lysozyme has been established its role in determining the bacterial ecology of the oral cavity is not clear.

Lactoperoxidase

It has been known for a number of years that a factor exists in milk, tears and saliva which can inhibit the growth and acid formation of some bacteria. Subsequently the substance was identified as an enzyme called lactoperoxidase. Lactoperoxidase oxidizes thiocyanate (SCN⁻) in the presence of hydrogen peroxide which is formed by many oral organisms. This anti-bacterial system is known to be inhibitory towards lactobacilli and some streptococci. The reaction proceeds as follows:

$$H_2O_2 + SCN^- \xrightarrow{\text{peroxidase}} OSCN^- + H_2O.$$

The mechanism of bacterial inhibition is due to the ability of hypothiocyanite (OSCN⁻) to oxidize thiol groups which leads to inactivation of many bacterial enzymes.

Although the mechanism by which the lactoperoxidase system may inhibit bacterial growth has been clarified, the clinical significance of the finding is unknown. The amount of hydrogen peroxide in vivo is too low for optimal inhibition by the lactoperoxidase system. Practical efforts to prevent caries and plaque formation by the use of hydrogen peroxide-generating enzymes to enhance the efficiency of the lactoperoxidase system have been described with positive results [*Hoogendoorn* et al., 1977].

Lactoferrin

The bacteriocidal effect of lactoferrin is due to its strong iron-binding capacity thereby removing iron from solution and making it unavailable as an essential bacterial nutrient. Lactoferrin has been shown to be antagonistic to *S. mutans*. The practical implication of this finding on caries prevalence is unknown.

Immunoglobulins

There are two principal immunological mechanisms involved in protection against infectious diseases. One involves production of antibodies (humoral immunity) whilst the other involves cells (cell-mediated immunity). Antibodies may be produced by plasma cells in lymph nodes for secretion into the general circulation (systemic immunity) or they may be produced by plasma cells associated with various secretory tissues, such as the salivary and mammary glands (local immunity). The antibodies produced by plasma cells of the systemic system are of five classes termed IgG, IgA, IgE, IgD and IgM of which IgG predominates. However, the predominant immunoglobulin class in saliva is IgA in a modified form – secretory immunoglobulin A or S-IgA [*Tomasi*, 1976] described below. The route of antigen administration may determine whether systemic or local immunity predominates. The best illustration of this is furnished by the action of the different polio vaccines. The basis of the Salk vaccine is a killed virus given intramuscularly which stimulates the production of IgG and IgA. The Sabin oral vaccine is a live, attenuated virus which causes an S-IgA response. Both vaccines are effective against polio virus.

Salivary immunoglobulin A differs from its serum counterpart in that it mostly exists as a dimer of IgA to which are attached 2 other molecules, one being termed secretory component and other J chain. Recent evidence suggests that secretory component is attached entirely to one of the 2 IgA molecules whilst the J chain is attached to both. All polymeric antibody molecules contain 1 J chain. Salivary IgA and J chains are synthesized by plasma cells located in the salivary glands. The secretory component is synthesized by the acinar cells and is attached while the dimeric IgA-J chain complex passes through the acinar cells on route to the saliva [*Brandtzaeg*, 1975]. Salivary IgA is particularly resistant to proteolytic enzymes, apparently due to its association with secretory component.

The existence of a local antibody system in plasma cells located in the salivary glands, which can be stimulated to produce S-IgA, is of great interest because of the potential for producing a local response to an antigen. It is known that ingestion of inactivated *S. mutans* cells by germ-free rats elicits salivary antibody formation as does consumption of large numbers of *S. mutans* cells by human subjects [*McGhee* et al., 1978]. There is, however, little evidence that this secretory response lasts longer than several months. The concentration of salivary IgA is approximately 4 mg/100 ml in stimulated submandibular and parotid saliva. However, its concentration is considerably higher in the secretions of minor salivary glands and reaches levels of about 30 mg/100 ml. These secretions are in close proximity to the teeth and may be of significance even though they account for only about 8% of the total volume of mixed saliva.

Animal experiments suggest that both systemically and locally produced antibodies may operate to protect against caries. The latter involves the local immune mechanism via the saliva and the other involves gingival crevicular fluid which is derived from plasma [*Lehner*, 1978]. This system is explained in more detail in vol. 2, chapter 12.

Other Salivary Proteins with Protective Functions

Glycoproteins

Glycoproteins are covalent complexes of protein and carbohydrate. They are usually classified according to the nature of the linkage of the carbohydrate side chain bound to the protein molecule. Based on the carbohydrate-protein linkage, the two major types of glycoproteins are the mucinous and serous glycoproteins. In the mucinous glycoproteins, the linkage is O-glycosidic between galactosamine and serine or threonine. In the serous type glycoproteins the linkage is between glucosamine and asparagine. In saliva the serous type glycoproteins include amylase, ribonuclease, immunoglobulins and the proline-rich glycoproteins.

The most important glycoproteins in saliva that have a protective function are the mucinous type. Mucin has been isolated from human submandibular, sublingual and palatal saliva. No mucins have been identified in human parotid saliva which contains serous glycoproteins only. Purified mucin from human submandibular saliva has a molecular weight in the 500,000–1 million range. About 70–85% of the dry weight of mucin consists of carbohydrate, and the protein core has high content of serine, threonine, proline, glycine and alanine. The carbohydrate side chains have been found to vary considerably in structure from one to another. The carbohydrates may be sulfated through an ester linkage of the amino sugars thereby imparting a negative charge to the molecule. Sialic acid, a common terminal carbohydrate constituent of mucins, is also negatively charged at neutral pH.

Mucins, because of their large molecular weight and complex structure, possess important properties. In solution, they occupy a large volume because of the hydrophilic carbohydrate side chains that cause an extension of the polymer and decreased mobility of the water molecules. The solutions, therefore, have a very high viscosity and form a protective hydrated coating on epithelial surfaces. Mucin prevents dehydration of the mucous membranes, and acts as a lubricant aiding in chewing, swallowing and in speech. In some people, certain of the mucins in whole saliva possess either A, B or O blood group activity and the ability to secrete these substances is inherited as a Mendelian dominant. The major source of these blood group substances appears to be the minor mucous glands and they are occasionally of forensic importance.

Salivary Agglutinins

Recent evidence indicates that some of the salivary glycoproteins can interact specifically with microorganisms. It has been demonstrated by *Gibbons and Spinell* [1970] that salivary glycoproteins can cause an aggregation of various strains of oral microorganisms. These salivary glycoproteins are different from salivary immunoglobulins and from serous glycoproteins. The exact structural nature of the interaction is poorly understood; however, the ability of specific macromolecules of saliva to agglutinate microorganisms has important biological implications. Agglutination of microorganisms could either result in their rapid removal from the oral cavity when the saliva is swallowed or, if the agglutinated microorganisms are more adherent, could promote their colonization of epithelial and dental surfaces. These phenomena are discussed further in chapter 5.

Salivary Proteins which Inhibit Formation of Hydroxyapatite

Several salivary proteins bind calcium and/or inhibit formation of hydroxyapatite. These proteins are statherin and a group of proline-rich proteins.

Statherin

Statherin, a polypeptide of molecular weight 5,380, consists of 43 amino acids and has a concentration in saliva of 2–6 μM [*Schlesinger and Hay*, 1977]. Statherin, in addition to inhibiting formation of hydroxyapatite, also prevents precipitation of calcium phosphate salts from supersaturated solutions by adsorbing onto early crystal nuclei. The physiological advantages of the presence of salivary statherin are that saliva can be supersaturated with respect to hydroxyapatite, thus facilitating remineralization of early carious lesions, without the spontaneous precipitation of calcium phosphate which would otherwise occur. In vitro, statherin is selectively adsorbed on enamel surfaces and this inhibits the continued formation of hydroxyapatite crystals on the enamel surface from the calcium and phosphate ions in saliva. The inhibition is due to the ability of the statherin to block crystal growth of calcium phosphate.

Proline-Rich Proteins

A number of proteins have been isolated from saliva which are characterized by a high content of proline varying from about 25–40% of the total number of amino acid residues. These proteins have been divided into basic, acidic and glycosylated proline-rich proteins and they all appear to possess extensive structural homology. They constitute about 70% of the total protein of parotid saliva with the acidic proline-rich fraction alone accounting for about 28%. A number of basic and acidic proline-rich proteins have been isolated by different workers. The acidic proteins were first described by *Bennick and Connell* [1971] and *Oppenheim* et al. [1971] and 2 of these, labeled A and C, have subsequently been characterized by *Bennick* [1982]. Both are linear polypeptides and protein C contains protein A plus an additional length of peptide at the C terminus. These proteins contain two types of calcium-binding sites involving phosphoserine and aspartic acid which are located at the N-terminal, relatively proline-poor regions of the protein. They inhibit hydroxyapatite formation and constitute a substantial amount of the protein extracted from newly formed pellicle in vivo.

While the roles of these proteins have not been completely elaborated, there is some evidence that acidic proline-rich proteins act to maintain the ionic calcium concentration in saliva by binding or releasing calcium in response to an increase or decrease, respectively, in total calcium concentration. They may also be involved in the prevention of ectopic mineralization, such as calculus, in the oral cavity and in the preservation of the integrity of mineralized tooth substance as they are readily absorbed by hydroxyapatite and at least the acidic proline-rich proteins are constituents of the salivary pellicle.

The Acquired Salivary Pellicle

A thoroughly clean tooth will, within seconds of exposure to saliva, acquire an amorphous, proteinaceous membrane called the acquired pellicle which originates from the adsorption of several salivary proteins upon the hydroxyapatite surface of enamel. This is of great clinical relevance as, following the acid-etch procedure, it is essential to prevent contact of the etched enamel with saliva prior to placement of a composite resin. Otherwise the salivary proteins will tend to fill up the defects in the newly etched surface.

Pellicle thickness varies from about 100 nm after 2 h to about 400 nm after 24–48 h [*Lie*, 1979]. The salivary pellicle usually has three structural features (fig. 9/5). The subsurface component penetrates a small distance into the pores and demineralized spaces of enamel, and has a dendritic appearance. Next is a component of several microns in thickness which uniformly forms on the surface of the tooth. A suprastructure of variable thickness forms over the surface pellicle. While some bacteria may be present, the initial salivary pellicle is predominantly bacteria-free. The adsorbed salivary coating becomes highly insoluble with time, probably due to denaturation of proteins. The coating becomes rapidly populated by mixed bacterial aggregates which grow in numbers and coalesce, to form the bacterial dental plaque which is discussed in chapter 5.

Mechanism of Salivary Pellicle Formation

There is no dispute that salivary proteins are the major constituents of the acquired coating following cleansing of teeth. What is not clearly understood is the mechanism by which proteins are adsorbed on enamel surfaces and which salivary proteins are selectively involved in the process.

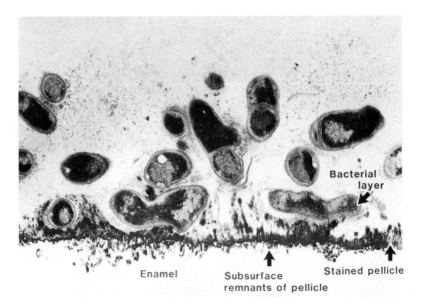

Fig. 9/5. Electron micrograph of stained organic salivary pellicle and early plaque on the surface of a demineralized tooth (courtesy, *M. Listgarten*). ×32,800.

In chapter 4 the important properties of surface apatite crystals of enamel and their interaction with solutions are discussed. The surface of apatite crystals is hydrophilic, highly charged and readily adsorbs proteins. A practical application of this property of hydroxyapatite is its wide use in chromatographic columns for the separation of proteins and nucleic acids. The negatively charged groups in the macromolecules, i.e. carboxyl, phosphate, and sulfate, as well as those with positive charges (amido and guanido groups) are bound to the hydroxyapatite by electrostatic bonding. Since the tooth surface is composed almost entirely of charged molecules the adsorption of salivary protein is most easily explained by this property of enamel. Binding of both positive and negative groups by surface enamel is possible since phosphate and calcium ions impart both acidic and basic properties to the enamel surface.

Composition of the Salivary Pellicle
Salivary proteins vary widely in their composition and charge properties. Saliva is in contact with hydroxyapatite crystallites of surface enamel which also vary in composition, hydration and surface charge. It

follows that there is a great variability in the interaction of the saliva and the surface of enamel. The salivary proteins that are known to be present in the pellicle, and some that have not been directly demonstrated but have a high affinity for hydroxyapatite are:

–   Acidic, proline-rich proteins (PRP).
–   Glycoproteins.
–   Serum proteins, enzymes, immunoglobulins.

Both statherin and acidic PRP are selectively adsorbed to hydroxyapatite [*Hay*, 1973]. Newly formed pellicle contains as much as 35% acidic PRP. This is reduced significantly in older samples of pellice presumably due to proteolytic breakdown of the absorbed protein [*Bennick*, 1982]. These proteins contain phosphate groups which interact with enamel, forming ionic bonds. Removal of the phospate groups from the molecule affects the binding but does not abolish it.

Statherin has a high affinity for hydroxyapatite and in all probability is a constituent of salivary pellicle although it has not been directly demonstrated. As with other salivary proteins, statherin is degraded by salivary proteases.

Sulfated glycoproteins have been demonstrated in the acquired pellicle in monkeys [*Rölla and Embery*, 1977]. These proteins are known to interact with microorganisms. Their presence in plaque may have significance in selectivity of the colonization of bacteria in plaque.

Salivary pellicle contains various serum proteins including immunoglobulins (IgA, IgG and IgM) and as many as 10 different proteins have been identified using immunofluorescent techniques. Enzymatic activities indicating the presence of amylase, lysozyme, neuraminidase, and lactoperoxidase have been detected in pellicle. The antibacterial substances may affect the microbial composition of the pellicle.

The total pellicle (acid-soluble and acid-insoluble) has a high proportion of glycine, serine and glutamic acids; and a low content of sulfur and aromatic amino acids [*Mayhall*, 1970; *Sönju and Rölla*, 1973]. In freshly formed (2-hour) pellicle, the absence of muramic and diaminopimelic acid indicates that significant amounts of bacterial cell wall components are not present.

Properties and Functions of Pellicle
The salivary pellicle on surface apatite alters the properties of the enamel surface. This coating exhibits the following properties:

–   It acts as a lubricant to prevent premature wear of the enamel during mastication.

- It reduces the rate of demineralization of tooth surface by acidic foods and drinks.
- It acts as a semipermeable membrane and reduces ion mobility but the movement of water is unaffected. This property is probably important in prevention of initial cavitation and in the formation of subsurface demineralization of incipient lesions (chapter 10).
- It reduces mobility of calcium and phosphate ions from the enamel surface to the fluid environment. This may be accomplished by the binding of calcium at the hydroxyapatite surface by acidic proline-rich salivary proteins.
- It forms the surface for bacterial colonization and may influence the formation of the microbial dental plaque (discussed in chapter 5).
- It prevents the continued enlargement of the tooth surface by crystal growth of hydroxyapatite which would tend to occur in saliva supersaturated with respect to that salt.

Small Organic Molecules in Saliva

Low concentrations of naturally occurring amino acids, urea and peptides are found in saliva. Of these compounds the most significant is urea, the nitrogenous end product of protein metabolism. It is a small molecule and readily penetrates capillary walls. The concentration of urea in saliva is 13–30 mg/100 ml and significantly correlates with the concentration of urea in blood [*Nikiforuk* et al., 1956]. Urea in saliva is rapidly metabolized by bacteria leading to the formation of ammonia and carbon dioxide with a net production of base. This source of base may be important for the pH-rise phase of the Stephan curve. At one time a dentifrice was marketed containing urea and ammonium phosphate. The rationale for this was that ammonium ion was believed to inhibit the growth of *Lactobacillus acidophilus*. Clinical studies evaluating these dentifrices failed to demonstrate any therapeutic benefits and these products are no longer marketed.

A tetrapeptide with the sequence glycine-glycine-lysine-arginine has been isolated from saliva [*Kleinberg* et al., 1977]. It has been shown that this peptide, named sialin, is converted into ammonia and putrescine and thus reduces the pH drop, and eventually converts it into a pH rise, when salivary bacteria are incubated in vitro with low concentrations of glucose. At the concentrations present in saliva, sialin has no detectable effect if the sugar concentration is greater than 0.1–0.2%. It cannot therefore be effective in restoring the plaque pH to neutrality after the drop caused by sugar consumption. To neutralize completely the acid produced from 1 mol to sucrose (342 g), 0.5 mol (208 g) of sialin would have to be degraded. It is obvious that the amount of sialin that would be required to neutralize acids produced by food does not make the addition of the compound to cariogenic foods a practical procedure.

Glucose in Saliva

Fortunately, an endogenous source of carbohydrates in saliva, such as glucose, is lacking. Fasting plasma may contain about 80 mg of glucose per 100 ml while salivary glucose is less than 1 mg/100 ml but this may be supplemented slightly by some of the sugars released from salivary glycoproteins by bacterial enzymes. High salivary glucose levels would, of course, be intolerable in that this would provide a continuous source of cariogenic substrate for glycolytic bacteria.

Functions of Saliva

The various inorganic and organic constituents of saliva are involved in a variety of important functions. These are summarized in point form.

-   Digestion and tasting:
    Solids must be solubilized in saliva before the taste buds can be stimulated for taste sensations.
    The low concentrations of sodium, chloride and glucose and the low buffering capacity of unstimulated saliva make it ideal for tasting low concentrations of salty, sweet, acid or bitter substances.
    Amylase is the major digestive enzyme of saliva, which assists in the oral clearance of starch-containing foods.
    Mucinous and serous secretions, by lubricating oral structures, play an important role in mastication, deglutition and phonation.
-   Protective:
    Saliva performs many significant protective functions. Saliva not only buffers extreme acid changes in the oral cavity but plays an important role in buffering of acid foods and acids produced by bacterial plaques.
    Antibacterial enzymes and substances such as lysozyme, S-IgA, lactoperoxidase, and lactoferrin may be important as determinants of the oral bacterial ecology.
    Of great importance is the physical cleansing by saliva in the form of washing, dilution and clearance from the oral cavity of food debris and bacteria.
    Ca^{2+} and PO_4^{3-} concentrations constitute an important natural defense mechanism in protecting teeth against dissolution and in permitting remineralization of slightly etched enamel.

The mucinous secretions are important in protecting the oral mucous membranes against dehydration.
– Excretory:
Several different types of compounds are excreted in saliva, and these include some alkaloids, antibiotics, alcohol, and viruses. However, some of these substances may be reabsorbed after being swallowed. Heptitis B virus is found in saliva; the high incidence of hepatitis in some dental groups is attributed to the presence of the virus in the saliva of a significant percentage of patients.
Because of excretory functions, saliva may serve as a secretion that may be used as a diagnostic tool for such systemic conditions as Tay-Sachs disease, hyperaldosteronism, cystic fibrosis and digitalis poisoning.
– Water balance:
About 700–800 ml of saliva is secreted daily and swallowed. This is significant in conserving water.
Saliva plays an important role in thermoregulation in some species such as the dog, which have no sweat glands and is necessary for suckling in such species as the rat.

Additional Reading

Dawes, C.: The chemistry and physiology of saliva; in Shaw, Sweeney, Cappuccino, Meller, Textbook of oral biology, p. 593 (Saunders, Toronto 1978).
Ferguson, D.B. (ed.): The environment of the teeth. Front. oral Physiol., vol. 3 (Karger, Basel 1981).
Kleinberg, I.; Ellison, S.A.; Mandel, I.D. (eds): Saliva and dental caries (Information Retrieval, New York 1979).

References

Abelson, D.C.; Mandel, I.D.: The effect of saliva on plaque pH in vivo. J. dent. Res. *60*: 1634 (1981).
Bennick A.: Salivary proline-rich proteins. Mol. cell. Biochem. *45*: 83 (1982).
Bennick A.; Connell, G.: Purification and partial characterization of four proteins from human parotid saliva. Biochem. J. *123:* 455 (1971).
Brandtzaeg, P.: Immunoglobulin systems of oral mucosa and saliva; in Dolby, Oral mucosa in health and disease, p. 137 (Blackwell, Oxford, 1975).
Dawes, C.: The effects of flow rate and duration of stimulation on the concentrations of protein and the main electrolytes in human parotid saliva. Archs oral Biol. *14*: 277 (1969).
Dawes. C.: Circadian rhythms in human salivary flow rate and composition. J. Physiol., Lond. *220*: 529 (1972).

Dawes, C.: Salivary secretion; in Cohen, Kramer, Scientific foundations of dentistry, p. 516 (Heinemann, London 1975).

Dawes C.: A mathematical model of salivary clearance of sugar from the oral cavity. Caries Res. *17*: 321–334 (1983).

Dreizen, S.; Brown, L.R.; Daly, T.E.; Drane, J.B.: Prevention of xerostomia-related dental caries in irradiated cancer patients. J. dent. Res. *56*: 99 (1977).

Ericsson, Y.: Clinical investigations of the salivary buffering action. Acta odont. scand. 17: 131 (1959).

Gibbons, R.J.; Spinell, D.M.: Salivary-induced aggregation of plaque bacteria; in McHugh, Dental plaque, p. 207 (Livingstone, Edinburgh 1970).

Grøn, P.: Saturation of human saliva with calcium phosphates. Archs oral Biol. *18*: 1385 (1973).

Grøn, P.; Hay, D.I.: Salivary calcium and phosphate interactions; in Shaw, Sweeney, Cappuccino, Meller, Textbook of oral biology, p. 617 (Saunders, Toronto 1978).

Hay, D.I.: The interaction of human parotid salivary proteins with hydroxyapatite. Archs oral biol. *18*: 1517 (1973).

Hoogendoorn, H.; Piessens, J.P.; Scholtes, W.; Stoddard, L.A.: Hypothiocyanite ion; the inhibitor formed by the system lactoperoxidase-thiocyanate-hydrogen peroxide. Caries Res. *11*: 77 (1977).

Jenkins, G.N.; Edgar, W.M.: Distribution and forms of F in saliva and plaque. Caries Res. *11*: suppl. 1, p. 226 (1977).

Keller P.J.; Kaufman, D.L.; Allan, B.J.; Williams, B.L.: Further studies on the structural differences between the isoenzymes of human parotid α-amylase. Biochemistry, N.Y. *10*: 4867 (1971).

Kleinberg, I.; Kanapka, J.A.; Craw, D.: Effect of saliva and salivary factors on the metabolism of the mixed oral flora, in Stiles, Loesche, O'Brien, Microbial aspects of dental caries, vol. II, p. 433 (Information Retrieval, Washington 1977).

Lehner, T.: A vaccine against dental decay. New Scient. *78*: 216 (1978).

Lie, T.: Morphologic studies on dental plaque formation. Acta odont. scand. *37*: 73 (1979).

Llory, H.; Dammron, A; Gioanni, M.; Frank, R.M.: Some population changes in oral anaerobic microorganisms, *Streptococcus mutans* and yeasts following irradiation of the salivary glands. Caries Res. *6*: 298 (1972).

Mayhall, C.W.: Concerning the composition and source of the acquired enamel pellicle of human teeth. Archs oral Biol. *15*: 1327 (1970).

McGhee, J.R.; Mestecky, J.; Arnold, R.R.; Michalek, S.M.; Prince, S.J.; Babb, J.L.: Induction of secretory antibodies in humans following ingestion of *Streptococcus mutans*, in McGhee, Mestecky, Babb, Secretory immunity and infection. Adv. exp. med. Biol., vol. 107, p. 177 (1978).

Merritt, A.D.; Kahn, R.C.: The human α-amylases. Adv. hum. Genet. *8*: 135 (1978).

Nikiforuk, G.; Jackson, S.H.; Cox, M.A.; Grainger, R.M.: Some blood and salivary nonprotein nitrogen constituents in children, and dental caries. J. Pediat. *49*: 425 (1956).

Oppenhcim, F.G., Hay, D.I.; Franzblau, C.: Proline-rich proteins from human parotid saliva. I. Isolation and partial characterization. Biochemistry, N.Y. *10*: 4233 (1971).

Rölla, G.; Embery, G.: Sulfated glycoproteins in the acquired pellicle and in plaque from *Macaca fascicularis* demonstrated with labeled sulfate. Scand. J. dent. Res. *85*: 237 (1977)

Schlesinger, D.H.; Hay, D.I.: Complete covalent structure of statherin, a tyrosine-rich acidic peptide which inhibits calcium phosphate precipitation from human parotid saliva. J. biol. Chem. *252*: 1689 (1977).

Shannon, I.L.: Biochemistry of fluoride in saliva. Caries Res. *11*: suppl. 1, p. 206 (1977).

Sönju, T.; Rölla, G.: Chemical analysis of the acquired pellicle formed in two hours on cleaned human teeth in vivo. Caries Res. *7:* 30 (1973).

Suddick, R.P.; Hyde, R.J.; Feller, R.P.: Salivary water and electrolytes and oral health; in Menaker, The biologic basis of dental caries, p. 132 (Harper & Row, New York 1980).

Tatevossian, A.; Gould, C.T.: The composition of the aqueous phase in human dental plaque. Archs oral Biol. *21:* 319 (1976).

Tomasi, T.B.: The immune system of secretions. Fdns Immunol. ser. (Prentice-Hall, Englewood Cliffs 1976).

Wah Leung, S.: A demonstration of the importance of bicarbonate as a salivary buffer. J. dent. Res. *30:* 403 (1951).

10 The Caries Process – Morphological and Chemical Events

In the previous chapters we have considered the epidemiology of dental caries, the essentiality of the host (tooth), oral flora, and local substrate in the caries process and the role of saliva in modifying these primary factors. The reader, by now, should have a substantial knowledge of the nature of tooth substance, the metabolism of mircoorganisms involved in caries, and the dietary determinants of dental caries. With this background, we now turn to the mechanisms whereby mineralized dental tissue is destroyed by the caries process. The approach shall be to first describe the morphological features and subsequently the chemical events involved in the formation of an incipient carious lesion in enamel. A description of salient features of caries of dentin and cementum is also presented.

The Incipient Carious Lesion in Enamel

The first discernible clinical sign of dental caries is the white spot, so-called because of the loss of translucency of the affected area. The white spot is most easily observed when the enamel is thoroughly dried (see chapter 1 for discussion of clinical aspects of the initial lesion). Clinically, no cavitation is evident but the surface may be rougher than normal enamel as assessed by a dental probe. The white spot is most frequently detected in the gingival area of the buccal or labial surfaces of the clinical crown of a tooth. Brown discoloration may become superimposed on white spots particularly if the lesion becomes arrested with time. The discoloration is extrinsic, resulting from the diffusion of organic material into the large pores characteristic of white spots. Incipient lesions are also very common on proximal, subcontact sites. These areas are not easily detected during a clinical examination since they are hidden from view by the adjacent contacting tooth; however, they are commonly observed on extracted teeth. Incipient interproximal lesions can be detected on a bite-wing radiograph as a small, cone-shaped radiolucent area in the outer enamel (fig. 10/1).

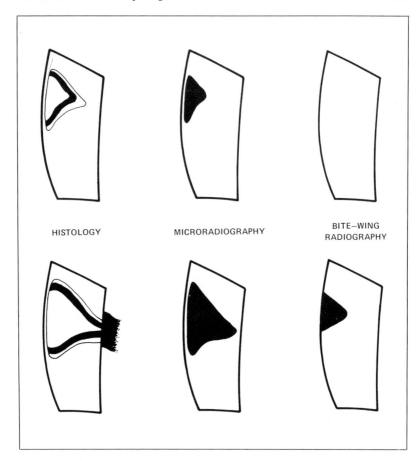

Fig. 10/1. Diagram to show the size of an enamel lesion when viewed by different techniques. In the top, the true extent of the lesion is shown histologically. Its size as observed by radiographic techniques is shown to the right. Such a lesion extending two thirds of the enamel thickness would not be observed on a clinical bite-wing radiograph. The larger lesion on the bottom of the diagram extends into the dentin. However, a clinical bite-wing radiograph gives the impression that the lesion is confined to the outer third of the enamel [from *Silverstone*, 1982, with permission].

At this stage, the incipient lesion may be arrested or even reversed by remineralization if an effective preventive program is enacted (more on remineralization in vol. 2, chapter 3). Restoration of an incipient lesion is an elective procedure which is generally not recommended except in cases of unusually high caries susceptibility.

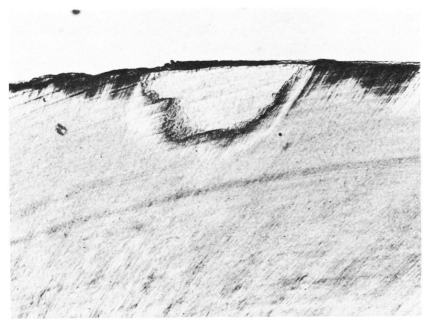

Fig. 10/2. Longitudinal ground section through a small enamel lesion. The section is examined in quinoline by transmitted light. The lesion shows a translucent zone over the entire advancing front. Superficial to this a dark zone can be seen, surrounding the body of the lesion. The striae of Retzius are enhanced in the body of the lesion, × 60 [from *Silverstone* et al., 1981, with permission].

Histological Features

A radiographically detectable initial enamel lesion when examined histologically will show the carious process penetrating to the underlying dentin, although the dentinal tissue is not invaded by bacteria. The relationship between lesion size as determined by different techniques is shown in figure 10/1. In the top diagram it can be seen that an enamel lesion penetrating two thirds of the depth of the enamel is not visible when examined by bite-wing radiography. Only when the lesion has penetrated into the underlying dentin can it be detected on the bite-wing radiograph. At this stage, radiographically the lesion is confined to the enamel only [*Silverstone*, 1982]. A carious lesion on the smooth surface of enamel is conical in shape with its broad base on enamel and the apex toward the dentin (fig. 10/2). When the lesion reaches the enamel-dentin junction it spreads laterally along the junction, thus undermining normal enamel.

In the case of fissure caries the initial lesion does not start at the base but on the lateral walls of the fissure as two smooth surface lesions that eventually fuse at the base of the fissure (fig. 10/3). The direction of the enamel prisms causes the carious lesion to broaden as it approaches dentin tissue and then to spread laterally at the enamel-dentin junction.

Light microscopy studies of carious lesions of enamel without cavitation have revealed four distinct zones (fig. 10/4) which represent varying degrees of hard tissue transformation [*Silverstone*, 1977]. Starting from the advancing front of the lesion these zones are classified as:

– A translucent zone which is the advancing front of the lesion.
– A dark zone separating the translucent zone from the body of the lesion.
– The body of the carious lesion which is markedly radiolucent.
– A relatively intact enamel surface layer.

These zones should not be interpreted as distinct entities but represent a continuum of changes as caries progresses.

Many studies of carious enamel have involved the use of polarized light microscopy. A brief description of this method of studying the crystal structure and aqueous phase of enamel will help in discussing the zones of carious enamel [*Silverstone*, 1973].

Structure of Carious Enamel and the Image in Polarized Light

Human enamel consists of apatite crystals packed closely together, orientated with their long axes approximately parallel with the long axis of each prism. The mineral is referred to as being birefringent, that is it has the property of resolving a beam of plane polarized light into two beams, one out of phase with the other. This birefringence due to the mineral component of the tissue is referred to as negative 'intrinsic birefringence'.

During carious dissolution spaces are created by removal of minerals. This results in an increase in the pore volume of the tissue which when filled with a medium having a refractive index (RI) which differs from that of the mineral phase produces another type of birefringence. This type of birefringence is known as 'form birefringence' and is positive in sign. As the RI of the medium in the pores progresses further from that of the enamel (1.62), so the amount of form birefringence increases. Similarly, as the pores increase in size and number (increasing demineralization) the amount of form birefringence will also increase.

Therefore, the observed birefringence seen in the polarizing microscope is due to a summation of the negative intrinsic birefringence of the mineral component, and the positive form birefringence due to the pores and the medium they contain. By measuring birefringence, it is possible to

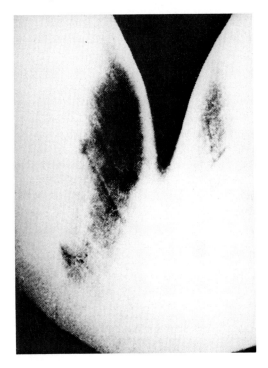

Fig. 10/3. Microradiograph of fissure caries showing the bilateral positioning of the lesion (courtesy *Silverstone*).

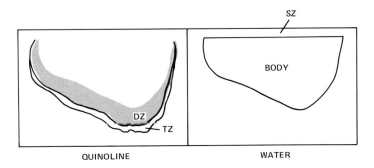

QUINOLINE   WATER

Fig. 10/4. Diagram to show the position of the four histological zones of enamel caries. All four zones cannot be observed in a single medium. Of the four classical histological zones, two are seen when the section is viewed in quinoline (R.I. 162) and the remaining two observed when the section is transferred to water. DZ = dark zone; TZ = translucent zone; SZ = surface zone.

calculate the internal pore volume in various areas of a lesion. For a more detailed description of polarized light and its uses and interpretation in enamel caries the reader is referred elsewhere [*Silverstone*, 1973].

The Translucent Zone

The advancing front of a carious lesion is represented by the translucent zone (fig. 10/2). The first discernible signs of enamel breakdown are seen in this area. This zone is not a consistent feature of enamel caries and is only seen when longitudinal ground sections of carious teeth are examined using agents such as quinoline or Canada balsam having a RI similar to enamel (RI – 1.62). Under these conditions approximately 50% of lesions show the appearance of a translucent zone [*Silverstone*, 1966]. Enamel alteration in this zone results in spaces or pores at junction sites such as the prism boundaries. The pores are large enough to admit quinoline resulting in essentially a structureless, translucent zone. Microdensitometric and chemical studies of this zone indicate some loss or mineral, and a resultant pore volume of about 1% as compared to 0.1% in normal enamel. The preferential removal of acid-labile moieties, such as carbonate and magnesium together with calcium and phosphate, is responsible for the increase in porosity [*Hallsworth* et al., 1973]. There is no evidence that organic material is removed or significantly altered in the translucent zone.

The Dark Zone

The dark zone lies deep to the body of the lesion and just superficial to the translucent zone (fig. 10/2). This zone is positively birefringent when the section is examined in quinoline with the polarizing microscope and has a pore volume of 2 – 4% (fig. 10/5). Mounting media such as quinoline or Canada balsam used in studying ground sections are unable to penetrate the small pores of this zone. This molecular sieving effect permits the micropores to remain filled with air. Light passing through this zone causes the brown discoloration of the dark zone. This is also the reason why the dark zone shows a reversal in its birefringence from negative to positive (fig. 10/5). Because of this phenomenon the dark zone is often referred to as the positive zone. When the section is examined in an aqueous medium having small molecules capable of penetrating the micropores, such as water, the dark zone is not visible (fig. 10/6). An enigma relating to the dark zone is why the pores are smaller than those seen in the translucent zone. Both

Fig. 10/5. Longitudinal ground section showing an enamel lesion examined in quinoline with the polarizing microscope. A well-marked dark zone can be seen at the advancing front of the lesion showing positive birefringence (courtesy *Silverstone*).

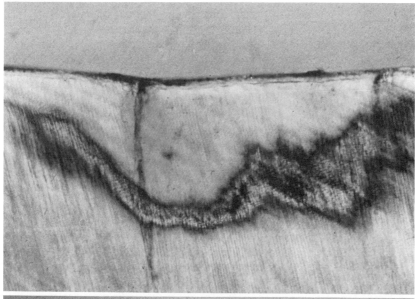

10/5

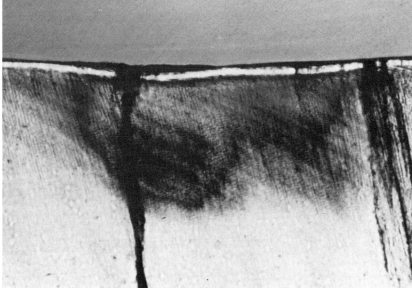

10/6

Fig. 10/6. Same lesion as in fig. 10/5 now examined in water with the polarizing microscope. Under these conditions the body of the lesion shows as an area of positive birefringence in sharp contrast to the surface zone which exhibits a negative birefringence (courtesy *Silverstone*).

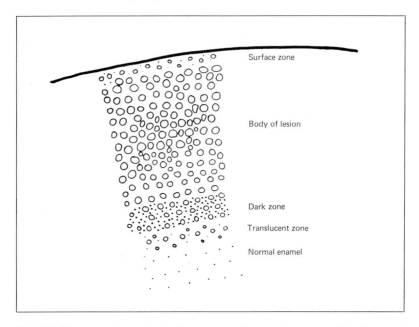

Fig. 10/7. Diagram to show the relative pore sizes in the various zones of the lesion and in normal enamel [from *Silverstone* et al., 1981, with permission].

zones represent mineral loss and a reasonable supposition is that the translucent zone at the advancing front of the carious lesion would be less demineralized and have a corresponding smaller pore size than the second zone, the dark zone. In experiments on the remineralization of enamel caries [*Silverstone and Poole*, 1968], it was shown that the dark zone increases in size, extending back into the area identified previously as the body of the lesion. This was the first clue as to the nature of the small pores in this region of the carious lesion. In further studies it was shown that the appearance of the dark zone was due to remineralization occurring at the advancing front of the lesion [*Silverstone*, 1977]. In addition, lesions without dark areas show normal dark zones at the appropriate histological site after exposure to synthetic calcifying fluids in vitro. The relative pore structure of the zones in a carious lesion is shown in figure 10/7.

The Body of the Lesion

Deep to the relatively unaffected enamel surface layer is the body of the carious lesion (fig. 10/4). Ground sections, when viewed in transmitted light, reveal enhanced striae of Retzius (fig. 10/2) and cross-striations in the

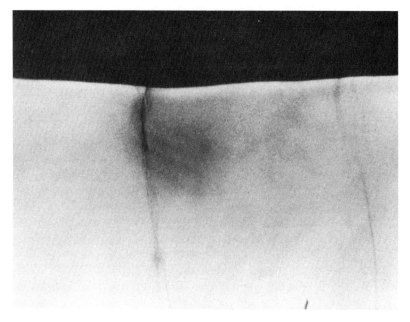

Fig. 10/8. Microradiograph of the lesion shown in fig. 10/5 and 10/6. The radiolucent subsurface region can be seen but is not comparable in size to that seen with the polarizing microscope (courtesy *Silverstone*).

enamel prisms. This zone, unlike normal enamel, is positively birefringent when examined in water (fig. 10/6), denoting a significant degree of mineral loss. *Silverstone* [1977] has shown that the body of the lesion has a minimum pore volume of 5% at its periphery and, even in a small subclinical lesion, there is a 25% pore volume. An increase in bound water and organic content follows the loss of mineral salts due to diffusion of saliva into this zone as caries progresses. Microradiographs confirm the radiolucent property of this zone (fig. 10/8). However, it can be seen from figure 10/8 that microradiography is a less sensitive technique than the use of polarized light microscopy (compare with fig. 10/5 and 10/6).

The Surface Zone

An important feature of the initial carious lesion is the presence of an apparently intact enamel surface overlying an area of subsurface demineralization. Quantitative studies of the surface layer, 20–100 μm thick, indicate that partial demineralization equivalent to about 1–10% loss of mineral salts has taken place. The surface zone has been defined as the zone of negative birefringence superficial to the positively birefringent body of the lesion seen when the section is examined in water (fig. 10/6) with the polarizing microscope [*Silverstone*, 1968]. Thus, the surface zone has a pore volume of less than 5% of spaces. It is important to realize that all four histological zones of the enamel lesion cannot be seen if the section is examined in a single medium.

Mechanism of Subsurface Lesion Formation in Incipient Caries

The mechanism by which a relatively sound outer enamel surface is preserved while the subsurface undergoes demineralization is intriguing and important in understanding the dynamics of enamel dissolution. Many research workers have developed experimental models which produce subsurface demineralization and which duplicate some of the morphological and biochemical aspects of an in vivo incipient lesion.

A common feature of studies that result in artificial caries-like lesions, including a relatively intact surface, involves a protective component which renders the surface enamel less soluble. In the earlier experiments the presence of colloids such as gelatin or hydroxyethyl cellulose in the acid solutions used to demineralize the enamel led to the formation of the various zones including an outer apparently intact zone. It was thought that the colloids adsorbed to the surface in the same way as salivary pellicle and protected the outer enamel from attack but allowed some acid to diffuse into the underlying enamel. Later, it was found that acid solutions almost saturated with calcium and phosphate ions also produced subsurface demineralization and an outer relatively intact layer which, under these conditions, seemed likely to be produced by reprecipitation of the calcium salts when the ions released from the enamel met the nearly saturated solvent. If the colloid solutions were dialyzed before use, they failed to produce a penetrating lesion from which it seemed that small ions such as phosphate and calcium in the colloids had protected the outer layer rather than an attachment of the colloid to the enamel surface. The explanation for this phenomenon is considered in detail later in this chapter. An initial carious lesion that is detected at the earliest clinical or radiographic stage with an intact surface and with no cavitation may have the potential for reversal and repair, if appropriate treatment is implemented.

Electron Microscopic Studies of Carious Enamel

Previous descriptions of the carious lesion using light microscopy are difficult to correlate with those of transmission electron microscopy since features like prism sheaths, interprismatic substance, cross-striations are

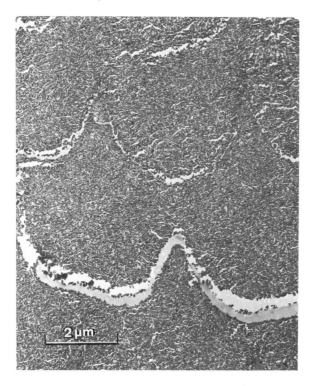

Fig. 10/9. Transmission electron micrograph through the body of a carious lesion cut transversely to prism direction. Prism junctions are marked by narrow channels. A diffuse demineralization is present throughout the tissue [from *Johnson*, 1967, with permission].

not observed at the ultrastructural level. Ultrastructural studies have been most valuable in clarifying the effects of caries on individaul enamel crystals.

Ultrastructural studies of enamel caries have shown that the intercrystalline space increases (fig. 10/9, 10/10). This can only happen if some mineral substance from the surface of enamel crystallites is removed or if there is selective dissolution of a separate amorphous calcium phosphate phase between crystals. The surface of crystals in a carious lesion show slight etching as evidenced by the irregularity of the margins (fig. 10/11). Evidence for the existence and removal of an amorphous intercrystalline phase is lacking. The most common crystal damage detected in electron microscopic studies is central or core defects due to preferential loss of minerals. This causes the enamel crystals to assume a hairpin appearance in

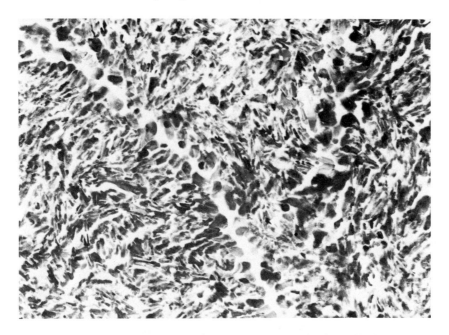

Fig. 10/10. Electron micrograph showing parts of two transversely sectioned prisms from carious enamel. Intercrystallite space containing embedding material can be clearly differentiated from artifact. A double row of enlarged, polyhedral crystals is present at the prism junction lining a channel which is largely artifact, but which does contain Araldite. This is seen where it formed a halo to crystals. The majority of crystals are irregular flattened hexagons with central deficiencies [from *Johnson*, 1967, with permission].

a longitudinal view (fig. 10/11). The finding is most easily explained on the basis of existence of lattice defects and/or different solubilities between the central core and the exterior of crystals. It is known that dislocations in the form of lattice defects increase in the core of crystals. Chemical reactivity increases at dislocation points, thus causing preferential loss of the crystal centers. It has also been suggested, but not proven, that there is a higher concentration of carbonate in the crystal center. Carbonate is preferentially dissolved in an acidic environment.

At the electron microscope level some enamel crystals at the periphery of the prism in the body of the lesion are often seen to be thicker and more electron-dense than in normal tissue (fig. 10/12). The larger crystals are thought to be formed in the process of recrystallization or remineralization. However, the remaining crystals within the lesion have been described as being smaller than those in sound enamel as a result of acid

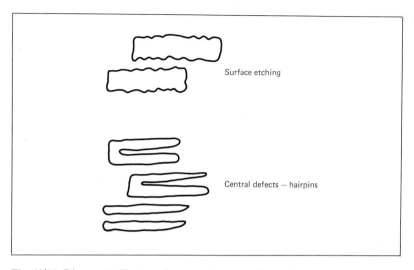

Fig. 10/11. Diagram to illustrate the two main types of crystal damage during carious dissolution (courtesy *Silverstone*).

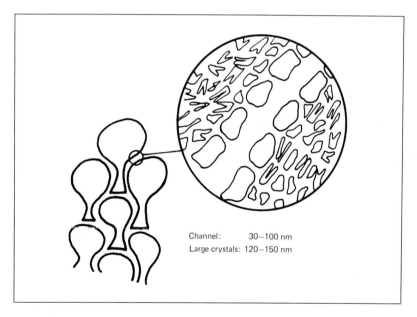

Fig. 10/12. Diagram to show the main features of enamel caries examined by transmission electron microscopy. These changes are seen in the advanced body of lesion (courtesy *Silverstone*).

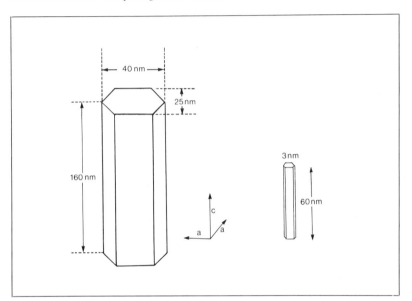

Fig. 10/13. Diagram to show the relationship between a typical crystal in human enamel (left) and the smaller crystal typical of dentin and bone (courtesy *Silverstone*).

dissolution. Figure 10/13 shows diagrammatically a typical crystal in human enamel and, to the right, a typical crystal in dentin or bone for comparison. The significant dimension is the greater diameter of the enamel crystal, which is approximately 40 nm.

Electron microscopic studies of carious lesions in enamel have shown clear effects on enamel crystallites. Currently it is difficult to correlate the chemical findings with ultrastructural observations on enamel crystals. It is known that there is a preferential removal of magnesium and carbonate from the translucent zone of enamel caries [*Hallsworth* et al., 1972]. It is not known whether magnesium is incorporated in the enamel crystal lattice or is on the crystal surface, or both. Nor is it known whether magnesium is linked with carbonate and, therefore, promotes dissolution. There is evidence that dissolution of carbonated apatites similar in composition to enamel is related to the concentration of carbonate [*Nelson and Featherstone*, 1983].

Recently a new microdissection technique coupled with high-resolution scanning electron microscopy has revealed ultrastructural features of the lesion not evident previously [*Silverstone*, 1983]. It was shown that the crystals in both the dark zone and the surface zone of the lesion are larger

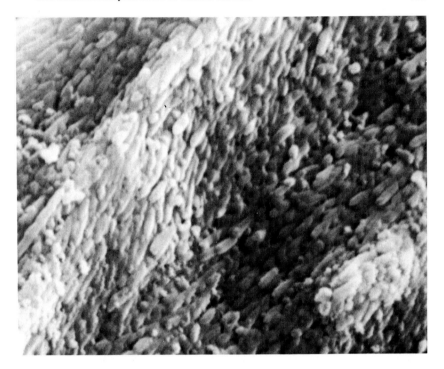

Fig. 10/14. High-resolution scanning electron micrograph from the dark zone of the enamel lesion. This specimen was produced by microdissection and coated with an ultrathin layer of platinum. Crystal diameters vary from 50 nm to in excess of 100 nm, being significantly larger than those in sound enamel (35 – 40 nm). This is direct evidence of crystal growth as a result of remineralization [*Silverstone*, 1983].

in diameter than those of sound enamel. Previously, with the exception of the single row of large crystals around the prism periphery in advanced lesions, all of the crystals in the enamel lesion were described as being significantly smaller than those of sound enamel. With this new technique, it has been shown that the crystals in sound enamel have a diameter of 35–40 nm, in the translucent zone there was a small decrease in size to 25–30 nm, and in the body of the lesion crystal diameters varied from 10 to 30 nm. However, in the dark zone, crystal diameters were found to be in the range 45–100 nm (fig. 10/14). The crystals in the surface zone were also seen to be larger than those of sound enamel being 40–75 nm in diameter. These size ranges were calculated on the basis of several hundred measurements in each of the zones of the lesion. This is the first direct observation

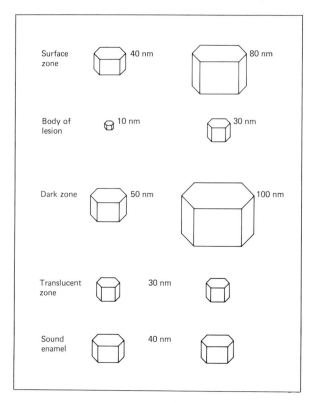

Fig. 10/15. Diagram to show the relative crystal diameters in a lesion of enamel caries compared to normal enamel as shown by microdissection coupled with high-resolution scanning electron microscopy [*Silverstone*, 1983].

Table 10/I. Approximate enamel composition comparing percentages on a weight basis and on a volume basis

Mineral crystals	Percent by weight	Percent by volume
Apatite $Ca_{10}(PO_4)_6(OH)_2$	92–94	
Carbonate CO_3^{2-} in crystal	2–4	
Na, Mg, K, Cl, Zn, etc.	about 1	
F	0.01–0.05	
	about 96 percent w/w	85–88 percent v/v
Water	2–3	6–10
Organic (protein and lipid)	about 1	2– 3

of remineralization occurring in the dark zone and the surface zone of the enamel lesion. This information substantiates previous evidence of re-mineralization occurring in these two zones as shown by polarized light studies [*Silverstone*, 1977]. Figure 10/15 shows diagrammatically the rela-tive crystal sizes in the four zones of the enamel lesion in relation to that of the sound enamel.

Enamel Caries Mechanism at a Chemical Level

During the past decade many aspects of the carious process have been clarified. The development of experimental models based on enamel dis-solution and the formation of incipient lesions in in vitro systems have led to a better understanding of the kinetics of enamel dissolution. This, in turn, has shed light on the variables that control this process and also on the mechanism by which substances, such as fluoride, repress caries. It is now possible to propose a caries mechanism which, while oversimplified, does provide the reader with a glimpse at what happens at a molecular level. First, some of the more important aspects of enamel chemistry and structure, and solubility of apatites will be reviewed.

Tooth enamel is composed of long thin crystallites of a hydroxyapatite-like mineral surrounded by a matrix of water and organic material (chapter 4). Enamel is a porous material and cannot be considered simply as a solid mass of hydroxyapatite. Hydroxyapatite, $Ca_{10}(PO_4)_6(OH)_2$, in its pure form is relatively low in solubility and low in reactivity. Enamel apatite, however, contains about 2–4% carbonate (CO_3^{2-}) and about 1% of metals other than calcium incorporated into the crystal structure (table 10/I). Therefore, enamel mineral should be considered as carbonated-apatite crystals incorporated in a water/protein/lipid superstructure which occupies about 15% by volume of enamel. These crystals are about 40 nm in dia-meter (approximately 1,000th of a hair's breadth) running from the outer enamel surface to the dentin, and nearly perpendicular to the surface [*Orams* et al., 1976]. The prisms, or enamel rods, are comprised of crystals clustered together, about 100 across, to give a diameter of about 4 μm as diagrammatically depicted in figure 10/16.

The protein and lipid [present in approximately equal quantities: *Odu-tuga and Prout*, 1974] together with a large proportion of the water form the diffusion channels through which chemical species must pass during enamel demineralization and remineralization.

Hydroxyapatite is readily soluble in acid under some conditions as are the related calcium phosphates; dicalcium phosphate dihydrate, DCPD, $CaHPO_4 \cdot 2H_2O$; tricalcium phosphate, TCP, $Ca_3(PO_4)_2$; and octacalcium

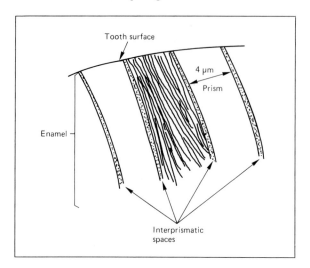

Fig. 10/16. Schematic diagram of enamel crystal and 'prism' arrangement to illustrate the diffusion channels and open porous structure [after *Featherstone*, 1980].

phosphate, OCP, $(Ca_8H_2(PO_4)_6 \cdot 5H_2O$, (fig. 10/17). However, before the carbonated-apatite crystals can dissolve acid must diffuse to the crystal surface through the porous matrix which surrounds the crystals and compete with the protein and lipid for active sites at the crystal surface. It is possible to reverse the dissolving step of the apatite crystals and actually regrow or 'remineralize' the crystal. Also, during dissolution a new chemical phase besides apatite may precipitate such as DCPD referred to in figure 10/17, depending on pH, calcium and phosphate concentrations and other chemical species present in the water phase immediately surrounding what is left of the dissolving crystals. All these events must be considered when thinking of the caries mechanism.

Studies on synthetic carbonated-apatites with similar chemical composition to dental enamel have shown that the rate of dissolution in weak acid is directly proportional to amount of carbonate present in the crystals [*Nelson and Featherstone*, 1983]. Fluoride present in the acid buffer markedly reduces this acid reactivity. Thus, the presence of fluoride during an acid challenge reduces the solubility rate at the crystal surfaces of enamel and this presumably is one significant cariostatic influence of fluoride in the plaque fluid [*Featherstone* et al., 1984].

Preferential loss of carbonate (CO_3^{2-}) and magnesium occurs during the early stages of dental caries in enamel (table 10/II). A high percentage of the CO_3^{2-} and Mg^{2+} originally present is lost during the first

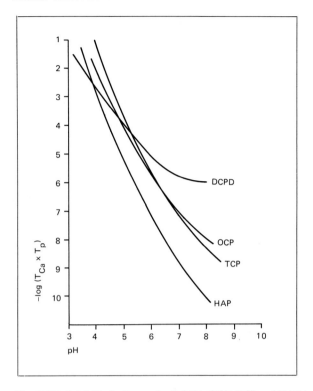

Fig. 10/17. Solubility isotherms for DCPD, OCP, TCP and HAP to illustrate the relative solubilities of each calcium phosphate as a function of pH and ion activity. Each line represents the position above which precipitation occurs, below which each salt dissolves [*Nancollas*, 1982].

Table 10/II. Typical values for the principal changes in early carious lesions in enamel [*Hallsworth* et al., 1972, 1973; adapted from *Williams and Elliott*, 1979]

Part of carious lesion	Loss of mineral percent by vol	Loss of magnesium percent by wt	Loss of CO_3^{2-} percent by wt
40 50 µm thick surface zone	10	not detectable[a]	
Body of lesion	24	20	[b]
Dark zone	6.3	12	
Translucent zone	1.2	12	19

[a] Both carious and sound surface enamel contain about 40% by weight less magnesium than normal interior enamel.
[b] The CO_3^{2-} content in the body of the lesion probably does not decrease much from that in the translucent zone [*Hallsworth*, private communication].

periods of acid attack. This, of course, is related to the presence of these ions in the apatite mineral, and they apparently form the site of preferential acid attack. Reversal of this dissolution step by recrystallization in between acid challenges produces less soluble crystalline material which incorporates less carbonate and more fluoride if fluoride is present in the immediate aqueous environment. Fluoride promotes this remineralization step and this mechanism is one of the principal cariostatic actions of the ion (see vol. 2, chapter 3).

The core of the enamel crystals and the surfaces probably contain carbonate-rich material which would explain the preferential dissolution of the central portion of the crystal and the surface etching which the electron microscope has revealed. It has been suggested [*Arends and Jongebloed*, 1977] that these areas of crystal disturbance are related to dislocations in the structure.

Plaque bacteria mainly produce the weak organic acids formic ($HCOOH$), acetic (CH_3COOH), lactic ($CH_3CH(OH)COOH$), and propionic (CH_3CH_2COOH) as by-products of carbohydrate metabolism [*Geddes*, 1975]. Because these are weak acids they can exist in an un-ionized form in equilibrium with their respective anion (e.g. lactate or acetate) and hydrogen ion.

$$HA \rightleftharpoons H^+ + A^-$$

This equilibrium is governed in each case by a unique dissociation constant, K_a for each acid. Hence the un-ionized form of each acid provides a storehouse of H^+ ions. The H^+ ion is the principal attacking species for the dissolution of enamel apatite, providing it can get to the crystal surfaces either by itself or be transported combined with the anion as the HA form, or un-ionized acid form. The anion, A^-, can also complex Ca^{2+} ions, more strongly in the case of lactate than the other acids listed above. *Gray* [1966, 1977] showed with in vitro enamel dissolution experiments that both these factors affected dissolution rates and resulted in subsurface lesion formation.

Recent studies by *Featherstone and Rodgers* [1981] using acetic and lactic acids alone, in combination, and at various pH values demonstrated the dependence of lesion formation on undissociated (un-ionized) acid concentration, [HA], and the degree of dissociation of the acid as it diffused. This latter factor is a function of K_a for each acid. Hence, lactic acid is a stronger acid than acetic acid, has less HL in solution than HA at a given pH, but dissociates more readily to produce H^+ and L^- as diffusion into enamel progresses. This diffusion takes place through the lipid/ protein/water phase and is somewhat similar to diffusion through other body membranes.

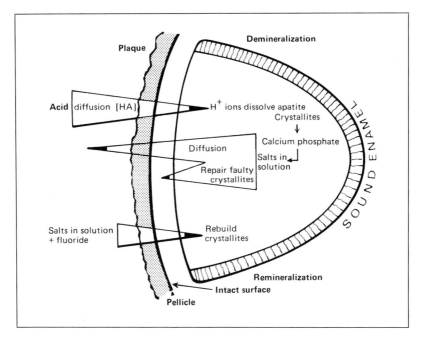

Fig. 10/18. Schematic illustration of acid attack of enamel apatite crystals by acid products from dental plaque, and the subsequent repair (remineralization) of faulty crystals by the calcium, phosphate, and fluoride in solution [modified after *Featherstone* et al., 1979].

From the above results it can be concluded that subsurface dissolution of enamel by acid media, similar to that produced by plaque plus sucrose in the oral environment, is governed by the following factors, schematically illustrated in figure 10/18.

– The overall reaction is diffusion controlled.
  The initial rate of reaction depends on how rapidly the hydrogen ions reach the enamel crystal surface.
– The principal source of hydrogen ions is the undissociated acid (HA). The rate of dissolution is affected by diffusion of the undissociated acid into the enamel as well as the concentration of hydrogen ions, at any point within the enamel.
– Concentration of the undissociated acid buffer is a function of the particular buffer and its dissociation constant.

- The initial rate of reaction is decreased by the presence in solution of the reaction products, such as calcium and phosphate ions, and fluoride.
- Reaction products precipitate, dissolve and reprecipitate depending on the above factors. This phenomenon is responsible for the observed dissolution of enamel and remineralization or formation of a new solid phase. Presumably, analogous reactions occur in the carious process in vivo.

The information about the morphological characteristics of carious lesions and the dynamics of enamel dissolution will now be combined and applied to the carious process. A simplified schematic illustration of the reactions involved in carious dissolution of enamel is shown in figure 10/19. The events and reactions may be described by the following model [*Featherstone* et al., 1979]:

- A protective organic film of strongly adsorbed protein, the acquired salivary pellicle, forms on the surface of enamel mineral. Acquisition of fluoride in surface enamel and loss of carbonate from the enamel surface may also contribute to the reduced solubility of the outer enamel surface.
- In the presence of a suitable carbohydrate substrate, such as sucrose, cariogenic plaque bacteria produce organic acids (lactic, acetic, propionic) localized within the plaque in juxtaposition to enamel. This is step 1 in figure 10/19.
- Production of these organic acids produces a concentration gradient that causes the hydrogen ions (H^+) and the undissociated acid (HA or HL, etc.) to diffuse into the enamel. This is step 2 in figure 10/19. As diffusion proceeds the undissociated acid molecules continually dissociate providing H^+ ions. These hydrogen ions are rapidly used up in the reaction with enamel, producing calcium and phosphate and promoting further acid dissociation.
- The undissociated HA and HL form a reservoir of hydrogen ions. Dissociation is dependent upon the pH and the concentration of undissociated molecules. As the HA and HL diffuse, dissociation into H^+, L^- and A^- occurs in an attempt to establish an equilibrium.
- The H^+, and to a lesser extent L^- and A^-, attack the apatite crystals particularly at vulnerable lattice points such as where CO_3^{2-} is present. This causes Ca^{2+}, OH^-, PO_4^{3-}, F^-, CO_3^{2-}, Na^+ and Mg^{2+} to be removed from the lattice and to diffuse to the solution phase between the crystals. This is step 3 in figure 10/19. Fluoride in solution markedly inhibits this dissolution stage of the process.
- These ions and their appropriate complexes ($CaHPO_4$, CaL^+,

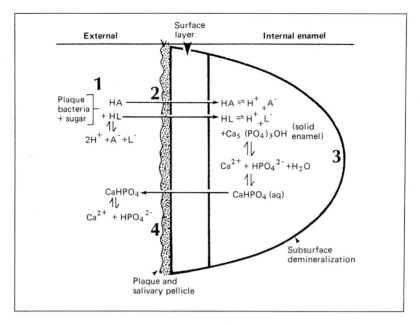

Fig. 10/19. Diagrammatic representation of simplified chemistry of subsurface demineralization proceeding after the 'intact' surface layer has been formed. $Ca_5(PO_4)_3OH$ is used to represent solid enamel crystals, which are more correctly a carbonated apatite (see text). All other species are aqueous ions or aqueous complexes in solution [modified after *Featherstone* et al., 1979].

$CaH_2PO_4^+$, etc.) will diffuse according to their concentration gradients through the newly enlarged pores of the carious enamel so that calcium and phosphate are lost to the external environment. Mineral loss, or demineralization, proceeds as long as sufficient acid is available. This is step 4 in figure 10/19.

- As more enamel dissolves and the concentration of the Ca^{2+} and PO_4^{3-} increases remineralization may occur on the surface of the existing crystals. New crystals may also form as $CaHPO_4$ or other phosphate phases. As more HA and HL diffuses and reaches a critical concentration it will cause some of the new crystal forms to dissolve as well as more enamel apatite crystals. These reactions mostly occur in the demineralized subsurface layers, particularly the body of the carious lesion which may be as much as 70% demineralized.
- As calcium and phosphate diffuse outwards remineralization becomes more and more likely as diffusion slows. This leads to the formation of an apparently 'intact' enamel surface layer, about 20–40 μm thick,

where the mineral content is higher than the body of the lesion (fig. 10/18). This is a remineralization phenomenon where damaged crystals have been repaired and an equilibrium eventually exists which maintains this surface layer but with some loss of minerals. The loss of ions to the plaque is balanced by deposition of ions diffusing outwards from the subsurface. This is somewhat analogous to a line of cars at the toll gate at a thruway exit, with cars entering and leaving continuously, but maintaining a steady line length at the gate.

– If subsurface dissolution continues and repair cannot keep pace with mineral loss this leads eventually to more extensive damage to crystal structure and cavitation.

– Dissolution of mineral salts eventually exposes the organic matrix of enamel and dentin to proteolytic enzymes of the oral flora.

– Proteolysis is important in the breakdown of dentin and cementum, less so in enamel as much of the protein is acid soluble and is lost.

At an incipient caries stage, and prior to cavitation, repair of a lesion may occur by remineralization. If the calcium and phosphate gradients are reversed and these species diffuse inwards rather than outwards then remineralization results. Crystal regrowth, or new precipitation, will also occur, of course, as the pH rises (see above, and fig. 10/18). Fluoride, if present at the crystal surface in the immediately adjacent water phase, promotes this remineralization by dramatically speeding up the process. There is now considerable evidence that one of the principal mechanisms of fluoride action is the enhancement of remineralization.

The reactions involved in the caries process also suggest many ways by which caries may be prevented or arrested. Among the most obvious methods are the following:

– Removal of substrate; substitution of substrate by noncariogenic sweetening agents such as xylitol; removal of plaque; interference with glycolytic bacterial metabolism. These procedures will reduce formation of organic acids and the diffusion of acids into enamel. There is an additional benefit from avoiding plaque acid formation by reducing the frequency of carbohydrate snacking.

– Development of more caries-resistant enamel by incorporation of fluoride ion during tooth maturation and remineralization; formation of fluorapatite-like material in surface enamel by topical fluoride applications.

– Maintaining a protective pellicle without the formation of thick, bacterial plaques, and maintaining an effective concentration of calcium and phosphate in the plaque fluid-pellicle-enamel surface interface by a satisfactory flow of fresh, well-buffered saliva.

–   Enhancement of the natural remineralizing action of saliva by regular
    and frequent administration of low levels of fluoride in drinking water,
    dentifrices and/or mouthrinses. These will also provide fluoride at the
    dissolution site at the time of acid challenge. Hence frequent availabil-
    ity of low concentrations of fluoride at the time of demineralization
    challenge by acid and the immediately ensuing remineralization step
    are major anticaries procedures.

The prevention of dental caries is covered in detail in volume 2.

Caries of Dentin

The pulp of the tooth and the adjoining dentin tissue should be viewed
as a single physiological complex. Both structures develop from the un-
differentiated mesenchymal cells of the dental papilla. The cellular common denominator of this complex is the odontoblast cell, located at the
periphery of the pulp at the predentin junction. Dentin is synthesized by
odontoblast cells. The long, tail-like odontoblastic processes are contained
within the mineralized canals which course through the dentin to the
dentino-enamel junction. Occasionally the process crosses the junction for
a short distance into enamel to form enamel spindles. The relationship of
the odontoblast to dentinal tissue is often compared to that of osteoblasts
and bone tissue. The odontoblastic processes possess a network of secondary branching anastomosing channels which go through foramen in the
peritubular walls of the canals. Stimuli that arise in the dentin travel down
the main and secondary odontoblastic processes and affect an extensive
area of dentin.

Progressing carious lesions penetrate the enamel, spread laterally
along the dentino-enamel junction and undermine the enamel. The lesion
invades the dentin following the direction of the dentinal tubules. This
pattern of invasion of dentin results in a cone-shaped lesion with its base at
the dentino-enamel junction and apex towards the pulp (fig. 10/20).

Microscopic Aspects of Dentinal Caries

A response to early enamel caries may be detected in pulpal tissue. An
inflammatory cell infiltration of the subodontoblastic layer indicates that
some stimuli reach the odontoblasts at this early stage. The changes in the
pulp and dentin depend upon the rate of progression of the lesion. The
advancing front of the carious process leads to demineralization, and is
subsequently followed by bacterial invasion. Changes in dentin and the
pulp are dependent upon the degree of demineralization and the numbers
of bacteria invading the tissue.

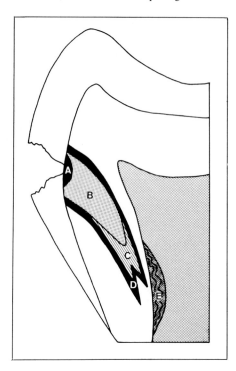

Fig. 10/20. Schematic drawing of the pathological process of dentinal caries depicting the zones generally seen in a light microscope examination. A = Zone of necrotic or decomposed dentin. B = Zone of bacterial invasion. C = Zone of demineralized dentin. D = Hypermineralized (sclerotic) zone. E = Reparative or secondary dentin layer (courtesy *Silverstone*).

The histopathology of bacterial invasions of dentin resulting in deep, active lesions has been extensively studied. The pathological process for descriptive purposes is usually divided into several zones, diagrammatically depicted in figure 10/20.

In an active carious lesion, the necrotic zone consists of disintegrating dentinal tubules, mixed oral flora and a structureless matrix degraded by proteolytic bacterial activity. This is the portion of the lesion that is readily removed by spoon excavators during cavity preparations. Beneath this necrotic zone is the infected layer where the organisms have penetrated the dentinal canals but no gross disintegration of the pericanalicular walls is evident (fig. 10/20). Next to the infected area is the zone of demineralization. In this zone, the mineral salts have been dissolved leaving a relatively intact tubular morphology. In the superficial layers of the demineralized zone a few bacteria may be found but in the deeper layer most of the tissue is sterile. This tissue, because of its consistency, is often called leathery dentin. The presense of a relatively intact although demineralized zone of dentin in the forefront of a dentinal caries attack has important clinical implications. In a conservative approach to the management of deep dentinal caries lesions, the necrotic and the infected portion of the dentin is removed but the demineralized zone in dentin is left behind. Complete removal of such tissue is not essential since it may lead to the exposure of the pulp. In a procedure called indirect pulp capping, a thin layer of calcium hydroxide is spread over this nonnecrotic, softened dentin and a restoration with a good marginal seal is placed over the calcium hydroxide capping. This often leads to the formation of secondary dentin and a normal pulpal response.

A deep dentinal caries lesion which progresses at a slow rate leads to the formation of a sclerotic zone beneath the demineralized area. The tubular lumens in the sclerotic zone are narrower than normal and may be occluded by crystallites. It is conjectured that as minerals are solubilized in the advancing demineralization front the concentration of calcium and phosphate increases and they are redeposited. It is possible that some of the recrystallization may be brought about by a specific odontoblastic action during the periods of caries arrest. The dentinal canals in the sclerotic zone may become completely obliterated by intraluminal calcification. The permeability of this zone is decreased and the level of mineralization increased beyond that in normal tissue. This, when accompanied by deep pigmentation and a relatively hard polished dentinal surface is indicative of arrested dentinal caries. Beneath the sclerotic zone the odontoblast may deposit a further layer of reparative dentin or secondary dentin. This not only thickens the dentin in the vicinity but also results in the odontoblasts advancing further into the pulp chamber away from the lesion front.

The pulp has great resiliency and reparative powers to cope with a carious attack. In a chronic lesion progressing at a slow rate, arrested dentinal caries may result. However, where the lesion is deep with no sign of arrest, it is important from a clinical standpoint to recognize that the pulp may be successfully protected if the necrotic, affected dentin is scrupulously removed and the intact morphologically demineralized dentin is treated with calcium hydroxide. This sealing off of the lesion from additional pathogenic bacteria enables the pulpal elements to form secondary dentin.

Caries of Cementum

The carious process in the cementum is similar to that occurring in the dentin. Clinically lesions develop as saucer-shaped. The location of cementum caries is usually in those areas where gingival recession has been severe and where self-cleansing properties are poor. Microradiographs of initial cementum caries indicates that subsurface demineralization also occurs in this tissue. In addition, densely mineralized surfaces have been observed, indicative of a remineralization process analogous to what has been called the sclerotic dentin.

References

Arends, J.; Jongebloed, W.L.: Dislocations and dissolution in apatites: theoretical considerations. Caries Res. *11:* 186 (1977).

Featherstone, J.D.B.: Chemistry and physiology of dental caries. Chem. N.Z. *44:* 21 (1980).

Featherstone, J.D.B.; Duncan, J.F.; Cutress, T.W.: A mechanism for dental caries based on chemical processes and diffusion phenomena during in vitro caries simulation on human tooth enamel. Archs oral Biol. *24:* 101 (1979).

Featherstone, J.D.B.; Rodgers, B.E.: Effect of acetic, lactic and other organic acids in the formation of artificial carious lesions. Caries Res. *15:* 337 (1981).

Featherstone, J.D.B.; Shields, C.P.; Khademazad, B.; Oldershaw, M.D.: Acid reactivity of carbonated-apatites with strontium and fluoride substitutions. J. dent. Res. *62:* 1049 (1983).

Featherstone, J.D.B.; Glena, R.; Shields, C.P.: Reactivity of carbonated-apatite in the presence of fluoride and/or strontium. J. dent. Res. *63:* 184 (1984).

Geddes, D.A.M.: Acids produced by human dental plaque metabolism in situ. Caries Res. *9:* 98 (1975).

Gray, J.A.: Kinetics of enamel dissolution during formation of incipient caries-like lesions. Archs oral Biol. *11:* 397 (1966).

Gray, J.A.: Chemical events during cariogenesis; in Rowe, Proc. Symp. Incipient Caries of Enamel (University of Michigan and Dent. Res. Inst., 1977).

Hallsworth, A.S; Robinson, C.; Weatherell, J.A.: Mineral and magnesium distribution within the approximal carious lesion of dental enamel. Caries Res. *6:* 156 (1972).

Hallsworth, A.S; Weatherell, J.A.; Robinson, C.: Loss of carbonate during the first stages of enamel caries. Caries Res. *7:* 345 (1973).

Johnson, N.W.: Some aspects of the ultrastructure of early human enamel caries seen with the electron microscope. Archs oral Biol. *12:* 1,505 (1967).

Nancollas, G.H. (ed.): Phase transformation during precipitation of calcium salts; in Biological mineralization and demineralization, p. 79 (Springer, Berlin 1982).

Nelson, D.G.A.; Featherstone, J.D.B.: Effect of carbonate and fluoride on the dissolution behaviour of synthetic apatites. Caries Res. *17:* 200 (1983).

Odutuga, A.A.; Prout, R.E.S.: Lipid analysis of human enamel and dentine. Archs oral Biol. *19: 729 (1974)*.

Orams, H.J.; Zybert, J.J.; Phakey, P.P.; Rachinger, W.A.: Ultrastructural study of human dental enamel using selected-area argon-ion-beam thinning. Archs oral Biol. *21:* 663 (1976).

Silverstone, L.M.: The primary translucent zone of enamel caries and of artificial caries-like lesions. Br. dent. J. *120:* 461 (1966).

Silverstone, L.M.: The surface zone in caries and in caries-like lesions produced in vitro. Br. dent. J. *125:* 145 (1968).

Silverstone, L.M.: The structure of carious enamel, including the early lesion; in Melcher, Zarb, Oral sciences reviews, No. 3, p. 100 (Munksgaard, Copenhagen 1973).

Silverstone, L.M.: Structural alterations of human dental enamel during incipient carious
    lesion development; in Rowe, Proc. Symp. Incipient Caries of Enamel (University of
    Michigan and Dent. Res. Inst., 1977).
Silverstone, L.M.: The relationship between the macroscopic, histological and radiographic
    appearance of interproximal lesions in human teeth: an in vitro study using an artificial
    caries technique; in Radiation exposure in pediatric dentistry. Pediatr. Dent. *3:* spec.
    issue 2, 414 (1982).
Silverstone, L.M.: Remineralization and enamel caries: significance of fluoride and effect on
    crystal diameters; in Leach, Edgar, Demineralization and remineralization of teeth, p.
    185 (IRL Press, Oxford 1983).
Silverstone, L.M.; Johnson, N.W.; Hardie, J.M.; Williams, R.A.D.: Dental caries: aetiolo-
    gy, pathology and prevention (Macmillan, London 1981).
Silverstone, L.M.; Poole, D.F.G.: Modification of the histological appearance of enamel
    caries after exposure to saliva and a calcifying fluid. Caries Res. *2:* 87 (1968).
Williams, R.A.D.; Elliott, J.C.: Basic and applied dental biochemistry (Churchill-
    Livingstone, Edinburgh 1979).

Appendix

Highlights in Dental Caries Research

This is a list of significant clinical and laboratory findings relating to dental caries starting from the 17th century when the discovery of the microscope permitted the first visualization of microorganisms recovered from tooth surfaces.

van Leeuwenhoek, A. **1683** Described the presence of minute animacules in scrapings from teeth. He also discovered dentinal tubules.	**1728** *Fauchard, P.* Founder of dentistry, published first edition of a classic textbook on dentistry.
Erdl **1843** Described filamentous parasites in surface membranes of teeth.	**1867** *Magitot, E.* Demonstrated dissolution of tooth substance by fermentation products of sugar. In his book Treatise on Dental Caries he supported the chemical theory of tooth decay.
Underwood, A.S. and Miles, W.J. **1881** Described presence of micrococci in histological sections of carious dentin.	
Leber, T. and Rottenstein, J.B. **1883** First to describe caries as due to acids.	**1890** *Miller, W.D.* Demonstrated essential relation between oral bacteria, acid and caries. Proposed the chemico-parasitic (i.e. the acid) theory of dental caries. Published his epoch-making volume Micro-Organisms of the Human Mouth in 1890.
Black, G.V. **1891** Promulgated scientific cavity preparation and the concept of extension for prevention.	
Williams, J.L. **1897** Demonstrated the bacterial plaque on enamel surfaces and described caries of enamel.	**1900** *Sieberth, O.* First isolated streptococci from carious dentin.
Eager, J.M. **1901** Mottled (fluorosed) enamel described for first time in residents of Italy.	**1915–** *Kligler, I.J., Howe, P.R. and Hatch* **1917** Reported the presence of acidogenic bacteria in carious lesions and were first to specify that lactobacilli may be involved.
Black, G.V. and McKay, F.S. **1916** Widespread finding of mottled enamel in the U.S.A. and that the cause was to be sought in the drinking water. Mottled teeth are associated with "no more caries than normal teeth".	**1924** *Clark, J.K.* Isolated *Streptococcus mutans* from carious lesions.

Mellanby, M.   **1929** | **1931**   *Churchill, H.V.. and Smith, M.C.*
Described the role of vitamin D in enamel hypo-   Fluoride discovered to be the specific cause of
plasia and hypothesized a correlation between   mottled enamel.
tooth structure and caries prevalence.

                                                            1933   *Hadley, P.*
                                                            Described the salivary lactobacillus count.

                                                            1939   *Fosdick, L.*
Stephen, R.M.   **1940**   Introduced the concept of critical pH at which
Determined hydrogen ion concentration on   enamel dissolves in the saliva-plaque environ-
plaque surface and carious lesion.   ment.

Bibby, B.   **1942**
Introduced topical fluorides for caries prevention.

Dean, T.H.   **1942**
Determined that a concentration of fluoride in a
communal water of 1 ppm resulted in optimal   **1944**   *Williams, N.B.*
caries benefits and insignificant fluorosis.   Immunized humans using Lactobacilli.

Qualitative relation established between the   **1945**   Controlled water fluoridation initiated in Brant-
concentration of fluoride in drinking water, the   ford, Canada; Grand Rapids, Michigan and
severity of mottled enamel (fluorosis) and dental   Newburgh, New York, USA.
caries prevalence.

Gustafsson, B.E.   **1954** | **1954**   *Orland, F.*
and co-workers   Showed that caries did not develop in caries-
Published the Vipeholm Study which clarified   susceptible, germ-free rats maintained on a
determinants of cariogenicity of diets.   cariogenic diet.

                                                            1960   *Keyes, P.*
                                                            Demonstrated that dental caries is a transmissi-
                                                            ble disease in laboratory aniamls.

                                                            1960   *Fitzgerald, R.J. and Keyes, P.*
                                                            Reported that the transmissible bacterial factor
                                                            in animal caries was a streptococcus (later iden-
                                                            tified as *S. mutans*).

Gray, J.A.   **1962** | **1962–** *Hardwick, J.L.; Leach, S.A.; Dawes, C. and*
First quantitative description of the carious   **1965**   *Jenkins, G.N.*
process in physico-chemical terms.   Found high levels of fluoride in dental plaque;
                                                            studied relationship to fluoride in water.

                                                            1964   *Muhler, J.C.*
                                                            Developed the first fluoridated dentifrice con-
Koulourides, T.; Feagin, F. and Pigman, W.   **1965**   taining stannous fluoride.
Reported remineralization of enamel by saliva.
                                                            1967   *Cueto, E. and Bunocore, M.G.*
                                                            First report of successful sealing of highly sus-
Turku Studies of sugars, especially xylitol, on **1975**   ceptible pit and fissure areas with an adhesive
dental health.   polymeric resin.

1965	**1983[1]**

Some major components of dental plaque matrix found to be bacterial polysaccharides.

Preferential colonization of animals and adherence of *S. mutans* to teeth enhanced to polymers synthesized from sucrose.

S. mutans associated numerically with existent lesions, incipient lesions and onset of lesions in humans.

Laboratory animals immunized against caries following vaccination by *S. mutans* cells.

Vaccination with purified proteins including cell wall antigens and glucosyl transferases of *S. mutans* found to confer caries protection in laboratory animals.

Extracellular polysaccharide (especially glucan) synthesis by *S. mutans* in presence of sucrose.

S. mutans group of bacteria found to comprise several serotypes, genotypes, biotypes. Serotypes related to specific cell wall antigens. Predominance of certain types in human mouth recognized.

Humans produce salivary antibodies after swallowing encapsulated *S. mutans* vaccine.

Major pathways of sugar transport and metabolism in cariogenic bacteria elucidated.

Chemotherapy aimed at decreasing *S. mutans* levels shown to decrease caries activity.

1960's – present

A dramatic decline in caries prevalence in the western world observed in both fluoridated and non-fluoridated communities. Decline is attributed to the widespread use of fluorides in different regimens, especially in fluoridated dentifrices and to a lesser extent to dietary changes including use of sugar substitutes.

---

[1] The above findings relating to microbiology emanated from several laboratories and involved many investigators making it difficult to associate the development of a specific concept with single individuals. Past research was often a solo effort, not so current findings which often have many intertwining branches. Much of this research is considered in detail in Chapters 5 and 6.

Subject Index